Better Homes and Gardens®

QUICK & EASY
DIET RECIPES

BETTER HOMES AND GARDENS® BOOKS

Editor Gerald M. Knox
Art Director Ernest Shelton
Managing Editor David A. Kirchner
Editorial Project Managers James D. Blume, Marsha Jahns, Rosanne Weber Mattson

Department Head, Cook Books Sharyl Heiken
Associate Department Heads Sandra Granseth, Rosemary C. Hutchinson, Elizabeth Woolever
Senior Food Editors Marcia Stanley, Joyce Trollope
Associate Food Editors Linda Henry, Mary Major, Diana McMillen, Mary Jo Plutt, Martha Schiel, Linda Foley Woodrum
Test Kitchen Director, Sharon Stilwell; Photo Studio Director, Janet Herwig; Home Economists: Jean Brekke, Kay Cargill, Marilyn Cornelius, Jennifer Darling, Maryellyn Krantz, Lynelle Munn, Dianna Nolin, Marge Steenson

Associate Art Directors Neoma Thomas, Linda Ford Vermie, Randall Yontz
Assistant Art Directors Lynda Haupert, Harijs Priekulis, Tom Wegner
Graphic Designers Mary Schlueter Bendgen, Mike Burns, Brian Wignall
Art Production Director, John Berg; Associate, Joe Heuer; Office Manager, Michaela Lester

President, Book Group Jeramy Lanigan
Vice President, Retail Marketing Jamie L. Martin
Vice President, Administrative Services Rick Rundall

BETTER HOMES AND GARDENS® MAGAZINE
President, Magazine Group James A. Autry
Editorial Director Doris Eby
Editorial Services Director Duane L. Gregg
Food and Nutrition Editor Nancy Byal

MEREDITH CORPORATION OFFICERS
Chairman of the Executive Committee E. T. Meredith III
Chairman of the Board Robert A. Burnett
President Jack D. Rehm

QUICK AND EASY DIET RECIPES
Editors Mary Jo Plutt, Martha Schiel, Joyce Trollope, Linda Foley Woodrum
Editorial Project Manager Marsha Jahns
Graphic Designer Harijs Priekulis
Electronic Text Processor Paula Forest
Contributing Photographers de Gennaro Studios, Mike Dieter, M. Jensen Photography, Inc., Scott Little, Kathy Sanders
Contributing Food Stylists Marilyn Cornelius, Kathleen E. German, Pat Godsted, Carol Grones, Janet Herwig, Mable Hoffman, Bonnie Rabert
Contributing Nutrition Consultants Roberta L. Duyff, M.S., R.D.; Sue Roberts, M.S., R.D./L.D.

On the cover: Shrimp Fettuccine (see recipe, page 51); Papaya Ice (see recipe, page 178)

Our seal assures you that every recipe in *Quick and Easy Diet Recipes* has been tested in the Better Homes and Gardens® Test Kitchen. This means that each recipe is practical and reliable, and meets our high standards of taste appeal.

"*I* really need to go on a diet, but right now I'm too busy. I don't have much time to cook, let alone prepare special diet meals." Sound familiar? The editors of Better Homes and Gardens® Books know that having enough time is a problem, and so is dieting. That's why we created this exciting cookbook for both the serious dieter and the casual calorie counter.

In it you'll find easy-to-understand answers to some common questions about calories, weight control, time-saving preparation techniques, and more. Choose the topics you want to learn more about. Then, page through chapter after chapter of delectable recipe ideas. Discover quick-to-fix, easy, and make-ahead recipes, as well as a selection of microwave recipes. For every recipe, you'll find the calorie count and a convenient timetable so you can fit low-calorie cooking into your busy schedule. Look for the super-fast recipes marked "20 minutes or less." Then, turn to the last chapter for a fantastic 14-day meal plan.

Start using this book today for tastier, easier dieting. What have you got to lose!

Contents

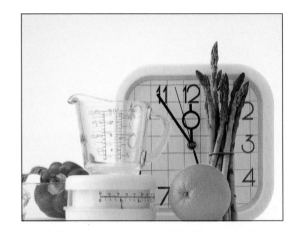
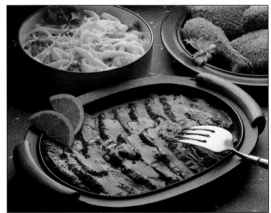
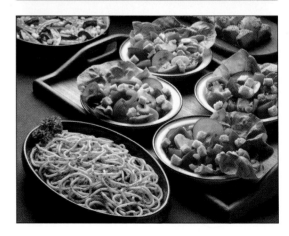

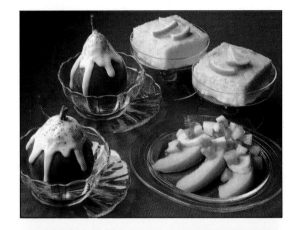
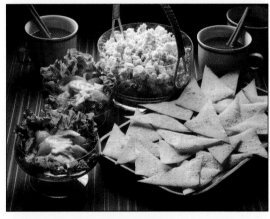
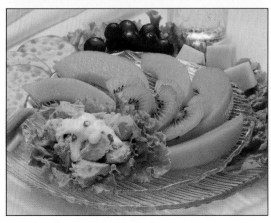

When You Want to Diet... But You're Short on Time

The battle of the telltale bulge and the race against the clock are two mealtime challenges many of us face each day. We're here to help.

Read over the dieting and timesaving information on the next several pages. You'll find the answers to some of your biggest dieting and meal preparation questions.

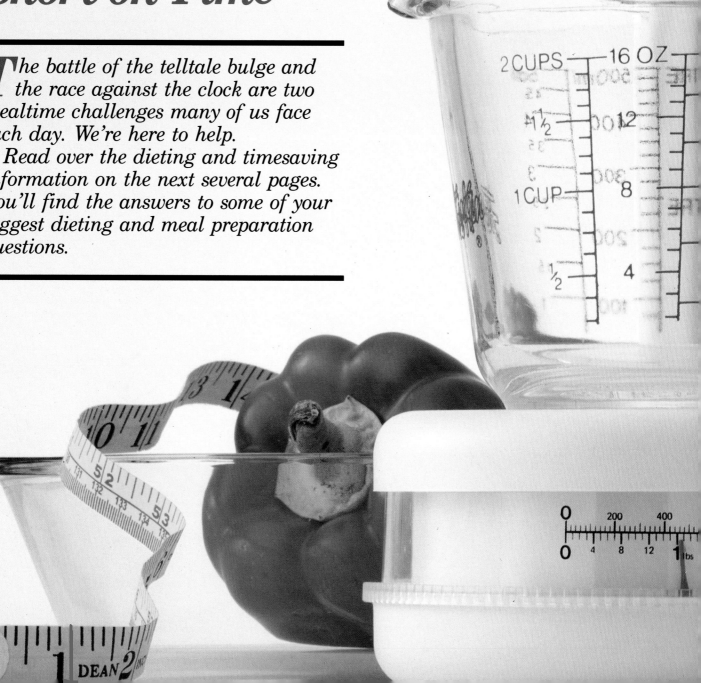

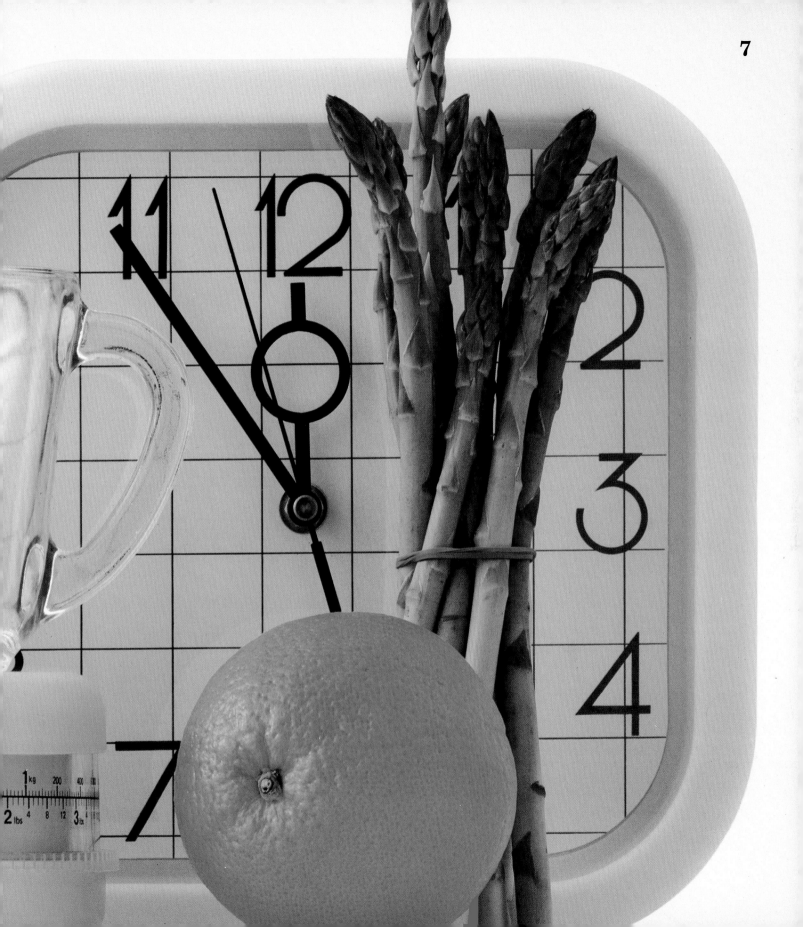

When You Want to Diet...

Get the facts before you begin dieting. What do you need to know? On the following pages you'll find basic nutrition information and ideas for meal planning, as well as tips on calories and weight control.

Nutrition Basics

Q **What is good nutrition?**

A Simply put, nutrition is how food affects the body. Being well-nourished means consuming nutrients in the amounts your body needs for optimal health—not too much, yet not too little.

Your strategies for good nutrition are shown in your eating habits. And, the evidence is you—how you look and how you feel. Good nutrition plays a key role in your total well-being.

Q **What are the various nutrients, and what do they do?**

A Nutrients are the substances in food that nourish your body. As the food you eat is digested, nutrients are released and carried to every cell of your body. That's where nourishment takes place.

More than 40 nutrients essential to your health belong in one of six categories—protein, carbohydrate, fat, vitamins, minerals, or water. Each group of nutrients—in fact, each specific nutrient—performs distinct functions:

Protein builds and repairs your body tissue. It's a nutrient essential for growth.

Carbohydrate and fat are your body's main energy sources, although protein supplies energy as well.

Vitamins, minerals, and water all regulate body processes, each in different ways. For example, vitamin A keeps your eyes healthy and helps them adjust to the dark. The B vitamins (thiamine, riboflavin, and niacin) help your body produce energy. Vitamin C helps you resist infection and keeps your gums and blood vessels healthy.

Two minerals, calcium and phosphorus, build strong bones and healthy teeth. Iron, another mineral, is a component of blood and helps carry oxygen to every one of your body's trillions of cells. And water, another nutrient, is part of all your body fluids.

Q **What about fiber?**

A Although it is a carbohydrate, fiber is not a nutrient. Sound confusing? Fiber, which is the tough, stringy part of plant cells, doesn't nourish your body because it isn't broken down fully during digestion. That's the key to its usefulness. Think of fiber as a broom. Its bulk helps "sweep" the intestine, aiding both digestion and elimination.

Q **What are calories, and where do they come from?**

A Calories measure energy, both the energy in food and the energy your body uses for exercise and for the physical functions that keep you alive.

Calories come from the food you eat. They aren't nutrients, although some people think so. Instead, three of the six nutrients provide calories. Carbohydrate and protein yield four calories per gram, and fat yields nine calories per gram. Although not a nutrient, alcohol contributes calories, too—about seven calories per gram.

Q Why does the caloric count of foods vary so much?

A Because the nutrient value of foods varies, each food provides a different number of calories. Fat, for example, has more than twice the calories per gram that protein and carbohydrate do. So foods high in fat tend to be high in calories. High-fiber foods tend to be low in calories. Fiber can't be fully digested and most high-fiber foods are also low in fat.

Look for these clues to a food's caloric count. Low-calorie foods tend to be thin and watery, crisp but not greasy-crisp, or bulky. High-calorie foods tend to be oily or greasy-crisp, sweet and gooey, thick and smooth, or alcoholic. Serving size also affects the caloric count. The bigger the serving, the more calories.

Q Does everyone have the same nutritional needs?

A Everyone needs the same nutrients, but in different amounts. Both age and sex influence nutritional requirements. Teenagers, for example, need the most nutrients, because they're growing rapidly. And, after childhood, males generally need more than females, largely because of body size. Both pregnant and nursing women need more than other women their age, as well.

Nutrient guidelines—by age and sex and for pregnancy and nursing—have been established by a scientific panel of the National Research Council. These guidelines, called the Recommended Dietary Allowances (RDAs), list specific amounts of 17 essential nutrients you need each day, including protein, 10 vitamins, and six minerals. The RDAs also include a recommended calorie intake, as well as safe and adequate ranges for 12 other nutrients.

The RDAs are guidelines that, if followed, meet the needs of most people. But they aren't etched in stone. Each person is unique—you're unique. So your specific nutrient needs might differ somewhat from the RDAs. Your own requirements even change a little from day to day.

The U.S. Recommended Daily Allowances (U.S. RDAs), used for product labeling, are based on the RDAs. They're less precise, because only a single figure is used for each nutrient, instead of specific figures for each sex and age group. With a few exceptions, the U.S. RDAs are the highest recommended allowance for each RDA.

Calories and Weight Control

Q How does my body use calories?

A Your body needs calories for three purposes: (1) metabolism, or body processes such as breathing and heartbeat, which keeps you alive; (2) physical activity; and (3) digestion of food.

The equations for weight control are simple. You maintain your body weight when you eat the same number of calories you burn. When you eat more than your body needs, you gain weight. And when you eat less, you lose. Although you can't change your metabolic rate much, you can change how many calories you burn through physical activity.

Q How much should I weigh?

A There's no one ideal weight for height. The most desirable weight for you depends on your body frame. Today's health experts also know that body composition (the amount of body fat and muscle mass) indicates whether people need a diet and exercise regimen. Evaluate yourself in several ways:
• Do a mirror test. If you see bulges and flab, you probably need to trim down and firm up.
• Give yourself a pinch test to estimate your body fat composition. With your thumb and index finger, pinch the skin on the back of your arm, thigh, or waist. Gently pull the skin away from the muscle so you only pinch skin and fat. If you pinch ½ to 1 inch, your level of body fat is probably normal. If you pinch less than ½ inch, you may be underweight. More suggests excess body fat. Do the pinch test in several places; most people carry their weight unevenly. A doctor or dietitian can measure body composition more precisely.
• Use a height-weight table (page 17) to find the desirable weight for your height and body frame. But remember, these tables are only guidelines.

Q How many calories do I need?

A That depends on you—your age, your body size, and your activity level, among other factors. The RDA for calories has been estimated for people who don't get much exercise. But because energy needs vary among people, calorie recommendations are also given as a range:

AGE	WOMEN	MEN
19–22	2,100 (1,700–2,500)	2,900 (2,500–3,300)
23–50	2,000 (1,600–2,400)	2,700 (2,300–3,100)
51–75	1,800 (1,400–2,200)	2,400 (2,000–2,800)
76+	1,600 (1,200–2,000)	2,050 (1,650–2,450)

Estimate your calorie needs (for weight maintenance) with this simple calculation:
1. Determine the calories you burn per pound: inactive, 12 calories per pound; lightly active (office work with a 20-minute walk), 14 calories per pound; moderately active (office work with 30 minutes of aerobic exercise), 20 calories per pound; extremely active, 25 calories per pound. (These examples represent typical energy expenditures.)
2. Multiply calories you burn per pound by your current weight in pounds to estimate daily calorie needs.

To lose weight, cut back on your caloric intake, burn more calories through exercise, or do both. Be careful not to restrict food intake too much. It's difficult to get all the nutrients needed in a diet with fewer than 1,200 calories. And diets below 800 calories may be hazardous, unless supervised by a doctor.

Q Why do some people seem to need more calories than others do?

A Nutritionists don't completely understand why some people can eat much more than others, and still stay at a desirable weight. Yet some things are clear.
• People who are more physically active need more calories. They need calories to power exercise. And a lean, muscular body seems to require more calories than a body of the same weight that has less muscle and more body fat.

• People with a large body frame need more calories to sustain their weight than smaller people do. That's one reason most men tend to need more calories than women do.
• During pregnancy and breast feeding, a woman needs more calories to sustain the needs of her infant as well as her own body.
• Metabolic rates slow as people get older. For every decade of life, your metabolic rate drops by about 10 percent. So you need fewer calories to keep body processes going.

Q How do I know just how many calories I'm consuming?

A Estimate your caloric intake by keeping a food record for three to seven typical days.
Record *everything* you eat and drink, including amounts, for each 24-hour period. Then look up the calories for each serving, using a calorie guide (pages 232–235) and the nutrition labels on packaged foods. Remember, recipes in this book list calories per serving, too. Now find the total for each day. When you've totaled each day, add them up and divide by the number of days you recorded to figure your average.

Q How many pounds can I safely lose each week?

A First of all, check with your doctor before starting a diet program. If you get the OK, don't try to lose weight too fast! Slow, sustained weight loss— one or two pounds per week—is the safest and usually the most effective way to reach your weight goals.
A pound of body fat equals about 3,500 calories. So by cutting out just 500 calories per day, you can lose one pound a week. Or cut 1,000 calories per day, and lose about two pounds a week.
Crash or fad diets sound alluring because they promise quick, dramatic weight loss. But they usually fail, at least in the long run. Initial weight loss is mostly water loss, which is quickly regained when the diet is over.

People who lose weight on one fad diet after another may do their bodies more harm than good. They may lose what they need most to look trim—muscle mass. Without exercise, the body uses muscle mass before body fat for energy when calories are restricted. Severe calorie restriction can cause other serious health problems, such as dehydration, fatigue, kidney problems, even death.

Q What diet plan makes the most health sense?

A The best diet for weight loss is a balanced diet that follows the four food-group guidelines. (Refer to the food groups pictured on pages 12–15.) For women, that can translate to as few as 1,200 to 1,400 carefully chosen calories a day, and for men, about 1,600 calories.

A variety of low-calorie, nutrient-dense foods can provide all the nutrients you need, without excess calories. So eat more fruits, vegetables, and whole-grains. High-fiber foods tend to be low in calories. Eat less fat and fatty foods and less sugar and sweets. And drink fewer alcoholic beverages.

Plan a weight-loss diet to match your own food likes, needs, and life-style. You won't stick to the diet if it isn't right for you.

Q How can exercise help me lose weight?

A You can lose weight by dieting alone. But it's easier, faster, even more fun to lose if you both diet *and* exercise. After all, exercise burns calories. Even a gradual increase in everyday activity, such as brisk walking, can make a difference. A brisk half-hour walk burns about 150 calories. But the harder and longer you exercise, the more calories you use. Thirty minutes of jogging uses 250 to 300 calories, and 45 minutes burns at least 375.

With regular exercise, you don't need to diet as strenuously to achieve the same weight goals. As a result, you're more likely to consume all the nutrients you need. Suppose you planned to lose two pounds a week by trimming 1,000 calories from your daily diet.

Instead, trim 750 calories and burn 250 calories more in exercise.

Exercise has four other body-trimming advantages: (1) Vigorous exercise produces extra body heat, which causes the body to burn calories at a faster rate for several hours. (2) A firm, lean body looks trimmer than a body with excess fat, even when body weight is just the same. (3) A muscular body burns calories at a faster rate than a body with more body fat. (4) And exercise may lower the body's set point, or the weight the body tends to return to naturally.

Q How can I maintain my desirable weight?

A Once you achieve your desirable weight, you want to maintain it comfortably. Weigh yourself each week, not more. Continue eating a balanced diet but try increasing portion size some. If you would continue eating at the same level needed for weight loss, you would continue losing weight.

The key to maintenance is to eat the same number of calories that your body burns. As soon as pounds creep back on, adjust your calorie intake or activity level. Try to make exercise a habit so you don't need to watch calories. Control and moderation are dietary guidelines to follow for a lifetime.

Planning What to Eat

Q What guidelines can I use when planning low-calorie menus?

A Variety, balance, and moderation—these are the three rules of good nutrition. No one food provides all the essential nutrients. Instead, *variety* ensures that your diet provides the 40 or more nutrients you need for good health.

You also need *balance* for good health. A balanced diet contains essential nutrients in recommended amounts. There's no undue emphasis on one type of food or nutrient.

Moderation means: Don't eat one or more foods in excess. Calorie control is part of a moderate diet.

Bread/Cereal Food Group

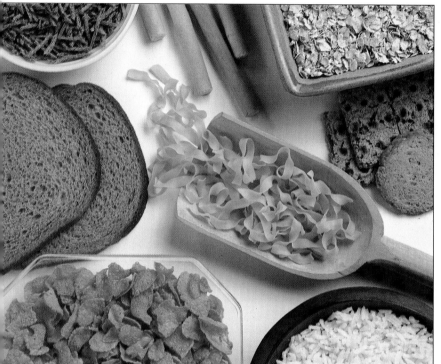

Plan to have 4 servings daily from foods in this group, which include whole grain and enriched breads and cereals, rice, and pasta. A typical serving size consists of 1 slice bread; ½ to ¾ cup cooked cereal, pasta, or rice; or 1 ounce ready-to-eat cereal. Foods in this group provide thiamine, niacin, and iron. Some are good fiber sources, as well.

Q **What are the four food-group guidelines?**

A The four food groups translate the scientific language of nutrients and RDAs into easy menu planning and food selection guidelines, guidelines that ensure both variety and balance. If your daily diet meets food-group recommendations, it is likely to provide nutrients in the amounts you need for good health. (Refer to the food groups pictured on pages 12–15. You'll find the recommended daily servings for each group and the serving sizes.)

Q **How nutritious is each food group?**

A Each food group contributes different important nutrients to the diet. So, by balancing your meals to provide the recommended amounts of each group, you get both a nutritious and a varied diet. Foods within each food group contain similar amounts of key nutrients. That's why they're grouped together. And that's why you can substitute one food for another within each food group. Besides the key nutrients, foods contain many other nutrients essential for health.

Q **How do sweets, fats, and alcoholic beverages fit into the food groups?**

A They don't, not in any of the four food groups. They are sometimes referred to as a fifth food group, however. The reason? Although they contain either carbohydrates or fats or both, they don't contain significant amounts of nutrients found in any of the other groups. Instead, they contribute mostly calories. So they're often called "empty-calorie" foods.

For people who can afford the calories, small amounts of fats and sweets do add flavor and interest to meals and snacks, but not much nutrition. They're extras. For good health, don't substitute empty-calorie foods for those in the four food groups.

Q How can I plan nutritious, low-calorie meals?

A Start your meal planning by selecting the main dish. Then, add side dishes, a beverage, and possibly a dessert to round out the meal, working with foods from each of the four food groups.

When planning a full day's menu, consider the food groups and include the recommended quantities for each group: the right number of servings in the recommended serving size. Your personal needs and preferences determine which foods to choose. But variety among and within each food group ensures a diet with the essential nutrients.

When you're watching calories, plan menus that include low-calorie foods from each food group. Instead of whole milk, have skim milk; instead of fried chicken, have baked chicken. And limit the amount of fats, sweets, and alcoholic beverages.

Q Do I have to eat three meals each day?

A There's nothing nutritionally sacred about eating three meals a day. Four, five, or six mini-meals also can provide all the nutrients you need, as long as you follow food group guidelines.

Q What nutrition guidelines promote health?

A The U.S. Department of Agriculture has established Dietary Guidelines for Americans based on the best scientific information available. Follow these guidelines as you choose and prepare foods for good health.

1) *Eat a variety of foods.* Variety may be the "spice of life," and it's also essential for good nutrition and good health. Each day, your body needs the 40 or more nutrients that only a varied diet provides. Most foods have more than one nutrient. But no one food has them all. To get the nutrients your body needs, in ample amounts, eat a varied diet.

Milk/Cheese Food Group

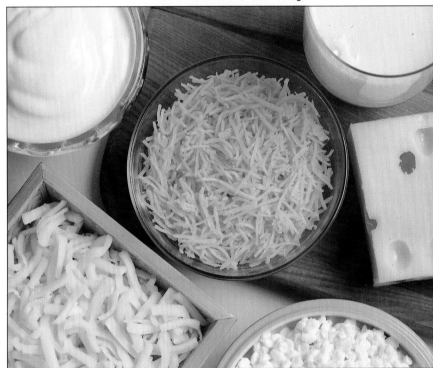

Serving sizes of this food group vary. They depend on age and, for a woman, whether she is pregnant or a nursing mother. For children under 9, provide 2 to 3 servings daily; children 9 to 12 and pregnant women need 3 servings daily. Teenagers and nursing mothers need 4 servings daily. Serve other adults 2 servings each day. A serving size consists of 8 ounces milk or yogurt, 1⅓ ounces hard cheese, or 2 cups cottage cheese. These foods are major sources of calcium, but they also add riboflavin, protein, and other vitamins to the diet.

Meat/Meat Substitutes Food Group

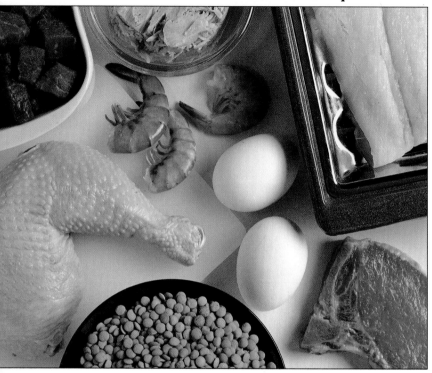

Meat/Meat Substitutes Food Group

You'll need two servings daily from foods in this group. A serving size consists of 2 to 3 ounces lean cooked meat, poultry, and fish (without bones); 2 eggs; or 1 to 1½ cups cooked legumes or lentils. Nutrients supplied by foods in this group include protein, iron, thiamine, and niacin. Suggested foods are beef, veal, pork, lamb, poultry, fish, shellfish, eggs, nuts, and legumes.

2) *Maintain desirable weight.* Maintaining your most desirable weight makes good health sense. Being too fat increases the chance of developing serious health conditions. In this book you'll find recipes and tips that will help you achieve and maintain your own best weight.

3) *Avoid too much fat, saturated fat, and cholesterol.* Most Americans eat more fat than they really need. About 37 percent of calories come from fat, 46 percent from carbohydrate, and 16 percent from protein. A suggested amount of fat in the diet is 30 to 33 percent of total daily calories. Eating less fat and more complex carbohydrates (starch and fiber) makes good health sense.

4) *Eat foods with adequate starch and fiber.* Grain products, dry beans, vegetables, and fruits are sources of starch and fiber. These foods have many virtues. Besides providing energy, they are good sources of vitamins and minerals. Many provide protein and fiber, and they're usually low in fat and cholesterol.

5) *Avoid too much sugar.* In one form or another, sugar is present in many foods you eat. Fruit, for example, contains sugar naturally. During processing, sugar is added to some foods. And table sugar, added in food preparation, is a common form.

Sugar itself has useful functions. It's a source of calories, or energy. The problem is that many people eat too much, too often. Diets full of high-sugar foods often have too many calories for people who must watch their weight. In addition, table sugar and many high-sugar foods have few other nutrients. For good health, avoid too much.

6) *Avoid too much sodium.* Sodium is an essential nutrient, necessary for maintaining the balance of fluids that help nutrients pass into your cells and wastes pass out. Where does sodium come from? From food, of course. About one-third is naturally present in food. About one-third comes from processed foods. The salt shaker provides the rest.

Most Americans get more sodium than they need. The average person consumes about 5,000 milligrams daily, but nutrition professionals say that 1,100 to 3,300 milligrams each day is enough.

7) *If you drink alcoholic beverages, do so in moderation.* Alcoholic beverages are high in calories and low in nutrients. In fact, they're empty-calorie beverages. Moreover, heavy drinking is associated with serious health conditions. If you're pregnant, avoid alcohol altogether, because even moderate amounts may cause birth defects and other problems during pregnancy.

Other Questions

Q What happens if I don't get all the nutrients I need?

A That depends on how deficient your diet is and for how long.

When you're undernourished, your body just doesn't work as well. And you can often see and feel the difference. You may be irritable, depressed, or nervous. You're more susceptible to colds and other infectious diseases. Cuts and sores heal more slowly. And you may tire easily after just a little exercise. Over the years, a poor diet takes its toll on your bones, your teeth, the fitness of your whole body.

The effects of a poor diet are more dramatic among severely malnourished people, such as anorexics, who starve themselves to become thin. Stunted growth, brain damage, severe wasting, even death are among the results.

Q Will extra vitamins or minerals give me more energy or keep me healthier?

A Neither vitamins nor minerals supply energy. And extra amounts—more than the RDAs— have no added health benefits for most people. Actually, too much of some nutrients can be as harmful as consuming too few!

Over time, megadoses, or large doses, of the fat-soluble vitamins A, D, E, and K are stored in the body. Although having extra on hand may sound healthful, actually these excess stores can cause health problems. Too much vitamin A, for example, can cause blurred vision, skin problems, headaches,

Vegetable/Fruit Food Group

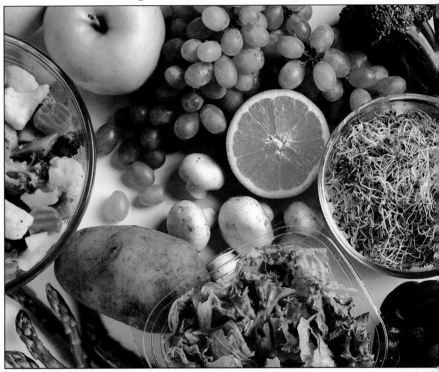

*F*our servings are needed each day, including one vitamin C-rich food (such as citrus fruit). One vitamin A-rich food (such as carrots, broccoli, or cantaloupe) should be served at least every other day. A serving size consists of ½ cup of fruit or vegetable, 1 medium orange or potato, ½ grapefruit, 4 ounces citrus juice, or 1 lettuce wedge. Nutrients provided by this group include vitamins A and C. This group also adds fiber to the diet.

and brain damage. Weakness, nausea, and constipation are early signs of too much vitamin D.

Large doses of water-soluble vitamins—B vitamins and vitamin C—can cause trouble, too, although the water-soluble vitamins aren't stored in the body. For example, excreting excess amounts of vitamin C puts a strain on the kidneys.

Food usually isn't the source of vitamin or mineral overdose, however. Nutrient supplements, often in the form of pills, are the common culprit. As a precaution, take supplements only under the direction of a physician. And avoid those with high nutrient doses: more than 100 percent of RDAs.

Q If I take a vitamin/mineral supplement, do I need to eat a balanced diet?

A Supplements can augment the diet. But they can't replace food. No supplement or combination of supplements can provide the 40 or more nutrients you need for good health. Only food in a balanced diet does that.

If you eat a balanced diet, you probably don't need supplements at all. Carefully chosen meals and snacks from the four food groups provide most healthy people with all the nutrients they need. There are some exceptions, however. Because adequate iron is hard to get from the diet, many women benefit from an iron supplement. During pregnancy, doctors usually prescribe iron and folic acid supplements to prevent anemia. And calcium supplements often are recommended for postmenopausal women to protect against osteoporosis.

Q Is snacking OK?

A Snacks can be nutritious. Carefully chosen, they provide many nutrients you need each day. In fact, snacks can fill the gaps in your day's nutrient intake. If you missed citrus juice for breakfast, enjoy an orange for a midmorning snack. Just watch out for empty calories when you snack.

Nutrient Information

Q How can ingredient lists and nutrition labels help me with food decisions?

A Both the ingredient list and nutrition information on a food label give you clues to what's inside the package.

Ingredients are listed in order by weight, from the largest amounts listed first to the smallest amounts listed last. Nutrition information on the label lets you know the nutrients provided by a single serving. You'll find the serving size, number of servings, calorie count, and gram weights of protein, carbohydrate, fat, and sodium. Sometimes the cholesterol content is listed. Other nutrients are listed by percentage of the U.S. Recommended Daily Allowances (U.S. RDAs).

Not all products are nutrition-labeled, but if a nutrition claim is made, or if a product contains added nutrients, this information must be on the label.

Q How can I use the nutrient information provided in this cookbook?

A The recipes in this book were created for the calorie-conscious cook. To help with menu planning, you'll find a nutrition analysis of each recipe.

Keep track of the calories, protein, carbohydrate, fat, cholesterol, sodium, and potassium in your menus. In each recipe we've published, you'll find the amounts of these nutrients by gram weight per individual recipe serving.

This is how the nutrition information accompanying the recipes was calculated:
• When ingredient options appear in the recipe, we used the first ingredient choice for the analysis.
• We omitted optional ingredients from the analysis.
• We based the nutrition analysis on the first serving size if a recipe gives variable serving sizes.
• When lean ground beef is an ingredient, we used 90% lean beef (10% fat) for the analysis.

Here are some simple guidelines based on the daily needs of females, 23 to 50 years old (in general, teenagers, pregnant women, and males need more calories): calories, 2,000; protein, 45–65 g; fat, 67 g; cholesterol, 300 mg; sodium, 1,100–3,300 mg; potassium, 1,875–5,625 mg.

IDEAL HEIGHT AND WEIGHT

	HEIGHT	SMALL FRAME	MEDIUM FRAME	LARGE FRAME
WOMEN	4'10"	102–111	109–121	118–131
	4'11"	103–113	111–123	120–134
	5'0"	104–115	113–126	122–137
	5'1"	106–118	115–129	125–140
	5'2"	108–121	118–132	128–143
	5'3"	111–124	121–135	131–147
	5'4"	114–127	124–138	134–151
	5'5"	117–130	127–141	137–155
	5'6"	120–133	130–144	140–159
	5'7"	123–136	133–147	143–163
	5'8"	126–139	136–150	146–167
	5'9"	129–142	139–153	149–170
	5'10"	132–145	142–156	152–173
	5'11"	135–148	145–159	155–176
	6'0"	138–151	148–162	158–179
MEN	5'2"	128–134	131–141	138–150
	5'3"	130–136	133–143	140–153
	5'4"	132–138	135–145	142–156
	5'5"	134–140	137–148	144–160
	5'6"	136–142	139–151	146–164
	5'7"	138–145	142–154	149–168
	5'8"	140–148	145–157	152–172
	5'9"	142–151	148–160	155–176
	5'10"	144–154	151–163	158–180
	5'11"	146–157	154–166	161–184
	6'0"	149–160	157–170	164–188
	6'1"	152–164	160–174	168–192
	6'2"	155–168	164–178	172–197
	6'3"	158–172	167–182	176–202
	6'4"	162–176	171–187	181–207

This table was issued in 1983 by the Metropolitan Life Insurance Company and is based on weights of policyholders with fewest illnesses and longest lives. Heights were measured in shoes with 1-inch heels, and weights with five pounds of indoor clothing (for men) and 3 pounds of indoor clothing (for women). These figures represent population averages; your ideal weight may differ.

But You're Short on Time

All too often, it seems as though there aren't enough hours in the day. If that's the case at your house, here are some shortcuts that will help save you time with your menu planning and meal preparations.

Planning

Q What can I do to prevent the last-minute dilemma of what to fix for a meal?

A Remember the familiar saying, "Plan ahead"? Well, that's a good way to avoid last-minute, meal-planning dilemmas.

Planning ahead means writing down your menus for a few days or a week at a time. With some planning, you won't waste precious minutes wondering what to serve and hoping you have everything. And you'll know that you're not repeating the same meal you served the day before.

Need another timesaving reason to plan ahead? Cook more than you need and count on having leftovers. Then, devise ways to use the planned leftovers for menus starring quick salads, stir-frys, or sandwiches. Be sure to set aside the planned leftovers before serving the meal so that you're not tempted to eat more than the portion size.

Q But, how can I plan low-calorie meals that are quick and easy?

A Use the recipes from this book, keeping your menu plans simple. Prepare only one or two foods from recipes, then fill in the rest of the meal with plain or purchased calorie-trimmed items. An easily cooked frozen vegetable or a tossed vegetable salad makes a simple menu addition.

Q What's the difference between quick and easy recipes in this book?

A Quick recipes are prepared in 45 minutes or less, from start to finish. Easy recipes are assembled quickly but take some time to cook or chill.

Q Can you give me some basic menu planning tips for quick, yet nutritious, meals?

A Keeping the four food groups and the number of servings in mind (see pages 12–15), start planning your menus around the main dish. Then, add a variety of foods to round out the meal.

Need some examples? For dinner, choose a one-dish meal, such as a casserole. That way, foods from more than one food group are combined in one dish and a good portion of the menu is planned.

Or, select a simple entrée, then add vegetables, an item from the bread group, and a fruit or vegetable salad. Don't forget to select a beverage. Skim milk is always a good, nutritious choice.

Consider what the foods will *look* like together. And, imagine what all the foods will *taste* like when they're served with each other.

Variety, balance, and moderation are important when planning menus, especially diet meals.

Q How else can I make meal preparation go more smoothly?

A Besides having a written menu and the necessary foods on hand, have a meal preparation schedule in mind: what should be started first, what next, and so on. With each recipe in the book, you'll find a preparation timetable that gives you an estimate of the time needed to prepare each recipe.

Q When should I plan to use make-ahead recipes?

A Make foods in advance for those days when you know you won't have time to prepare a full-fledged meal. Stockpile the freezer or refrigerate items ahead for especially easy meals. Check the make-ahead sections in this book for recipes.

Q What are some quick-cooking techniques that a dieter can plan to use?

A Stir-frying meat and vegetables in a large skillet or wok, using very little fat or a nonstick spray coating, is one speedy cooking method.

Another way to cook quickly is by broiling. Broiling lets the fat drip away from the meat during cooking, thus reducing calories.

Poaching in liquid is another method to cut calories. It takes just minutes to simmer fish, poultry, or eggs till done.

Q What about fitting a crockery cooker into my menu plans?

A Definitely use this appliance and let dinner cook itself. Your crockery cooker simmers the food during the day so you come home to dinner that's practically ready for the table. What could be easier! Check the index for several crockery cooker recipe suggestions.

Q What are some timesaving ingredients I can plan to use that will speed cooking?

A Buy ingredients in the form needed for a recipe. Opt for shredded or sliced cheeses; cut-up chicken; boned and skinned chicken breasts; cut-up meats, such as stew meat; frozen meat patties; canned fish, chicken, turkey, and ham; cooked meats from the deli; bread crumbs and croutons; bottled minced garlic; dried minced onion, garlic, and parsley flakes; frozen chopped onion, green pepper, and chives; frozen fruit juice concentrates; items from the salad bar; shredded cabbage and coleslaw mixtures; and bottled lemon juice.

Other items to purchase that will quickly round out your meals include: canned soups; quick-cooking rice and couscous; frozen and canned vegetables; fresh, canned (juice-pack), and frozen (unsweetened) fruits; low-fat dairy products; whole-grain breads; and low-calorie beverages.

Q Can you give me a list of foods to keep on hand for unplanned last-minute meals?

A Here are some foods you can use for emergency meals: eggs, low-fat cheese, skim milk, lean meat, pasta, rice, fruits and vegetables, lettuce and other salad greens, and whole-grain breads.

To prevent extra trips to the store, keep these staples on hand: flour, sugar, salt, pepper, herbs and spices, cornstarch, baking powder, baking soda, coffee, tea, cooking oil, margarine, calorie-reduced mayonnaise and salad dressings, prepared mustard, and instant beef and chicken bouillon granules.

Q Should I write out a shopping list?

A By all means. At the store, you'll not only save time, but you'll think twice about items not on your list—those items that don't fit on your diet.

Here are some additional shopping list hints:
• Make it a habit to list items when you're about to run out of them. That way you won't forget the item on your next trip to the store.
• Make out your grocery list when planning your menus so ingredients won't be missing when it's time to start cooking.
• After you've become familiar with your favorite store, write down your shopping list in the order that you walk through the store. You'll avoid backtracking for missed items.

Q How can I do my grocery shopping most efficiently?

A Select a store that carries all of the products you'll need. A one-stop supermarket generally carries everything from dairy products to fresh fish and meats to fresh fruits and vegetables to frozen foods. You'll save time by not having to drive to specialty food stores for individual items on your list.

A word of caution: It's best *not* to shop on an empty stomach. Everything looks good when you're hungry, especially when you're on a diet.

Keep the shopping trips to a minimum—once a week, if possible. You'll save time and maybe even some money and calories by limiting your shopping.

Become a label reader and learn as much as you can about the nutritional content of foods you buy.

Q What's the best time of the day to shop for groceries?

A After several trips to the store at various times during the week, you'll be able to identify the "off hours" for the store where you shop. Try to plan your shopping during those less busy times. Generally, Saturday mornings and right after work during the week are busy times.

Q What's the best way to handle foods when I get home?

A Store the foods properly in the refrigerator, in the freezer, or on the shelf. Consider the freezer for long-term storage and the refrigerator for perishable foods that will be used within a few days. Nonperishable staples can be stored in a cool, dry place.

Here are some additional storage tips:
• Cut up meats in the desired portions and wrap them properly before storing in the freezer.
• Store canned foods in a cool, dry place away from sunlight. Ideal storage temperature is between 50°F. and 70°F. If you store a can or two of fruit in the refrigerator, it will be ready for a quick salad with lettuce or a calorie-trimmed dessert.

Time to Cook

Q How can I streamline my cooking activities?

A Read the recipe before you begin. Then, gather all of the ingredients and equipment you'll need. Many of the recipe preparation and cooking steps in this book overlap one another so that the recipes can be prepared easily. While one part of the recipe is cooking or chilling, you can prepare another part of the recipe.

Q How can I use the recipe timings in this book?

A Use them as a guide for the amount of time to allow for preparing the recipe. Some of the recipes list both a preparation time and a cooking time. Others give a total preparation time, indicating that preparation and cooking times are added together.

Note the recipes marked "20 minutes or less." Select these recipes for especially quick dishes.

Times for make-ahead recipes include advance preparation time, meaning total preparation time before the food is chilled or frozen.

Q Besides freezing make-ahead recipes, can I use the freezer to help save time?

A Yes. Use it to keep frozen fruits, vegetables, and meats on hand. Make sure that any frozen food items are wrapped with moisture- and vaporproof wraps or placed in freezer containers, then sealed properly. Be sure to label the packages properly as well. Labeling with contents and date takes the guesswork out of identifying a package's contents and the length of time it's been in the freezer.

Need another timesaving use for the freezer? Use it to quick-chill foods. Remember to check the food frequently so that it only chills and doesn't freeze.

Q What are some other "make-ahead" tips that will save time when preparing a meal?

A Save time by chopping several onions or green peppers at once when you have the equipment out on your counter. Then, freeze the items for use in recipes. You also can snip chives and parsley in quantity, then store in the freezer.

Shredded or grated cheese is another ingredient you can prepare ahead to have on hand. When you're shredding cheese for one recipe, prepare more than you need and refrigerate the extra, tightly sealed.

Q Are there ingredient substitutions that I can make if I run out of something?

A There are many emergency substitutions to use in cooking. Some of them are listed below. (Calories may vary between the two products, so check the calorie chart on pages 232–235 for the differences.)
- 2 tablespoons all-purpose flour for 1 tablespoon cornstarch (for thickening)
- ¾ cup tomato paste plus 1 cup water for 2 cups tomato sauce
- ½ cup tomato sauce plus ½ cup water for 1 cup tomato juice
- ⅛ teaspoon garlic powder for 1 clove garlic
- 1 teaspoon onion powder *or* 1 tablespoon dried minced onion for 1 small onion
- 1 tablespoon prepared mustard for 1 teaspoon dry mustard
- 1 teaspoon dried herbs, crushed, for 1 tablespoon snipped fresh herbs
- 1 teaspoon instant bouillon granules dissolved in 1 cup water for 1 cup broth

Q How should I organize my kitchen so that I can cook most efficiently?

A Keep equipment near the place it's used most often. For example, store a cutting board close to the kitchen sink, where you cut up vegetables. Store cooking containers and utensils near the range.

Have a place for everything and keep everything in its place. That way you'll know just where to look for a necessary piece of equipment.

Use as few bowls and utensils as possible. It saves on cleanup.

Q What are some appliances that help save time in the kitchen?

A Blenders and food processors are ideal for chopping and combining foods in a jiffy.

The microwave oven is handy for thawing frozen foods quickly and cooking entire recipes. Check the microwave sections of this book for recipes. You also can use your microwave to shortcut parts of food preparation, such as warming, melting, and softening foods.

Q What about using equipment with nonstick finishes?

A The easy-care finishes on cooking equipment are great for dieters. By using pans with nonstick coatings, you can cut down on the amount of fat needed during cooking. Cleanup is easier, too.

Q What's a simple way to avoid monotony in a diet that includes quick-cooking foods?

A Perk up plain foods with herbs and spices. Start with ¼ teaspoon for each 4 servings. Because small amounts are generally used in recipes, herbs add few calories but plenty of flavor. So, use them often to add special interest to a dish.

To easily crush dried herbs, rub the dried leaves between the palms of your hands and drop them right into the cooking container.

Tips for Trimming Calories

Even small calorie savings add up when you're trying to lose weight. Apply these slimming techniques to recipes you cook regularly and you'll trim a few calories from many of your meals.

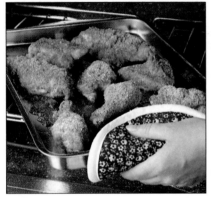

1 Fat-free oven "frying" gives a crispy crust to foods such as chicken and fish that traditionally are coated with a breading mixture. During skillet frying, those coatings absorb fat.

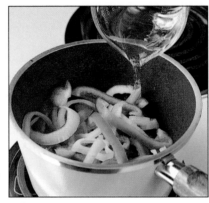

2 When a casserole or skillet-meal recipe calls for precooking vegetables, such as onions, green peppers, and celery, simmer them in a little water instead of sautéing in butter or oil.

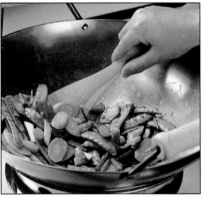

3 When stir-frying, spray a cold wok or skillet with nonstick spray coating, then preheat. After stir-frying the first batch, add a little cooking oil, if needed, to cook remaining ingredients.

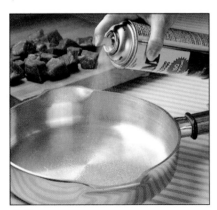

7 To keep meat from sticking without using fat, brown meat in a pan sprayed with nonstick spray coating. Use the spray on a cold pan following the label directions.

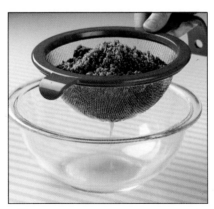

8 Thoroughly drain away the excess fat after browning ground meat. Use either a wire mesh strainer or a metal colander held well above the pool of accumulating fat.

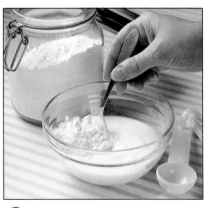

9 Low-fat yogurt makes a good substitute for sour cream. For thickened sauces, stir flour (2 tablespoons per cup of yogurt) into the yogurt before cooking to prevent curdling.

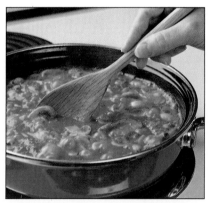

4 *Instead of thickening a sauce with flour or cornstarch, save a few calories by reducing the sauce to make it thicker. Do this by gently boiling the sauce to evaporate some of the liquid.*

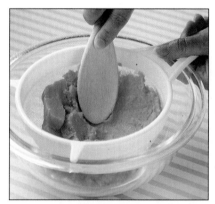

5 *Use cooked and pureed vegetables instead of conventional thickeners (cornstarch and flour) for sauces and soups. The bonus? You'll get the nutrients and flavor of the vegetable.*

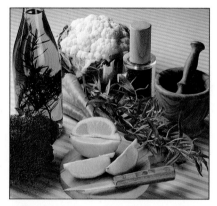

6 *Low-calorie vegetables are good dieters' choices, but skip the rich sauces. Instead, try lemon juice, flavored vinegars, garlic, and herbs and spices to accent the flavors of the vegetables.*

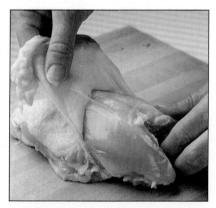

10 *Reduce the calories in chicken by removing all the skin from the pieces before cooking. Many of the calories are found in the skin and the fat just beneath the skin.*

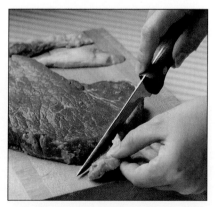

11 *For calorie-reduced meat dishes, start with the leanest cuts of meat available, such as round steak. Then, use a sharp knife to trim away separable fat before cooking.*

Calorie-Minded Main Dishes

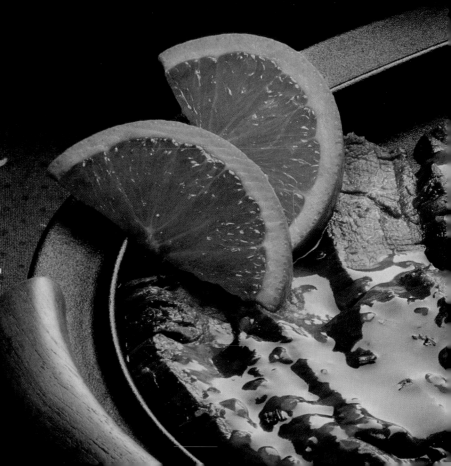

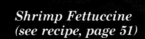

Shrimp Fettuccine
(see recipe, page 51)

Whittle away unnecessary calories from the meal's main dish, where many of the calories lurk. That's good advice, but how do you do it? Just select from the calorie-conscious meat, poultry, fish, and meatless recipes in this chapter.

As you thumb through the pages, get ready for some dieter's surprises. Pizza and pasta are only two of the many noteworthy dishes to fit your diet and schedule.

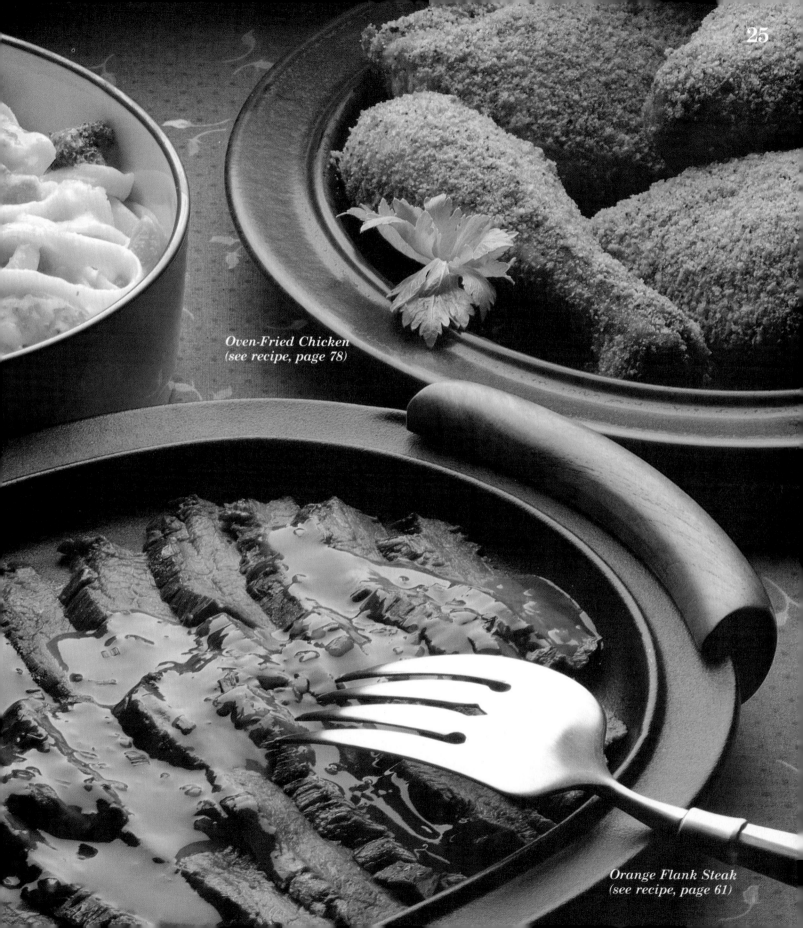

Oven-Fried Chicken
(see recipe, page 78)

Orange Flank Steak
(see recipe, page 61)

20 minutes or less

PICK-A-SAUCE POULTRY

Tantalize your taste buds with one of three tempting sauces.

Nonstick spray coating
4 boned skinless chicken breast halves *or* turkey breast tenderloin steaks (about 1 pound total)

■ Spray a *cold* large skillet with nonstick coating. Preheat skillet, then add the chicken or turkey. Cook over medium heat for 8 to 10 minutes or till tender and no longer pink, turning the pieces over occasionally to brown evenly. Transfer the chicken or turkey to a serving platter. Cover and keep warm.

■ While the poultry is cooking, measure the ingredients for one of the sauces below, if desired. Then cook sauce. Serve sauce over poultry. Makes 4 servings.

Marsala Sauce: Cut ½ cup seedless red *or* green *grapes* in half. Combine ¼ cup *marsala or dry sherry,* ¼ cup *water,* 1 teaspoon *cornstarch,* and ¼ teaspoon instant *chicken bouillon granules.* Add the grapes and marsala mixture to the skillet in which chicken was cooked. Cook and stir over medium-high heat till mixture is thickened and bubbly. Then cook and stir for 1 minute more. Spoon sauce over poultry. Makes 4 servings.

Indian Curry Sauce: To the hot skillet in which chicken was cooked add 1 teaspoon *margarine or butter* and ½ teaspoon *curry powder;* cook and stir for 30 seconds or till bubbly. Combine ½ cup plain low-fat *yogurt,* 2 tablespoons *skim milk,* 1 tablespoon all-purpose *flour,* 1 tablespoon *currants,* and ¼ teaspoon bottled minced *garlic or* dash *garlic powder.* Add to skillet. Cook and stir till thickened and bubbly. Then cook and stir for 1 minute more. Spoon sauce over poultry. Makes 4 servings.

Barbecue Sauce: In the hot skillet in which chicken was cooked combine ⅓ cup reduced-calorie *catsup,* 2 tablespoons frozen chopped *onion* (see tip, page 39), 1 tablespoon frozen chopped *green pepper* (see tip, page 39), 2 tablespoons *orange juice,* ½ teaspoon dry *mustard,* and ⅛ teaspoon *chili powder.* Cook and stir over medium heat till onion and pepper are tender. Spoon sauce over poultry. Makes 4 servings.

PER SERVING

Calories	125
Protein	26 g
Carbohydrate	0 g
Fat	1 g
Cholesterol	66 mg
Sodium	74 mg
Potassium	289 mg

TIMETABLE

Total preparation time: 15 minutes

Calories	36

Calories	40

Calories	20

TERIYAKI CHICKEN

Concerned about your sodium intake? Try sodium-reduced or light soy sauce—it has less sodium than regular soy sauce. Look for it in your supermarket.

4 boned skinless chicken
  breast halves *or* turkey
  breast tenderloin steaks
  (about 1 pound total)
2 tablespoons soy sauce
2 tablespoons sake *or*
  dry sherry
1 teaspoon dry mustard
½ teaspoon ground ginger
½ teaspoon bottled minced
  garlic *or* ⅛ teaspoon
  garlic powder
1 teaspoon sesame seed

■ Preheat the broiler. Meanwhile, place poultry in a plastic bag; set bag in a bowl. For marinade, in a small mixing bowl combine soy sauce, sake or dry sherry, mustard, ginger, and garlic. Pour marinade over poultry in bag. Marinate for 10 minutes at room temperature, turning bag occasionally. Drain poultry, reserving marinade.

■ Place poultry on the unheated rack of a broiler pan. Broil poultry 4 inches from the heat for 4 minutes. Brush with marinade, then turn poultry over and broil for 3 minutes more. Brush with marinade and sprinkle with sesame seed. Continue broiling for 1 to 2 minutes more or till poultry is tender and no longer pink. Makes 4 servings.

PER SERVING

Calories	131
Protein	26 g
Carbohydrate	0 g
Fat	2 g
Cholesterol	66 mg
Sodium	203 mg
Potassium	301 mg

TIMETABLE

Preparation time:
15 minutes

Cooking time:
8 to 9 minutes

CHICKEN ROMANO

Save time on cleanup: Combine the crumb mixture on a piece of waxed paper.

3 tablespoons fine dry
  bread crumbs
2 tablespoons grated
  Romano *or* Parmesan
  cheese
1 teaspoon dried parsley
  flakes
½ teaspoon dried basil,
  crushed
⅛ teaspoon garlic powder
¼ cup skim milk
4 boned skinless chicken
  breast halves *or* turkey
  breast tenderloin steaks
  (about 1 pound total)

■ Preheat the oven to 425°. Meanwhile, in a shallow dish combine bread crumbs, Romano or Parmesan cheese, parsley, basil, and garlic powder. Pour milk into another shallow dish.

■ Dip chicken or turkey pieces into milk, then roll them in the crumb mixture. Place coated pieces in an ungreased 13x9x2-inch baking pan.

■ Bake in the 425° oven for 10 to 12 minutes or till poultry is tender and no longer pink. To serve, transfer to a serving platter. Makes 4 servings.

PER SERVING

Calories	161
Protein	28 g
Carbohydrate	4 g
Fat	2 g
Cholesterol	70 mg
Sodium	154 mg
Potassium	329 mg

TIMETABLE

Preparation time:
10 minutes

Cooking time:
10 to 12 minutes

GARLIC THAI CHICKEN

In the tradition of Thailand's spicy stir-fry dishes, this packs a red pepper punch!

2 tablespoons soy sauce
1½ teaspoons bottled minced garlic *or* ½ teaspoon garlic powder
1 teaspoon sesame oil
½ teaspoon crushed red pepper
¼ teaspoon ground coriander
12 ounces boned skinless chicken breast halves
1½ cups quick-cooking rice *or* 1 cup quick-cooking couscous
8 green onions
Nonstick spray coating

■ In a medium mixing bowl combine soy sauce, garlic, sesame oil, red pepper, and coriander. Set aside. Cut chicken into about 1-inch chunks, then add it to the soy sauce mixture in the bowl. Toss lightly to coat, then set aside.

■ Cook rice according to package directions, *except* omit the margarine or butter. (Or, in a medium saucepan bring 1½ cups *water* and ¼ teaspoon *salt* to boiling. Add couscous. Cover and remove from heat. Let stand for 5 minutes.) While rice (or couscous) is standing, cut onions into about 1½-inch pieces. Spray a *cold* wok or large skillet with nonstick coating. Preheat wok or skillet over high heat.

■ Add *undrained* chicken mixture to hot wok or skillet. Stir-fry for 2 minutes; add onions. Continue to stir-fry chicken and onions for 2 to 3 minutes more or till chicken is no longer pink and onions are tender. Serve with hot rice or couscous. Makes 4 servings.

PER SERVING

Calories	252
Protein	23 g
Carbohydrate	32 g
Fat	2 g
Cholesterol	49 mg
Sodium	837 mg
Potassium	291 mg

TIMETABLE

Total preparation time: 25 minutes

FOIL-BAKED CHICKEN

Try a crisp lettuce wedge topped with low-calorie salad dressing to round out this meal-in-a-pouch.

4 boned skinless chicken breast halves *or* turkey breast tenderloin steaks (about 1 pound total)
1 medium tomato
¼ cup sliced pitted ripe olives
¼ cup frozen chopped onion (see tip, page 39)
1 tablespoon lemon juice
½ teaspoon celery salt
¼ teaspoon dried basil, crushed
¼ teaspoon dried marjoram, crushed
¼ teaspoon pepper
¾ cup finely shredded cheddar cheese (3 ounces)

■ Preheat the oven to 400°. Meanwhile, cut *four* 14x12-inch pieces of heavy foil. Place *1* piece of poultry on *each* piece of foil. Cut tomato into 8 slices, then place *2* slices atop *each* poultry piece. Drain olives and sprinkle *one-fourth* of the olives and frozen onion atop *each* poultry piece. Drizzle with lemon juice.

■ In a small bowl stir together celery salt, basil, marjoram, and pepper. Sprinkle mixture over poultry pieces. Bring up long edges of foil and, leaving a little space for expansion of steam, seal foil tightly with a double fold. Then fold short ends of foil to seal.

■ Bake foil packets in the 400° oven about 20 minutes or till poultry is tender and no longer pink. Carefully unseal packets. Sprinkle with the shredded cheese. To serve, remove to individual plates with a slotted spoon. Makes 4 servings.

PER SERVING

Calories	231
Protein	32 g
Carbohydrate	3 g
Fat	10 g
Cholesterol	88 mg
Sodium	495 mg
Potassium	386 mg

TIMETABLE

Preparation time: 20 minutes

Cooking time: about 20 minutes

CHICKEN AND VEGETABLES

Give this stir-fry dish a Mediterranean flavor by using one cup of quick-cooking couscous in place of the rice.

1½ cups quick-cooking rice
12 ounces boned skinless chicken breast halves *or* turkey breast tenderloin steaks
¾ cup chicken broth
2 tablespoons soy sauce *or* oyster sauce
1 tablespoon cornstarch
1 tablespoon dry sherry
1 teaspoon sugar
½ teaspoon sesame oil
½ teaspoon bottled minced garlic *or* ⅛ teaspoon garlic powder
¼ teaspoon ground ginger
  Nonstick spray coating
3 cups loose-pack frozen French-style green beans, broccoli, mushrooms, and red pepper *or* frozen green beans, broccoli, onions, and mushrooms

■ Cook rice according to package directions, *except* omit the margarine or butter. (Or, in a medium saucepan bring 1½ cups *water*, 1 tablespoon *margarine*, and ¼ teaspoon *salt* to boiling. Add 1 cup quick-cooking *couscous*. Cover and remove from heat. Let stand for 5 minutes.) Meanwhile, thinly slice chicken or turkey into bite-size strips; set aside.

■ For sauce, in a small mixing bowl stir together broth, soy sauce or oyster sauce, cornstarch, sherry, sugar, sesame oil, garlic, and ginger. Set sauce aside.

■ Spray a *cold* wok or large skillet with nonstick coating. Preheat wok or skillet over high heat; add frozen vegetables. Stir-fry over high heat about 3 minutes. Remove vegetables from wok. Add poultry to the wok. Stir-fry about 3 minutes or till tender and no longer pink. Push poultry from center.

■ Stir sauce, then add it to the center of the wok. Cook and stir till thickened and bubbly. Cook and stir for 1 minute more. Return vegetables to the wok. Toss gently to coat with sauce. Cook and stir for 1 minute more. Serve over hot rice (or couscous). Makes 4 servings.

PER SERVING

Calories	320
Protein	26 g
Carbohydrate	42 g
Fat	4 g
Cholesterol	49 mg
Sodium	1,447 mg
Potassium	493 mg

TIMETABLE

Total preparation time: 25 minutes

CHICKEN CREOLE

Cabbage that's already shredded is available in the produce section of the supermarket. It makes short work of this delicious one-dish meal.

12 ounces boned skinless chicken breast halves
2 cups shredded cabbage
½ cup frozen chopped green pepper (see tip, page 39)
⅓ cup frozen chopped onion (see tip, page 39)
1 cup quick-cooking rice
1 6-ounce can tomato paste
1 tablespoon chili powder
½ teaspoon sugar
½ teaspoon salt
  Several dashes bottled hot pepper sauce (optional)

■ Cut chicken into ½-inch cubes. In a large skillet combine chicken, cabbage, frozen green pepper, frozen onion, and 1½ cups *hot water*. Bring to boiling, then reduce heat. Cover and simmer about 5 minutes or till vegetables are nearly tender. *Do not drain.*

■ While the chicken mixture is cooking, cook rice according to package directions, *except* omit the margarine or butter.

■ Stir tomato paste, chili powder, sugar, salt, and hot pepper sauce, if desired, into chicken mixture in skillet. Return to boiling; reduce heat. Simmer, covered, for 3 minutes. Serve over rice. Makes 4 servings.

PER SERVING

Calories	244
Protein	24 g
Carbohydrate	33 g
Fat	2 g
Cholesterol	49 mg
Sodium	867 mg
Potassium	795 mg

TIMETABLE

Total preparation time: 25 minutes

TACO CHICKEN-STUFFED TOMATOES

Keep cans of chicken chilled in your refrigerator for cool, refreshing salads anytime.

2 7-inch flour tortillas
2 5-ounce cans chunk-style chicken
2 cups shredded cabbage
¼ cup plain low-fat yogurt
¼ cup reduced-calorie mayonnaise
   or salad dressing
2 teaspoons chili powder
¼ teaspoon dried minced onion
4 medium tomatoes
   Lettuce leaves *or* shredded cabbage
¼ cup finely shredded cheddar cheese

■ For tortilla chips, preheat the oven to 375°. Meanwhile, cut stack of tortillas into 8 wedges to make a total of 16 wedges (see photo 1). Spread wedges in a single layer on a baking sheet. Bake in the 375° oven about 10 minutes or till dry and crisp.

■ While tortilla wedges are baking, drain chicken. In a mixing bowl combine chicken, cabbage, yogurt, mayonnaise or salad dressing, chili powder, and onion. Toss lightly till well mixed. For tomato cups, cut out ½ inch of the core from *each* tomato (see photo 2). Invert tomatoes. For each, cut from top to, *but not quite through*, stem end, making 6 wedges.

■ For salads, line plates with lettuce or cabbage. Place tomatoes on plates. Spread wedges slightly apart; fill with chicken mixture. Top with cheese. Serve with tortilla wedges. Makes 4 servings.

PER SERVING		TIMETABLE
Calories	274	Total preparation time: 30 minutes
Protein	22 g	
Carbohydrate	15 g	
Fat	14 g	
Cholesterol	57 mg	
Sodium	559 mg	
Potassium	469 mg	

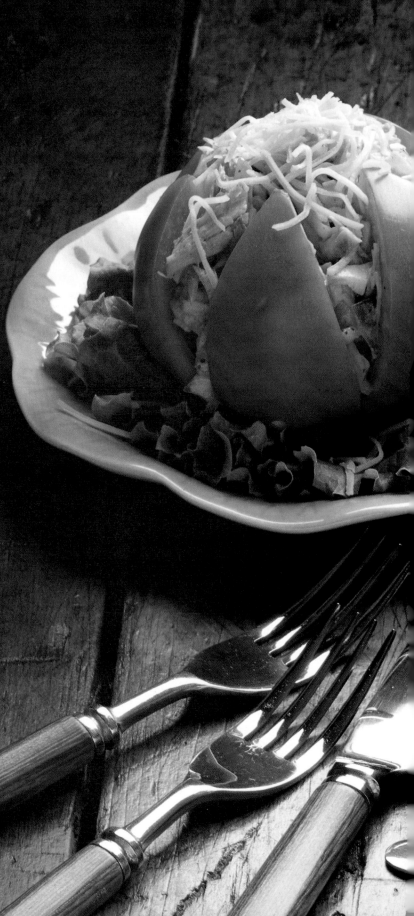

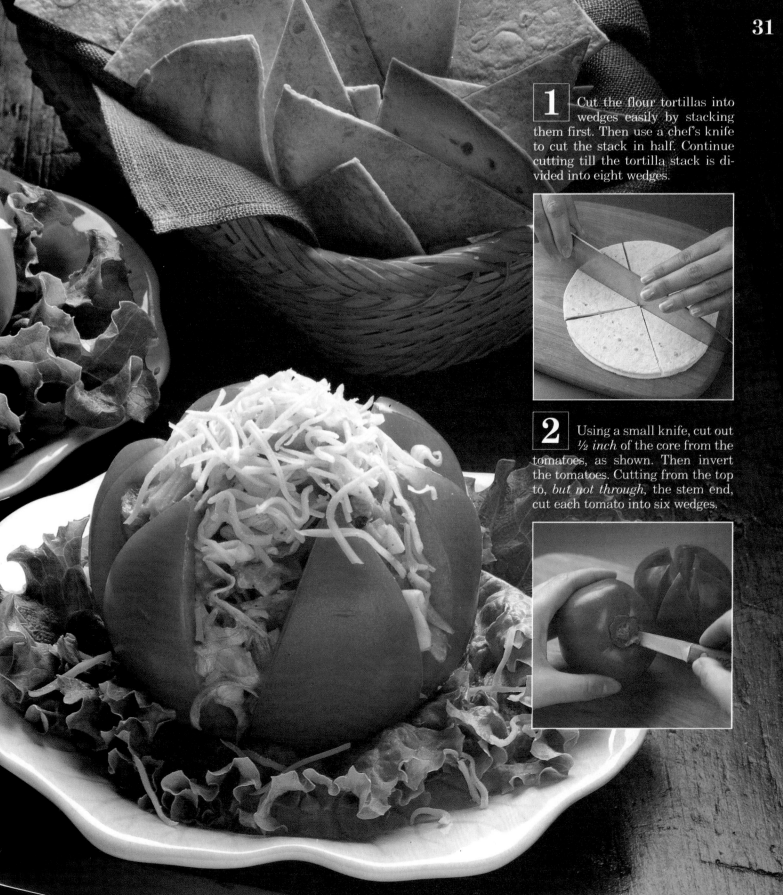

1 Cut the flour tortillas into wedges easily by stacking them first. Then use a chef's knife to cut the stack in half. Continue cutting till the tortilla stack is divided into eight wedges.

2 Using a small knife, cut out ½ *inch* of the core from the tomatoes, as shown. Then invert the tomatoes. Cutting from the top to, *but not through,* the stem end, cut each tomato into six wedges.

20 minutes or less

ITALIAN-STYLE TURKEY STEAKS

Add a fresh touch with a tomato rose and fresh herb sprig garnish.

2 ounces green noodles *or* fettuccine
2 teaspoons cooking oil
2 boneless turkey breast steaks (about 6 ounces total)
1 cup whole fresh mushrooms
1 8-ounce can stewed tomatoes
½ teaspoon dried minced onion
¼ teaspoon dried oregano, crushed
2 tablespoons grated Parmesan cheese

■ Cook pasta according to package directions, *except* use a large saucepan and 3 cups *hot water.*

■ While pasta is cooking, in a medium skillet heat oil till hot. Cook turkey steaks in hot oil about 2 minutes on each side or till browned. Meanwhile, cut mushrooms into fourths.

■ Remove turkey from skillet, reserving drippings. Cook mushrooms in drippings for 3 minutes. Remove skillet from heat and add *undrained* tomatoes, onion, and oregano. Return turkey to the skillet. Bring to boiling. Boil rapidly, uncovered, about 2 minutes or till liquid is slightly reduced and turkey is tender and no longer pink.

■ To serve, transfer turkey and sauce to a serving plate. Sprinkle Parmesan cheese over turkey steaks. Drain pasta. Serve turkey and sauce with pasta. Makes 2 servings.

PER SERVING

Calories	308
Protein	29 g
Carbohydrate	31 g
Fat	8 g
Cholesterol	58 mg
Sodium	991 mg
Potassium	722 mg

TIMETABLE

Total preparation time: about 15 minutes

INDIAN CHICKEN

Two 10-ounce packages of frozen asparagus spears make an elegant alternative to the broccoli spears.

4 boned skinless chicken breast halves *or* turkey breast tenderloin steaks (about 1 pound total)
½ cup plain low-fat yogurt
1 tablespoon all-purpose flour
2 tablespoons water
1 teaspoon curry powder
½ teaspoon bottled minced garlic *or* ⅛ teaspoon garlic powder
¼ teaspoon salt
¼ teaspoon dried finely shredded lemon peel
Dash paprika
2 10-ounce packages frozen broccoli spears
¼ cup peanuts

■ Preheat the oven to 400°. Place poultry in a shallow baking dish. Cover with foil and bake in the 400° oven for 20 to 25 minutes or till poultry is tender and no longer pink.

■ While the poultry is baking, combine yogurt and flour; set aside. In a saucepan stir together water, curry powder, garlic, salt, lemon peel, and paprika. Bring to boiling, then reduce the heat. Cover and simmer for 1 minute. Add yogurt mixture. Cook and stir till mixture is thickened and bubbly. Then cook and stir for 1 minute more.

■ Cook broccoli (or asparagus) according to package directions. Drain. Chop peanuts. To serve, arrange broccoli on a serving platter. Place poultry on top. Pour sauce over poultry. Top with chopped peanuts. Makes 4 servings.

PER SERVING

Calories	247
Protein	35 g
Carbohydrate	13 g
Fat	7 g
Cholesterol	68 mg
Sodium	255 mg
Potassium	790 mg

TIMETABLE

Total preparation time: 35 minutes

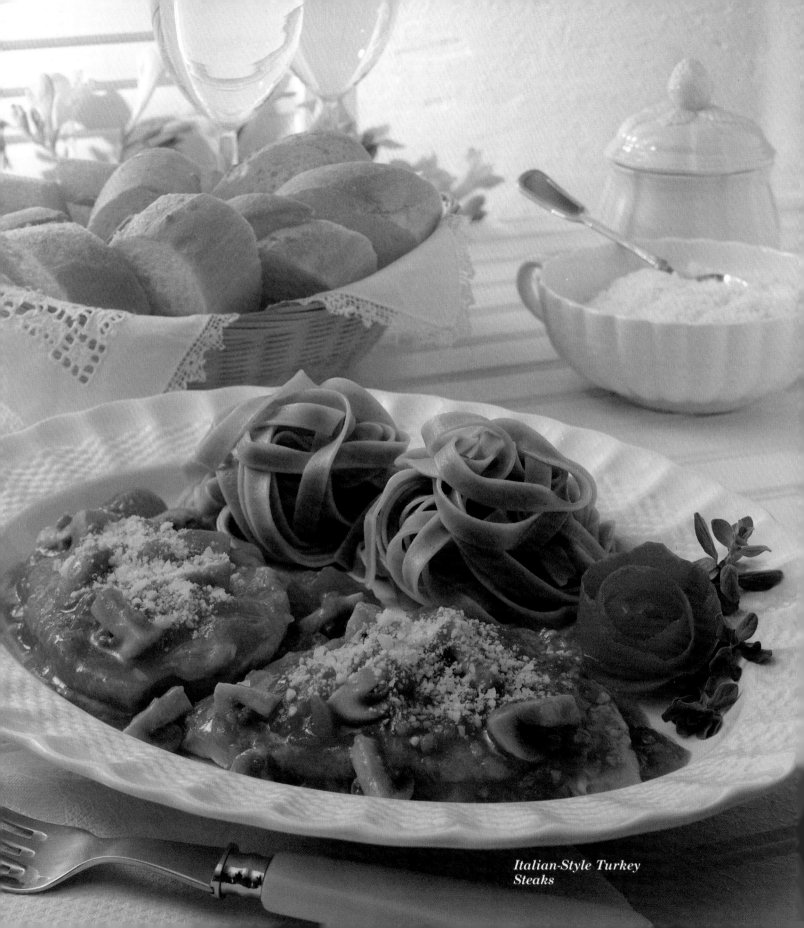

Italian-Style Turkey
Steaks

BROCCOLI-STUFFED TURKEY STEAKS

4 4-ounce turkey breast
   tenderloin steaks
1 10-ounce package frozen
   broccoli spears
1 2-ounce jar sliced
   pimiento
   Nonstick spray coating
1 cup skim milk
4 teaspoons cornstarch
1 teaspoon instant chicken
   bouillon granules
¼ teaspoon dried rosemary,
   crushed
2 ounces sliced American
   cheese
   Few dashes bottled hot
   pepper sauce (optional)

■ Preheat the oven to 350°. Meanwhile, place a turkey steak between 2 pieces of clear plastic wrap. Pound with the flat side of a meat mallet just enough to flatten slightly (about 8 inches long). Place frozen broccoli in a colander. Run *hot water* over broccoli just till spears can be broken apart. Drain well.

■ Place *one-fourth* of the broccoli across *each* turkey tenderloin steak. Drain pimiento. Place *one-fourth* of the pimiento strips atop broccoli. Fold turkey tenderloin steak over the broccoli.

■ Spray a 12x7½x2-inch baking dish with nonstick coating. Place stuffed turkey steaks in the baking dish. Cover with foil. Bake in the 350° oven about 30 minutes or till turkey is tender and no longer pink.

■ While turkey is baking, in a small saucepan combine milk, cornstarch, bouillon granules, and rosemary. Cook and stir over medium-high heat till thickened and bubbly. Then tear up the cheese while adding it to sauce. Add hot pepper sauce, if desired. Stir till cheese melts. To serve, transfer the turkey to a serving platter; pour sauce over stuffed tenderloins. Makes 4 servings.

PER SERVING

Calories	239
Protein	34 g
Carbohydrate	10 g
Fat	7 g
Cholesterol	83 mg
Sodium	413 mg
Potassium	664 mg

TIMETABLE

Preparation time:
15 minutes

Cooking time:
about 30 minutes

20 minutes or less

TURKEY SALAD IN A PITA

Visit a take-out salad bar to save preparation time for this recipe. Check the tip on page 137 for details.

1 10½-ounce can mandarin
   orange sections
   (water pack)
2 cups torn mixed salad
   greens (see tip, page 137)
¼ cup slivered almonds
¼ cup reduced-calorie
   buttermilk salad dressing
¼ teaspoon dried tarragon,
   crushed
2 large pita bread rounds
1 6-ounce package sliced
   fully cooked turkey breast

■ Drain mandarin orange sections.

■ In a large mixing bowl combine orange sections, salad greens, and almonds. Stir together buttermilk dressing and tarragon; pour over salad mixture and toss lightly to coat well.

■ To serve, cut pitas in half crosswise. Open pockets. Place *1½ or 2* slices of turkey breast in *each* pita half. Divide salad mixture among the 4 pocket halves. Makes 4 servings.

PER SERVING

Calories	255
Protein	16 g
Carbohydrate	30 g
Fat	8 g
Cholesterol	13 mg
Sodium	610 mg
Potassium	291 mg

TIMETABLE

Total preparation time:
about 15 minutes

SWISS-HAM CHICKEN 'N' NOODLES

8 ounces boned skinless
   chicken breast halves
3 ounces medium noodles
   (2¼ cups)
1 2½-ounce jar sliced
   mushrooms
2 slices low-fat fully cooked
   ham (about 2 ounces total)
2 ounces process Swiss
   cheese
1¼ cups skim milk
2 tablespoons all-purpose
   flour
2 teaspoons Dijon-style
   mustard
⅛ teaspoon onion powder
⅛ teaspoon pepper
   Frozen snipped chives
   (see tip, page 39)

■ In a large saucepan bring 3 cups unsalted *hot water* to boiling. Meanwhile, cut chicken into ½-inch cubes. Add chicken and noodles to water. Return to boiling; simmer for 5 to 7 minutes or till chicken and pasta are done. Drain chicken and pasta; keep warm.

■ While chicken and pasta are cooking, drain mushrooms and chop ham; set aside. Tear cheese into small pieces; set aside.

■ In a small saucepan combine ¼ *cup* of the milk and the flour. Stir in remaining milk, mustard, onion powder, and pepper. Cook and stir over medium-high heat till thickened and bubbly. Stir in mushrooms, ham, and cheese. Cook and stir for 1 minute more or till cheese melts and mixture is heated through.

■ Pour sauce mixture over hot chicken and pasta and toss lightly to coat. Transfer to a serving dish. Sprinkle with chives. Makes 4 servings.

PER SERVING

Calories	255
Protein	25 g
Carbohydrate	23 g
Fat	6 g
Cholesterol	73 mg
Sodium	555 mg
Potassium	432 mg

TIMETABLE

Total preparation time:
25 minutes

TURKEY PIZZA

This pizza isn't made to be picked up—use a knife and fork so you don't miss a bite of this dieter's delight.

½ pound ground raw
   turkey
½ teaspoon dried Italian
   seasoning, crushed
¼ teaspoon fennel seed
1 4-ounce can mushroom
   stems and pieces
   Nonstick spray coating
1 10-ounce package
   refrigerated pizza
   dough
1 8-ounce can pizza sauce
½ cup frozen chopped green
   pepper (see tip, page 39)
1 8-ounce package shredded
   mozzarella cheese (2 cups)
   Crushed red pepper
   (optional)

■ Preheat the oven to 425°. Meanwhile, break the ground turkey into large pieces while adding it to a large skillet. Cook turkey, Italian seasoning, and fennel seed over high heat till turkey is no longer pink. Drain off fat.

■ Drain mushrooms and set aside. Spray a 15x10x1-inch baking pan with nonstick coating. Unroll pizza dough and press it into baking pan. Spread dough with pizza sauce to within ¼ inch of crust edge. Sprinkle with cooked turkey, mushrooms, and frozen green pepper. Top with cheese.

■ Bake in the 425° oven for 14 to 17 minutes or till crust is golden. If desired, sprinkle with crushed red pepper. Makes 6 servings.

PER SERVING

Calories	300
Protein	24 g
Carbohydrate	28 g
Fat	10 g
Cholesterol	45 mg
Sodium	741 mg
Potassium	226 mg

TIMETABLE

Preparation time:
20 minutes

Cooking time:
14 to 17 minutes

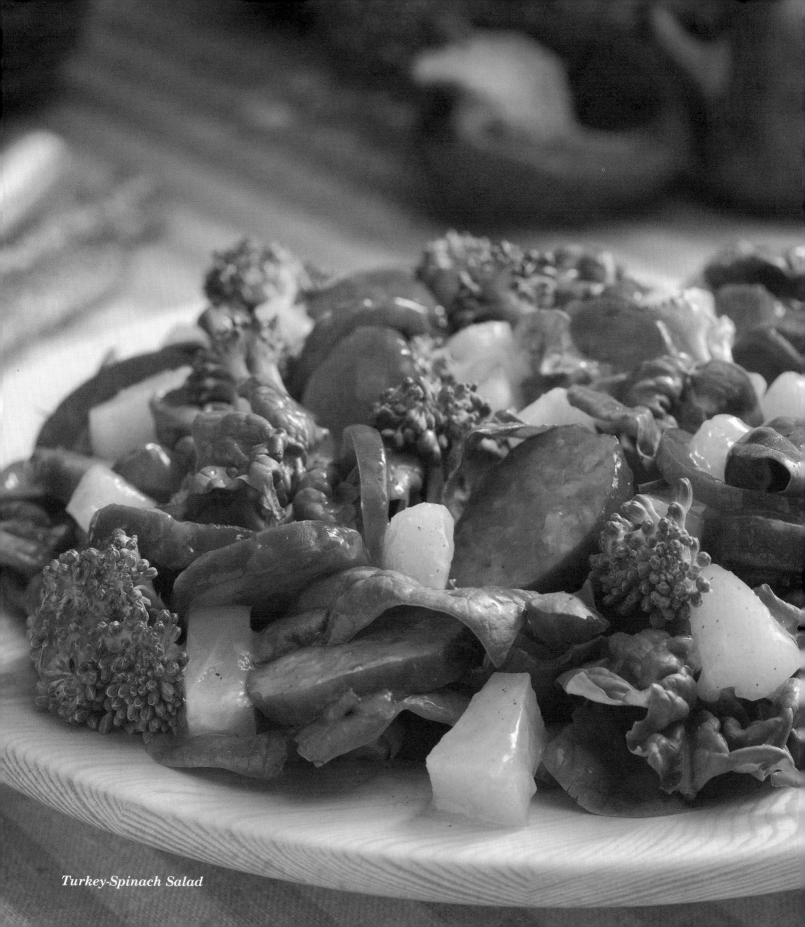

Turkey-Spinach Salad

TURKEY-SPINACH SALAD

Full-flavored, spicy, and chock-full of fruit and sausage chunks—what more could you ask of a whole-meal salad?

5 ounces fresh spinach
1 15¼-ounce can pineapple
    tidbits (juice pack)
1 tablespoon cornstarch
1 tablespoon lemon juice
¼ teaspoon ground ginger
⅛ teaspoon ground allspice
⅛ teaspoon pepper
12 ounces fully cooked
    smoked turkey sausage
1 small sweet red pepper
1½ cups broccoli flowerets

■ Clean and tear spinach into bite-size pieces (you should have about 4 cups). Arrange on *4* individual salad plates; set aside. Drain pineapple, reserving the juice. Add water to the reserved juice to equal *1 cup* liquid. In a bowl combine juice mixture, cornstarch, lemon juice, ginger, allspice, and pepper; set aside.

■ Cut turkey sausage into ¼-inch slices and cut pepper into thin strips; set pepper aside. In a large skillet cook and stir turkey sausage slices over medium heat till lightly browned. Stir pineapple juice mixture; add juice mixture, broccoli, and pepper strips to skillet. Cook and stir till thickened and bubbly, then cook and stir for 2 minutes more. Add pineapple tidbits and heat through. To serve, spoon hot sausage mixture over torn spinach on salad plates. Serves 4.

PER SERVING

Calories	261
Protein	16 g
Carbohydrate	24 g
Fat	12 g
Cholesterol	58 mg
Sodium	705 mg
Potassium	655 mg

TIMETABLE

Total preparation time:
25 minutes

20 minutes or less

CHICKEN FAJITAS

Some brands of tortillas will be more flexible if you wrap them in foil and heat them in a 350° oven about 8 minutes. Check the package for details.

2 tablespoons lemon juice
½ teaspoon garlic salt
½ teaspoon ground cumin
½ teaspoon dried oregano,
    crushed
2 dashes bottled hot pepper
    sauce
12 ounces boned skinless
    chicken breast halves *or*
    turkey breast tenderloin
    steaks
1 medium tomato
4 lettuce leaves
    Nonstick spray coating
¼ cup frozen chopped onion
    (see tip, page 39)
¼ cup frozen chopped green
    pepper (see tip, page 39)
4 7- to 8- inch flour tortillas
¼ cup plain low-fat yogurt
    (optional)

■ In a mixing bowl combine lemon juice, garlic salt, cumin, oregano, and hot pepper sauce. Slice poultry into thin bite-size strips; add it to the juice mixture in the bowl. Toss lightly to coat; set aside. Chop tomato and shred lettuce. Then set tomato and lettuce aside in serving bowls.

■ Spray a *cold* large skillet with nonstick coating. Preheat skillet over high heat. Add *undrained* poultry mixture, frozen onion, and frozen green pepper to the hot skillet. Cook and stir over high heat for 2 to 3 minutes or till poultry is tender and no longer pink and liquid has evaporated. Transfer meat mixture to a serving bowl.

■ To serve, let all assemble their own fajitas. For each fajita, spoon some of the poultry mixture across the center of a tortilla to within 1 inch of 1 side. Top with yogurt, if desired; tomato; and lettuce. Roll tortilla around meat and toppings. Makes 4 servings.

PER SERVING

Calories	173
Protein	22 g
Carbohydrate	17 g
Fat	2 g
Cholesterol	49 mg
Sodium	297 mg
Potassium	340 mg

TIMETABLE

Total preparation time:
20 minutes

20 minutes or less

GREEK-STYLE BURGERS

For an even fresher taste, use 2 teaspoons snipped fresh mint for the ¾ teaspoon dried mint—1½ teaspoons in the burger and the rest in the sauce.

¼ **cup fine dry bread crumbs**
¼ **cup frozen chopped onion (see tip, opposite)**
2 **tablespoons skim milk**
¾ **teaspoon dried mint, crushed**
¼ **teaspoon salt**
12 **ounces ground raw turkey**
Nonstick spray coating
1 **small tomato**
⅓ **of a small cucumber**
¼ **cup plain low-fat yogurt**
2 **tablespoons reduced-calorie mayonnaise** *or* **salad dressing**
2 **large pita bread rounds**

■ In a medium mixing bowl combine bread crumbs, frozen onion, milk, ½ *teaspoon* of the mint, and salt. Add ground turkey, then mix well. Shape mixture into four ½-inch-thick patties.

■ Spray a *cold* large skillet with nonstick coating. Cook patties over medium heat for 4 minutes. Turn patties and cook for 4 to 5 minutes more, or till no longer pink.

■ While patties are cooking, thinly slice the tomato; set aside. Remove seeds from cucumber; shred cucumber. In a small mixing bowl stir together cucumber, yogurt, mayonnaise or salad dressing, and the remaining mint.

■ To serve, cut pitas in half crosswise. Open pockets. Place patties and tomato slices into pockets. Spoon yogurt sauce on top of each patty in pita. Serves 4.

PER SERVING

Calories	277
Protein	26 g
Carbohydrate	30 g
Fat	5 g
Cholesterol	63 mg
Sodium	290 mg
Potassium	359 mg

TIMETABLE

Preparation time:
5 minutes

Cooking time:
8 to 9 minutes

20 minutes or less

CHICKEN-CORN CHOWDER

This creamy soup is off the shelf and on the table in 15 minutes flat!

1 **teaspoon instant chicken bouillon granules**
2 **ounces medium noodles**
1 **10¾-ounce can condensed cream of chicken soup**
1 **8¾-ounce can cream-style corn**
2 **tablespoons chopped pimiento**
1 **6¾-ounce can chunk-style chicken** *or* **1½ cups diced cooked chicken (see tip, page 109)**
Snipped parsley

■ In a large saucepan combine bouillon granules and 3 cups *hot water*. Bring to boiling. Break noodles slightly while adding them to the broth mixture in the saucepan. Return to boiling, then reduce heat. Cover and simmer for 5 minutes. *Do not drain.*

■ Stir in cream of chicken soup, corn, and pimiento. Bring to boiling, stirring constantly. Add *undrained* canned chicken or cooked chicken to saucepan. Heat the mixture through.

■ To serve, ladle soup into individual bowls. Garnish with parsley. Makes 4 servings.

PER SERVING

Calories	252
Protein	16 g
Carbohydrate	28 g
Fat	9 g
Cholesterol	49 mg
Sodium	1,111 mg
Potassium	241 mg

TIMETABLE

Total preparation time:
15 minutes

VEGETABLE-TURKEY POCKETS

1 medium cucumber
½ of a small tomato
1 medium carrot
3 slices fully cooked
   turkey breast
   (about 3 ounces total)
3 slices American cheese
⅓ cup reduced-calorie creamy
   Italian salad dressing
2 large pita bread rounds
¼ cup alfalfa sprouts
4 teaspoons sunflower nuts

■ Chop cucumber and tomato. Thinly bias-slice carrot. Cut turkey and cheese into bite-size strips.

■ In a medium mixing bowl combine cucumber, tomato, carrot, turkey, and cheese. Pour salad dressing over mixture in bowl. Toss lightly to coat.

■ To serve, cut pitas in half crosswise. Open pockets. Spoon *one-fourth* of the vegetable mixture into *each* pocket half. Top *each* with *one-fourth* of the sprouts and nuts. Makes 4 servings.

PER SERVING

Calories	277
Protein	16 g
Carbohydrate	28 g
Fat	11 g
Cholesterol	34 mg
Sodium	449 mg
Potassium	271 mg

TIMETABLE

Total preparation time:
20 minutes

CHICKEN-NOODLE AND VEGETABLE SOUP

2 14½-ounce cans chicken
   broth
1 medium carrot
1 stalk celery
8 ounces boned skinless
   chicken breast halves
¼ teaspoon dried rosemary,
   crushed
¼ teaspoon dried basil,
   crushed
   Dash poultry seasoning
1 ounce fine noodles (½ cup)

■ In a large saucepan bring broth to boiling. Meanwhile, thinly slice carrot and celery. Cut chicken into ½-inch cubes. Add carrot, celery, chicken, rosemary, basil, and poultry seasoning to broth; return mixture to boiling.

■ When broth boils, reduce heat. Add noodles. Cover and simmer for 5 to 7 minutes or till chicken is no longer pink and noodles are tender. Serves 3.

PER SERVING

Calories	178
Protein	25 g
Carbohydrate	11 g
Fat	3 g
Cholesterol	53 mg
Sodium	946 mg
Potassium	580 mg

TIMETABLE

Total preparation time:
15 minutes

INGREDIENT TIME-SAVERS

Frozen chopped vegetables or snipped herbs save recipe preparation time. Buy chopped onions, green peppers, and snipped chives already frozen. Or, when chopping onion, green onion, or green pepper, or snipping parsley, dill, basil, and chives, cut up extras. Then label and freeze them in airtight containers. (Fresh onions, peppers, parsley, and herbs also can be used in the recipes.)

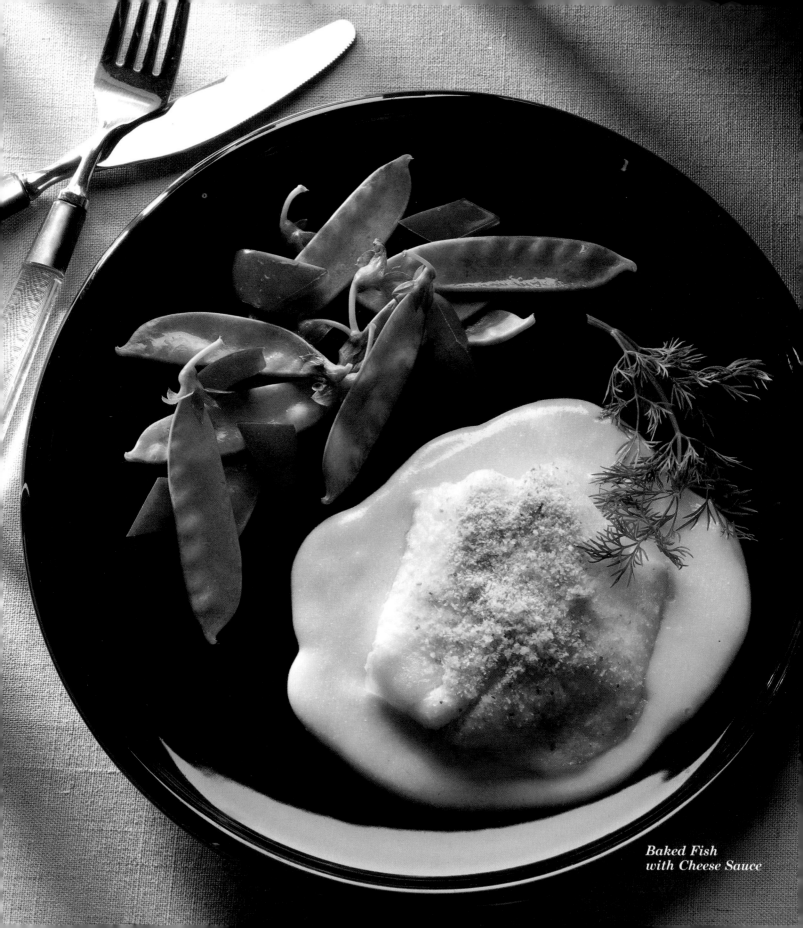

*Baked Fish
with Cheese Sauce*

BAKED FISH WITH CHEESE SAUCE

Nonstick spray coating
1 pound fresh skinless orange roughy, flounder, *or* sole fillets (½ to ¾ inch thick)
1 tablespoon margarine *or* butter
2 tablespoons fine dry bread crumbs
¾ cup skim milk
1 tablespoon all-purpose flour
½ cup shredded cheddar cheese (2 ounces)
1½ teaspoons Dijon-style mustard
Fresh dillweed (optional)

■ Preheat the oven to 400°. Meanwhile, spray a shallow baking dish with nonstick coating. Place fillets in dish, tucking under any thin edges.

■ Melt margarine or butter; brush on top of fish. Top with bread crumbs. Bake in the 400° oven for 10 to 15 minutes or till fish flakes easily with a fork.

■ While fish is baking, prepare sauce. In a small saucepan stir together milk and flour. Cook and stir over medium heat till thickened and bubbly. Add cheese and mustard. Cook and stir till cheese melts.

■ To serve, divide sauce among *4* individual serving plates. Place *1* portion of fish on *each* plate atop sauce. Garnish with dillweed and serve with steamed pea pods and sweet red pepper, if desired. Serves 4.

PER SERVING

Calories	206
Protein	22 g
Carbohydrate	6 g
Fat	8 g
Cholesterol	70 mg
Sodium	361 mg
Potassium	477 mg

TIMETABLE

Preparation time: 10 minutes

Cooking time: 10 to 15 minutes

20 minutes or less

SALMON-POTATO TOSS

If you like, quick-chill salad in the freezer for 5 minutes before adding greens. Tear the greens while salad chills; add them, toss lightly, and serve.

2 stalks celery
1 16-ounce can sliced potatoes
1 12½-ounce can boneless, skinless pink salmon
½ cup plain low-fat yogurt
¼ cup reduced-calorie mayonnaise *or* salad dressing
2 tablespoons frozen sliced green onion (see tip, page 39)
1 tablespoon chopped pimiento
1 tablespoon Dijon-style mustard
2 teaspoons celery seed
¼ teaspoon salt
⅛ teaspoon pepper
4 cups torn mixed salad greens (see tip, page 137)

■ Slice celery. Drain potatoes and salmon.

■ In a large mixing bowl or large salad bowl, stir together yogurt, mayonnaise or salad dressing, green onion, pimiento, mustard, celery seed, salt, and pepper. Add celery and potatoes. Toss lightly to mix. Then break salmon into large chunks while adding it to potato mixture. Add salad greens. Toss lightly to coat. Makes 4 servings.

PER SERVING

Calories	231
Protein	19 g
Carbohydrate	16 g
Fat	10 g
Cholesterol	27 mg
Sodium	850 mg
Potassium	769 mg

TIMETABLE

Total preparation time: 10 minutes

20 minutes or less

POACHED FISH WITH SAUCE

Some low-fat fish choices include cod, orange roughy, sole, flounder, and catfish fillets or halibut steaks.

1 pound fresh skinless fish fillets *or* steaks (no thicker than 1 inch)

■ To poach fish, measure thickness of fish. In a large skillet pour in enough *hot water* to half-cover the fish. Bring water just to boiling, then carefully add the fish. Return just to boiling, then reduce heat. Cover and simmer gently till fish flakes easily with a fork (allow 4 to 6 minutes per ½-inch thickness of fish).

■ Meanwhile, if desired, prepare 1 of the sauces below. Serve sauce over poached fish. Serves 4.

Dilly-Yogurt Sauce: Remove seeds and finely chop ½ of a small *cucumber* (you should have about ½ cup). In a small mixing bowl stir together the cucumber, ½ of an 8-ounce carton (½ cup) plain low-fat *yogurt*, 1 teaspoon *horseradish mustard*, ½ teaspoon dried *minced onion*, ½ teaspoon dried *dillweed*, and ⅛ teaspoon *salt*. Makes 4 servings.

Chili-Tomato Sauce: In a small saucepan combine one 8-ounce can stewed *tomatoes*, 1 teaspoon *cornstarch*, ½ teaspoon *chili powder*, ¼ teaspoon bottled minced *garlic* or dash *garlic powder*, and dash bottled *hot pepper sauce*. Cook and stir over medium-high heat till thickened and bubbly. Then cook and stir for 2 minutes more. Makes 4 servings.

PER SERVING

Calories	91
Protein	20 g
Carbohydrate	0 g
Fat	1 g
Cholesterol	42 mg
Sodium	78 mg
Potassium	431 mg

TIMETABLE

Total preparation time: about 10 minutes

Calories	22

Calories	18

EASY GUMBO SOUP

Choctaw Indians first dried sassafras leaves to make filé powder, a thickener popularized in Cajun gumbos, which adds a thyme-like flavor.

1   8-ounce can stewed
    tomatoes
1   6-ounce can vegetable
    juice cocktail
¼   cup frozen chopped
    green pepper (see tip,
    page 39)
½   teaspoon dried minced
    onion
¼   teaspoon Worcestershire
    sauce
⅛   teaspoon ground red
    pepper
1   5- or 6-ounce package
    frozen cooked shrimp
¼   cup quick-cooking rice
½   teaspoon filé powder
    (optional)

■ In a medium saucepan combine *undrained* tomatoes, vegetable juice cocktail, frozen green pepper, onion, Worcestershire sauce, ground red pepper, and ½ cup *water*. Bring mixture to boiling. Stir in frozen shrimp and *uncooked* rice. Return the mixture to boiling; remove from the heat. If desired, stir in the filé powder.

■ Let stand, covered, for 5 minutes or till rice is done. Stir before serving. Makes 2 servings.

PER SERVING

Calories	166
Protein	18 g
Carbohydrate	23 g
Fat	1 g
Cholesterol	89 mg
Sodium	714 mg
Potassium	634 mg

TIMETABLE

Total preparation time:
20 minutes

BROCCOLI-SOLE ROLL-UPS

1   10-ounce package frozen
    broccoli spears
4   3- to 4-ounce fresh skinless
    sole, flounder, *or*
    walleyed pike fillets
    (¼ to ½ inch thick)
¼   cup reduced-calorie
    mayonnaise *or* salad
    dressing
¼   cup plain low-fat yogurt
2   teaspoons Dijon-style
    mustard
    Frozen snipped chives
    (see tip, page 39)

■ Place frozen broccoli in a colander. Run *hot water* over vegetables just till thawed. Drain well. Meanwhile, in a large skillet place a wire rack or a large open steamer basket. Pour enough *hot water* to almost reach the rack. Bring water to boiling; reduce heat to a simmer.

■ While water is coming to a boil, prepare fish rolls. Place *one-fourth* of the thawed broccoli spears on one end of *each* fillet. Roll fillets around broccoli. If necessary, secure with wooden toothpicks. Carefully place rolls, seam side down, on the wire rack or steamer basket. Cover skillet. Steam about 10 minutes or till fish flakes easily with a fork.

■ For sauce, in a small saucepan stir together mayonnaise or salad dressing, yogurt, and mustard. Cook and stir just till heated through. *Do not boil.* To serve, using a wide-slotted spatula, transfer fish rolls to a serving platter. Discard toothpicks. Spoon sauce over rolls; sprinkle with frozen snipped chives. Serves 4.

PER SERVING

Calories	149
Protein	18 g
Carbohydrate	5 g
Fat	6 g
Cholesterol	38 mg
Sodium	253 mg
Potassium	566 mg

TIMETABLE

Total preparation time:
20 minutes

20 minutes or less

SWEET 'N' SOUR MONKFISH

Monkfish is a low-fat, firm-textured fish with a pleasant, mild flavor.

1   cup quick-cooking rice
8   ounces fresh skinless
    monkfish fillets *or* tuna
    steaks (¾ to 1 inch thick)
1   8-ounce can pineapple
    tidbits (juice pack)
1   tablespoon cooking oil
3   tablespoons soy sauce
1   tablespoon brown sugar
1   tablespoon vinegar
2   teaspoons cornstarch
½   teaspoon ground ginger
    Dash garlic powder
1   6-ounce package frozen
    pea pods

■ Cook rice according to package directions, *except* omit margarine or butter. Meanwhile, cut fish into 1-inch pieces. Drain pineapple, reserving juice.

■ Preheat a wok or large skillet over medium-high heat. Add oil to wok or skillet. Meanwhile, for sauce, in a small bowl combine reserved pineapple juice, soy sauce, brown sugar, vinegar, cornstarch, ginger, and garlic powder.

■ Add fish to the hot wok. Stir-fry over medium-high heat for 3 to 6 minutes or till fish flakes easily with a fork, being careful not to break up pieces. Push fish from center of wok or skillet.

■ Stir sauce, then add it to center of wok. Cook and stir till thickened and bubbly. Cook and stir about 30 seconds, then add pineapple and pea pods. Toss sauce lightly with ingredients. Cover and cook for 1 to 2 minutes more or till pea pods are heated through. Serve with hot rice. Makes 3 servings.

PER SERVING

Calories	382
Protein	24 g
Carbohydrate	51 g
Fat	9 g
Cholesterol	29 mg
Sodium	1,320 mg
Potassium	445 mg

TIMETABLE

Total preparation time: 20 minutes

VEGETABLE-TOPPED FISH

Go with the grain in the recipe, or substitute ⅓ cup quick-cooking rice for the bulgur and decrease the water to ¼ cup.

½   cup water
½   of a small tomato
⅓   cup bulgur
½   teaspoon instant chicken
    bouillon granules
½   pound fresh skinless orange
    roughy, flounder, *or* pike
    fillets (about ½ inch thick)
¼   teaspoon garlic salt
¼   teaspoon dried basil,
    crushed
1   cup loose-pack frozen
    broccoli, baby carrots,
    and water chestnuts *or*
    frozen cauliflower,
    broccoli, and carrots
2   tablespoons dry white wine

■ Preheat the oven to 450°. Meanwhile, bring water to boiling. Chop tomato; set aside. In a 10x6x2-inch baking dish combine bulgur and instant chicken bouillon granules. Pour boiling water over bulgur. Place fish on top of bulgur, tucking under any thin edges. Sprinkle with garlic salt and basil.

■ Place frozen vegetables and tomato atop fish; drizzle with wine. Cover tightly with foil. Bake in the 450° oven about 25 to 30 minutes or till fish flakes easily with a fork. Makes 2 servings.

PER SERVING

Calories	208
Protein	20 g
Carbohydrate	24 g
Fat	1 g
Cholesterol	55 mg
Sodium	477 mg
Potassium	609 mg

TIMETABLE

Preparation time: 10 minutes

Cooking time: 25 to 30 minutes

RICOTTA-STUFFED SOLE

There's nothing diet-tasting about these cheese-filled fish fillets smothered in a rich, thick tomato sauce!

½ cup low-fat ricotta cheese
2 tablespoons grated
    Parmesan cheese
1 tablespoon frozen sliced
    green onion (see tip,
    page 39)
¼ teaspoon dried Italian
    seasoning *or* dried basil,
    crushed
    Dash pepper
4 3-ounce fresh skinless sole
    or flounder fillets (about
    ½ inch thick)
½ cup spaghetti sauce
    with mushrooms
¼ cup shredded mozzarella
    cheese (1 ounce)

■ Preheat the oven to 375°. While oven is heating, in a small bowl combine ricotta cheese, Parmesan cheese, green onion, Italian seasoning or basil, and pepper. Place about *2 tablespoons* of the cheese mixture on 1 end of *each* fillet. Roll fillets around cheese mixture. If necessary, secure with wooden toothpicks. Place rolls, seam side down, in a 9-inch pie plate.

■ Bake fish rolls in the 375° oven for 20 to 25 minutes or till fish flakes easily with a fork. Drain off liquid. Spoon spaghetti sauce over fish rolls. Sprinkle with shredded mozzarella cheese. Bake for 2 to 3 minutes more or till the cheese is melted. Discard toothpicks before serving. Makes 4 servings.

PER SERVING

Calories	199
Protein	25 g
Carbohydrate	7 g
Fat	8 g
Cholesterol	56 mg
Sodium	494 mg
Potassium	434 mg

TIMETABLE

Preparation time:
10 minutes

Cooking time:
22 to 28 minutes

---

20 minutes or less

MACARONI-TUNA SOUP

Keep the tuna in big chunks by gently stirring it in just before you finish cooking the soup.

3 ounces tiny shell
    macaroni (¾ cup)
1 9-ounce can tuna
    (water pack)
1 14½-ounce can chicken
    broth
1 14½-ounce can stewed
    tomatoes
1 12-ounce can (1½ cups)
    tomato juice
¼ cup frozen chopped onion
    (see tip, page 39)
1 4-ounce can diced
    green chili peppers
1 to 1½ teaspoons chili
    powder
¼ cup finely shredded
    cheddar cheese (1 ounce)
    (optional)

■ Cook pasta according to package directions, *except* use a large saucepan and 4 cups *hot water*. Drain pasta and return it to the saucepan. Meanwhile, drain tuna.

■ Stir broth, *undrained* tomatoes, tomato juice, onion, chili peppers, and chili powder into drained pasta in saucepan. Bring to boiling. Then gently stir in tuna. Heat through. *Do not boil.*

■ To serve, ladle soup into individual soup bowls. If desired, sprinkle with cheese. Makes 4 or 5 servings.

PER SERVING

Calories	232
Protein	25 g
Carbohydrate	30 g
Fat	2 g
Cholesterol	40 mg
Sodium	1,225 mg
Potassium	789 mg

TIMETABLE

Total preparation time:
20 minutes

20 minutes or less

RICE-SHRIMP GUMBO

Gumbo, the Cajun version of French bouillabaisse, uses seafood and vegetables native to Louisiana.

½ cup frozen chopped onion (see tip, page 39)
½ cup frozen chopped green pepper (see tip, page 39)
¼ cup water
1 28-ounce can tomatoes
½ teaspoon bottled minced garlic *or* ⅛ teaspoon garlic powder
¼ teaspoon dried rosemary, crushed
¼ teaspoon paprika
¼ teaspoon pepper
1½ cups water
1 6¼-ounce package quick-cooking long grain and wild rice mix
1 16-ounce package frozen peeled and deveined shrimp
Several dashes bottled hot pepper sauce

■ In a large saucepan combine frozen onion, green pepper, and ¼ cup water. Bring mixture to boiling, then reduce heat. Cover and simmer for 3 to 5 minutes or till vegetables are tender.

■ While onion and pepper are cooking, cut up tomatoes. Add *undrained* tomatoes to onion mixture, along with garlic, rosemary, paprika, and pepper. Stir in 1½ cups water and *both* packets from rice mix. Bring mixture to boiling. Add frozen shrimp. Return to boiling, then reduce heat. Cover and simmer for 4 to 5 minutes or till rice is tender and shrimp turn pink. To serve, ladle gumbo into individual soup bowls. Pass hot pepper sauce. Makes 6 servings.

PER SERVING

Calories	136
Protein	17 g
Carbohydrate	15 g
Fat	1 g
Cholesterol	95 mg
Sodium	323 mg
Potassium	519 mg

TIMETABLE

Total preparation time: 20 minutes

---

20 minutes or less

SHRIMP 'N' PEA SALAD

When it comes time to line the plates, shredded lettuce makes an attractive, easy-to-eat alternative to whole lettuce leaves.

1 8-ounce package frozen cooked shrimp
1½ cups frozen peas
3 medium green onions
2 stalks celery
1 medium tomato
¼ cup peanuts
½ cup plain low-fat yogurt
¼ cup reduced-calorie mayonnaise *or* salad dressing
1 teaspoon curry powder
¼ teaspoon frozen, finely shredded lemon peel (see tip, page 66)
Lettuce leaves

■ Place frozen shrimp and peas in a colander. Run *cool water* over them just till thawed; drain well.

■ While shrimp and peas are thawing, slice onions and celery. Cut tomato into 8 wedges. Chop peanuts.

■ In a medium mixing bowl stir together yogurt, mayonnaise or salad dressing, curry powder, and lemon peel. Add shrimp, peas, onions, and celery. Toss lightly till ingredients are coated.

■ To serve, line plates with lettuce leaves. Spoon shrimp mixture onto the plates. Garnish with tomato wedges and chopped peanuts. Makes 4 servings

PER SERVING

Calories	223
Protein	19 g
Carbohydrate	15 g
Fat	10 g
Cholesterol	73 mg
Sodium	267 mg
Potassium	502 mg

TIMETABLE

Total preparation time: 20 minutes

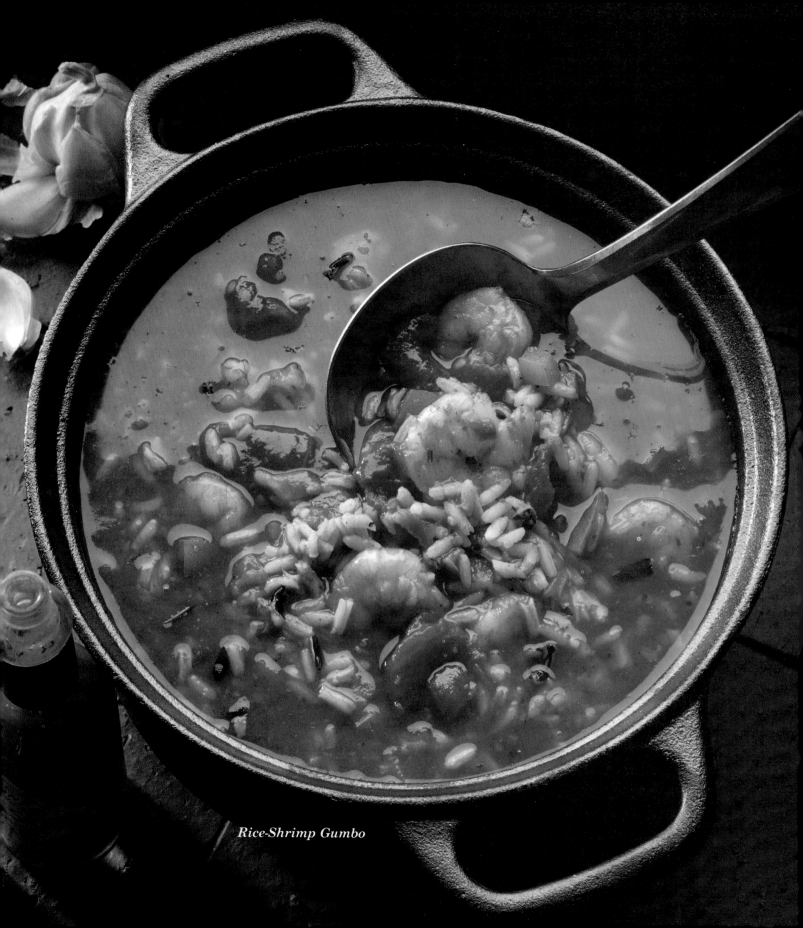

Rice-Shrimp Gumbo

SCALLOP KABOBS

Serve lemon wedges with the kabobs for a splash of color and a dash of flavor.

2 small zucchini (about 8 ounces total)
1 pound fresh scallops
⅓ cup reduced-calorie Italian salad dressing
8 cherry tomatoes

■ Preheat the broiler. Meanwhile, bias-slice zucchini into ½-inch pieces. In a medium saucepan combine the zucchini with enough *hot water* to cover. Bring to boiling; remove from heat. Let stand for 2 minutes; drain. Meanwhile, halve any large scallops; rinse and pat scallops dry.

■ Loosely thread scallops and zucchini alternately onto *eight* 6-inch skewers, leaving about ¼ inch of space between pieces. Brush kabobs lightly with some of the salad dressing.

■ Place kabobs on the unheated rack of a broiler pan. Broil 4 inches from the heat for 10 to 12 minutes or till scallops are opaque, turning several times and brushing with any remaining dressing. Add *1* cherry tomato to the end of *each* kabob. Makes 4 servings.

PER SERVING	
Calories	125
Protein	18 g
Carbohydrate	7 g
Fat	2 g
Cholesterol	41 mg
Sodium	298 mg
Potassium	634 mg

TIMETABLE

Preparation time:
15 minutes

Cooking time:
10 to 12 minutes

DILLY TUNA-ZUCCHINI PATTIES

½ of a small zucchini (about 3 ounces)
2 eggs
1 tablespoon dried minced onion
⅓ cup seasoned fine dry bread crumbs
1 tablespoon dried parsley flakes
½ teaspoon dried dillweed
⅛ teaspoon pepper
1 6½-ounce can tuna (water pack) *or* boneless, skinless pink salmon
1 small tomato, sliced (optional)

■ Preheat the broiler. Meanwhile, shred zucchini (you should have about ½ cup). In a medium mixing bowl beat eggs slightly. Add onion, then stir in zucchini, dry bread crumbs, parsley, dillweed, and pepper. Drain and flake tuna or salmon. Add fish to mixture and stir till combined.

■ Shape fish mixture into three ¾-inch-thick patties. Place fish patties on the unheated rack of a broiler pan. Broil patties 4 inches from the heat for 3 minutes. Carefully turn patties over and broil for 3 minutes more or till golden brown and hot. Top patties with tomato slices, if desired. Makes 3 servings.

PER SERVING	
Calories	187
Protein	23 g
Carbohydrate	11 g
Fat	5 g
Cholesterol	222 mg
Sodium	157 mg
Potassium	342 mg

TIMETABLE

Preparation time:
15 minutes

Cooking time:
6 minutes

SIMPLE SALMON SKILLET

For a richer color and just 34 additional calories per serving, substitute red or sockeye salmon for the pink salmon.

1 medium onion
1 9-ounce package frozen Italian-style green beans
2 tablespoons soy sauce
1 tablespoon cornstarch
½ teaspoon dry mustard
½ teaspoon frozen, finely shredded lemon peel (see tip, page 66)
1 15½-ounce can pink salmon
1 8-ounce can bamboo shoots

■ Slice onion and separate into rings. In a large skillet cook onion and frozen beans in ¼ cup *water* for 3 minutes. Meanwhile, in a small bowl combine soy sauce, cornstarch, dry mustard, lemon peel, and ½ cup *cold water;* set aside.

■ Drain salmon; remove skin and bones. Break salmon into chunks. Drain bamboo shoots. Stir cornstarch mixture and add to vegetable mixture in skillet. Cook and stir till mixture is thickened and bubbly. Stir in salmon chunks and bamboo shoots. Cover and cook for 2 minutes more or till mixture is heated through. Makes 4 servings.

PER SERVING

Calories	172
Protein	21 g
Carbohydrate	11 g
Fat	5 g
Cholesterol	30 mg
Sodium	848 mg
Potassium	495 mg

TIMETABLE

Total preparation time: 15 minutes

SALMON-FILLED TORTILLAS

1 8-ounce can whole kernel corn
3 ounces Monterey Jack cheese
2 teaspoons cornstarch
1 8-ounce carton plain low-fat yogurt
¼ cup canned chopped green chili peppers
1 tablespoon frozen snipped chives (see tip, page 39)
½ teaspoon ground coriander
1 6½-ounce can boneless, skinless pink salmon
4 7- to 8-inch flour tortillas
Paprika

■ Preheat the oven to 350°. Meanwhile, drain corn and shred cheese (you should have ¾ cup cheese). In a small saucepan stir cornstarch into ½ cup of the yogurt. Stir in corn, chili peppers, chives, and coriander. Cook and stir till mixture is thickened and bubbly. Stir in ¼ cup of the cheese till melted. Drain salmon and break up. Stir salmon into yogurt mixture.

■ Place *one-fourth* of the salmon mixture on *each* tortilla. Roll up tortillas and place, seam side down, in a lightly greased 10x6x2-inch baking dish. Cover with foil. Bake tortillas in the 350° oven about 20 minutes or till heated through.

■ To serve, sprinkle tortillas with remaining cheese and paprika and serve with the remaining yogurt. Makes 4 servings.

PER SERVING

Calories	270
Protein	18 g
Carbohydrate	27 g
Fat	10 g
Cholesterol	35 mg
Sodium	418 mg
Potassium	361 mg

TIMETABLE

Preparation time: 15 minutes

Cooking time: about 20 minutes

FAST PAELLA

Saffron is an expensive spice valued for the rich golden color and subtle flavor it imparts to foods. For a less costly alternative, choose turmeric.

1   9-ounce package frozen artichoke hearts
1   4.6-ounce package regular chicken-flavored rice mix
½   cup frozen chopped onion (see tip, page 39)
1   teaspoon bottled minced garlic *or* ¼ teaspoon garlic powder
⅛   teaspoon ground saffron *or* ground turmeric
⅛   teaspoon ground red pepper
1   8-ounce package frozen peeled and deveined shrimp
½   cup frozen peas
1   cup cubed cooked chicken (see tip, page 109)
1   medium tomato

■ In a large saucepan combine frozen artichoke hearts, rice mix, onion, garlic, saffron or turmeric, red pepper, and 1¼ cups *water*. Bring mixture to boiling, then reduce heat. Simmer, uncovered, for 10 minutes or till of desired consistency, stirring occasionally. Add frozen shrimp and peas. Cook about 6 minutes more or till shrimp turn pink, stirring occasionally. Add chicken; heat through.

■ While the rice mixture is cooking, chop tomato. Stir the tomato into rice mixture just before serving. Makes 4 servings.

PER SERVING

Calories	275
Protein	27 g
Carbohydrate	34 g
Fat	4 g
Cholesterol	116 mg
Sodium	866 mg
Potassium	321 mg

TIMETABLE

Total preparation time: 25 minutes

SEAFOOD CHOWDER

Nonfat dry milk is the secret to this rich and creamy dish.

1   cup frozen loose-pack hash brown potatoes
1   cup frozen whole kernel corn
½   cup frozen chopped onion (see tip, page 39)
½   cup frozen chopped green pepper (see tip, page 39)
2   teaspoons instant chicken bouillon granules
½   teaspoon dried basil, crushed
¼   cup nonfat dry milk powder
3   tablespoons all-purpose flour
1½ cups skim milk
1   8-ounce package frozen peeled and deveined shrimp
8   ounces bay scallops

■ In a large saucepan combine potatoes, corn, onion, green pepper, bouillon granules, basil, and 1 cup *water*. Bring to boiling, then reduce heat. Cover and simmer about 5 minutes or till vegetables are tender.

■ Stir together nonfat dry milk powder and flour. Stir in milk. Add milk mixture to vegetables.

■ Cook and stir over medium-high heat till thickened and bubbly. Stir in frozen shrimp and scallops. Return just to boiling, stirring frequently; reduce the heat. Simmer gently about 1 to 2 minutes more or till shrimp turn pink and scallops are opaque, stirring often. Makes 4 servings.

PER SERVING

Calories	252
Protein	29 g
Carbohydrate	31 g
Fat	2 g
Cholesterol	94 mg
Sodium	494 mg
Potassium	859 mg

TIMETABLE

Total preparation time: 25 minutes

SHRIMP FETTUCCINE

Garnish with tomato. (Pictured on the cover and on pages 24 and 25.)

3 ounces fettuccine
1 8-ounce package frozen peeled and deveined shrimp
2 cups loose-pack frozen broccoli, carrots, and onion *or* frozen broccoli carrots, and cauliflower
1 tablespoon margarine *or* butter
1 tablespoon cornstarch
½ teaspoon instant chicken bouillon granules
¼ teaspoon bottled minced garlic
⅛ teaspoon lemon-pepper seasoning
¾ cup skim milk
2 tablespoons dry white wine *or* skim milk
2 tablespoons finely shredded *or* grated Parmesan cheese

■ In a large saucepan cook pasta in 4 cups *hot water* for 8 minutes. Add shrimp and frozen vegetables. Return to boiling, then reduce heat. Simmer gently for 1 to 3 minutes or till shrimp turn pink and pasta is tender. Drain and leave in saucepan.

■ While shrimp and vegetables are cooking, in a small saucepan melt margarine or butter. Stir in cornstarch, bouillon granules, garlic, and lemon-pepper seasoning. Add ¾ cup milk. Cook and stir over medium-high heat till thickened and bubbly. Cook and stir for 2 minutes more. Stir in wine or 2 tablespoons milk. Pour over pasta mixture. Toss to combine. Top with Parmesan cheese. If desired, garnish with tomatoes and parsley. Makes 3 servings.

PER SERVING

Calories	291
Protein	23 g
Carbohydrate	34 g
Fat	6 g
Cholesterol	116 mg
Sodium	306 mg
Potassium	523 mg

TIMETABLE

Total preparation time: 25 minutes

20 minutes or less

SEAFOOD-PASTA SALAD

Save even more time by using the salad-style crab-flavored fish pieces. The pieces are already bite-size and ready to use.

¾ cup corkscrew macaroni
16 ounces crab-flavored fish sticks
1 10½-ounce can mandarin orange sections (water pack)
4 cups torn mixed salad greens (see tip, page 137)
2 tablespoons frozen sliced green onion (see tip, page 39)
1 8-ounce carton orange low-fat yogurt
1 tablespoon frozen orange juice concentrate
¼ cup sliced almonds

■ Cook the macaroni according to package directions, *except* use a large saucepan and 3 cups *hot water*. (If fish is frozen, place fish in a colander. Run *cool water* over fish just till thawed.) Drain macaroni, then transfer it to a large bowl of *ice water*. Let stand for 2 minutes. Drain well and remove unmelted ice.

■ While macaroni is cooling, cut crab-flavored fish sticks into 1-inch pieces. Drain oranges.

■ In a large salad bowl combine pasta, crab-flavored fish, oranges, salad greens, and green onion. Stir together yogurt and orange juice concentrate; pour atop pasta-salad greens mixture. Toss lightly to coat. To serve, spoon onto 4 individual serving plates. Sprinkle almonds over salads. Makes 4 servings.

PER SERVING

Calories	331
Protein	33 g
Carbohydrate	31 g
Fat	8 g
Cholesterol	105 mg
Sodium	493 mg
Potassium	775 mg

TIMETABLE

Total preparation time: about 20 minutes

HAMBURGER STRATA

Are your taste buds demanding lasagna, but you think you don't dare indulge? Phooey! Satisfy 'em with a serving of this lasagna taste-alike.

½ **pound lean ground beef**
½ **cup frozen chopped onion
   (see tip, page 39)**
2 **cups plain croutons**
1 **7-ounce can whole kernel
   corn**
1 **8-ounce can tomato sauce**
½ **cup shredded mozzarella
   cheese (2 ounces)**
2 **eggs**
½ **cup skim milk**
¾ **teaspoon dried Italian
   seasoning, crushed**

■ Preheat the oven to 325°. Meanwhile, break the ground meat into large pieces while adding it to a skillet. Add the frozen onion. Cook meat and onion over high heat till meat is brown and onion is tender. Drain off fat.

■ Place *1 cup* of the croutons in an ungreased 10x6x2-inch baking dish. Drain corn; spoon corn evenly atop croutons. Spoon meat mixture over corn; spoon tomato sauce atop. Sprinkle with cheese. Top with remaining *1 cup* croutons.

■ In a mixing bowl beat eggs lightly. Stir in milk and Italian seasoning. Pour over layers in dish. Cover with foil. Bake in the 325° oven about 25 minutes or till a knife inserted off center comes out clean. Let stand for 5 minutes before serving. Makes 4 servings.

PER SERVING

Calories	335
Protein	24 g
Carbohydrate	28 g
Fat	13 g
Cholesterol	186 mg
Sodium	911 mg
Potassium	558 mg

TIMETABLE

Preparation time:
15 minutes

Cooking time:
about 25 minutes

Standing time:
5 minutes

PRESTO PASTA 'N' RICE

Heat-and-eat pasta or rice are only as far away as your freezer and microwave oven.

Simply cook the pasta or rice according to the package directions. (Rinse and drain pasta well.) Place freezer bags in 6-ounce custard cups; place ½-cup single-serving portions of pasta or rice into the freezer bags. Seal, label with contents and date, then freeze till firm. Remove custard cups. (Pasta and rice will keep up to 6 months in the freezer.)

To reheat one serving, place pasta or rice in a microwave-safe bowl. Cover loosely with waxed paper. Micro-cook on 100% power (high) for 1 to 2 minutes or till hot.

BEEF SOFT SHELLS

These simple sandwich packets are ready in about 20 minutes.

2   **7- to 8-inch flour tortillas**
4   **ounces lean ground beef**
¼   **cup frozen chopped onion (see tip, page 39)**
¼   **cup taco sauce**
¼   **teaspoon chili powder**
½   **cup shredded cheddar cheese (2 ounces)**
2   **small lettuce leaves**

■ Preheat the oven to 350°. Meanwhile, wrap tortillas in foil. Place in the oven and heat about 8 minutes or till tortillas are warm.

■ While the tortillas are heating, break ground meat into large pieces while adding it to a medium saucepan. Add frozen onion. Cook meat and onion over high heat till meat is brown and onion is tender. Drain off fat. Stir in *2 tablespoons* of the taco sauce and the chili powder.

■ To serve, spoon *half* of the beef mixture onto *each* tortilla near 1 edge. Top with *half* of the cheese and *1* lettuce leaf. Fold edge nearest filling up and over filling just till mixture is covered. Fold in the 2 sides envelope fashion, then roll up. Serve immediately with remaining taco sauce. Makes 2 servings.

PER SERVING

Calories	290
Protein	21 g
Carbohydrate	18 g
Fat	15 g
Cholesterol	70 mg
Sodium	411 mg
Potassium	279 mg

TIMETABLE

Total preparation time:
20 minutes

QUICK BURGER TORTILLAS

1   **slice white bread**
3   **tablespoons skim milk**
¾   **pound lean ground beef**
¼   **cup canned chopped green chili peppers**
¼   **teaspoon salt**
4   **7- to 8- inch flour tortillas**
½   **cup salsa**

■ Preheat the broiler. Meanwhile, place slice of bread in a large mixing bowl. Pour milk atop. Let stand for 5 minutes to soften bread. Add ground beef, chili peppers, and salt. Mix well. On waxed paper shape meat mixture into 4 oval patties 5 inches long and ¾ inch thick.

■ Place patties on the unheated rack of a broiler pan. Broil patties 3 to 4 inches from the heat for 6 minutes. Turn patties over and broil for 6 to 8 minutes more or till desired doneness.

■ While meat is broiling, warm tortillas, if desired, and salsa. To serve, place *1* meat patty onto *each* tortilla near 1 edge. Dollop with salsa. Fold edge nearest patty up and over to overlap patty. Fold 2 opposite sides of tortilla so they overlap on top of patty. Begin eating from open end. Makes 4 servings.

PER SERVING

Calories	239
Protein	20 g
Carbohydrate	20 g
Fat	8 g
Cholesterol	60 mg
Sodium	420 mg
Potassium	288 mg

TIMETABLE

Preparation time:
15 minutes

Cooking time:
12 to 14 minutes

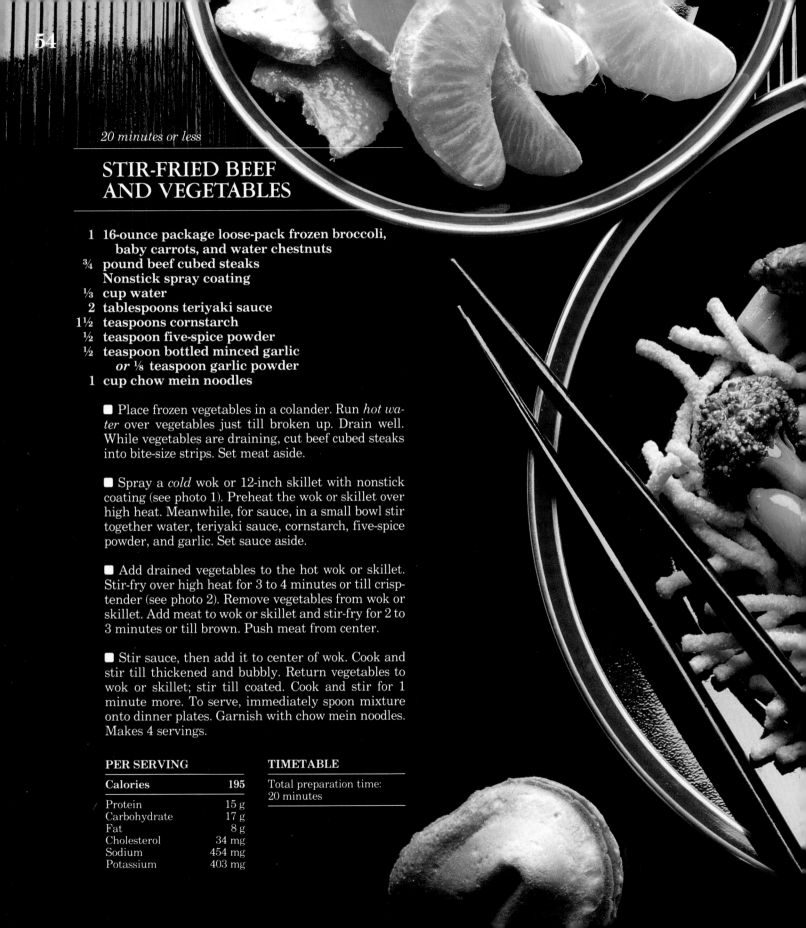

20 minutes or less

STIR-FRIED BEEF AND VEGETABLES

1	16-ounce package loose-pack frozen broccoli, baby carrots, and water chestnuts
¾	pound beef cubed steaks
	Nonstick spray coating
⅓	cup water
2	tablespoons teriyaki sauce
1½	teaspoons cornstarch
½	teaspoon five-spice powder
½	teaspoon bottled minced garlic *or* ⅛ teaspoon garlic powder
1	cup chow mein noodles

■ Place frozen vegetables in a colander. Run *hot water* over vegetables just till broken up. Drain well. While vegetables are draining, cut beef cubed steaks into bite-size strips. Set meat aside.

■ Spray a *cold* wok or 12-inch skillet with nonstick coating (see photo 1). Preheat the wok or skillet over high heat. Meanwhile, for sauce, in a small bowl stir together water, teriyaki sauce, cornstarch, five-spice powder, and garlic. Set sauce aside.

■ Add drained vegetables to the hot wok or skillet. Stir-fry over high heat for 3 to 4 minutes or till crisp-tender (see photo 2). Remove vegetables from wok or skillet. Add meat to wok or skillet and stir-fry for 2 to 3 minutes or till brown. Push meat from center.

■ Stir sauce, then add it to center of wok. Cook and stir till thickened and bubbly. Return vegetables to wok or skillet; stir till coated. Cook and stir for 1 minute more. To serve, immediately spoon mixture onto dinner plates. Garnish with chow mein noodles. Makes 4 servings.

PER SERVING		TIMETABLE
Calories	**195**	Total preparation time: 20 minutes
Protein	15 g	
Carbohydrate	17 g	
Fat	8 g	
Cholesterol	34 mg	
Sodium	454 mg	
Potassium	403 mg	

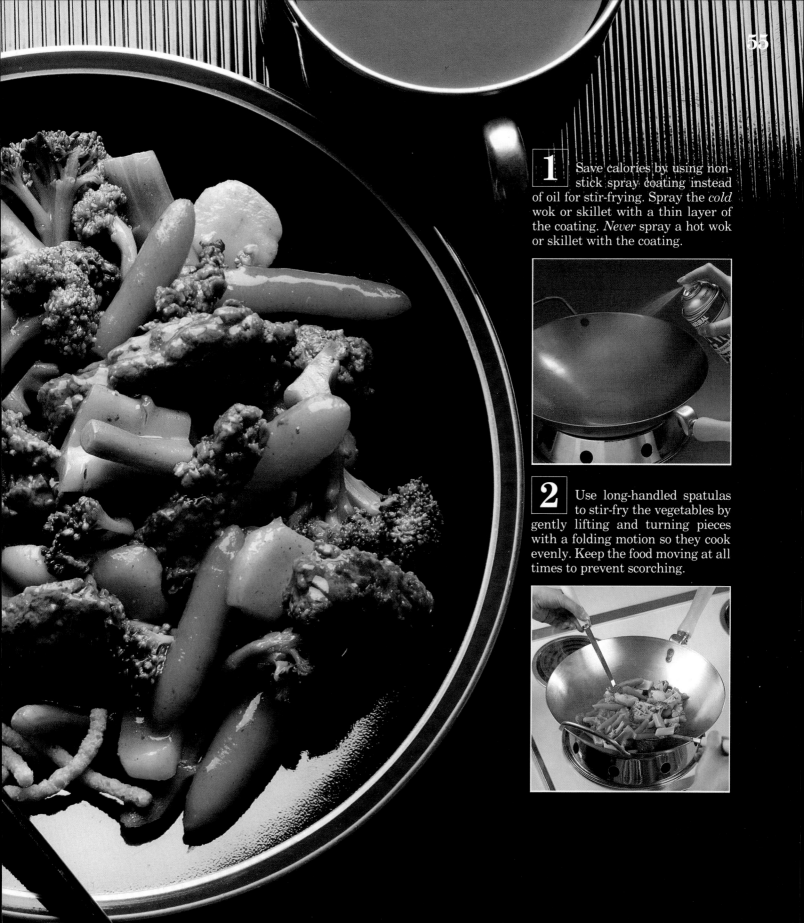

1 Save calories by using non-stick spray coating instead of oil for stir-frying. Spray the *cold* wok or skillet with a thin layer of the coating. *Never* spray a hot wok or skillet with the coating.

2 Use long-handled spatulas to stir-fry the vegetables by gently lifting and turning pieces with a folding motion so they cook evenly. Keep the food moving at all times to prevent scorching.

BEEFY PASTA SALAD

Change the personality of this main-dish salad to fit your mood—try bow tie, wagon wheel, or even elbow macaroni.

¾ cup corkscrew macaroni (2 ounces)
⅓ cup reduced-calorie mayonnaise *or* salad dressing
⅓ cup plain low-fat yogurt
1 tablespoon prepared horseradish
1 tablespoon frozen snipped chives (see tip, page 39)
½ teaspoon Worcestershire sauce
Dash garlic powder
6 ounces lean cooked beef
1 medium tomato
4 large lettuce leaves
½ cup frozen peas

■ Cook macaroni according to package directions, *except* use a large saucepan and 3 cups *hot water.*

■ While pasta is cooking, stir together the mayonnaise or salad dressing, yogurt, horseradish, chives, Worcestershire sauce, and garlic powder. Cover and chill while preparing rest of salad.

■ Trim fat from beef and cut meat into julienne strips; place in a large mixing bowl. Chop and seed tomato; add to beef. Place lettuce on plates.

■ Drain pasta and transfer it to a large bowl of *ice water.* Let stand for 2 minutes. Then drain well and remove unmelted ice cubes. Add drained pasta and frozen peas to mixing bowl with meat. Pour dressing over pasta mixture. Toss gently till ingredients are well coated. Serve salad on lettuce-lined plates. Makes 4 servings.

PER SERVING

Calories	232
Protein	17 g
Carbohydrate	17 g
Fat	11 g
Cholesterol	40 mg
Sodium	454 mg
Potassium	311 mg

TIMETABLE

Total preparation time: 30 minutes

QUICK-COOKING STEAK STEW

Some supermarkets sell meat already cut for stir-fries—perfect for this full-flavored stew.

½ pound boneless beef top round steak
⅛ teaspoon pepper
Nonstick spray coating
1 14½-ounce can beef broth
1 9-ounce package frozen cut green beans
½ of a 12-ounce package (1½ cups) frozen hash brown potatoes with onion and peppers
½ of a 15-ounce can (1 cup) herbed tomato sauce
1 tablespoon cornstarch
½ teaspoon sugar

■ Trim fat from meat. Thinly slice meat across the grain into bite-size strips. Sprinkle with pepper. Spray a *cold* large saucepan with nonstick coating. Cook meat in saucepan over medium heat until meat is evenly browned.

■ Add beef broth. Bring mixture to boiling, then reduce heat. Cover and simmer for 10 minutes. Meanwhile, place frozen beans and potatoes in a colander. Run *hot water* over beans and potatoes just till thawed. Drain thoroughly.

■ Add beans and potatoes to saucepan. Return to boiling. Simmer, covered, for 5 to 8 minutes more or till beans are tender. Meanwhile, stir together tomato sauce, cornstarch, and sugar. Stir into the meat-vegetable mixture. Cook and stir till mixture is thickened and bubbly. Cook and stir for 2 minutes more. Makes 3 servings.

PER SERVING

Calories	243
Protein	23 g
Carbohydrate	28 g
Fat	5 g
Cholesterol	46 mg
Sodium	826 mg
Potassium	854 mg

TIMETABLE

Total preparation time: 35 minutes

GARDEN BURGERS

1 egg white
3 tablespoons water
1 slice bread
½ teaspoon dried oregano, crushed
¼ teaspoon salt
   Dash pepper
1 pound lean ground beef
½ of a small cucumber
½ cup tomato sauce
1 teaspoon frozen snipped chives (see tip, page 39)
¼ teaspoon dried oregano, crushed

■ Preheat the broiler. Meanwhile, in a medium mixing bowl beat the egg white and water together till combined. Tear bread into soft crumbs into the bowl. Stir in ½ teaspoon oregano, salt, and pepper. Add beef, then mix well. Shape the meat mixture into four ¾-inch-thick patties.

■ Place patties on the unheated rack of a broiler pan. Broil patties 3 to 4 inches from the heat for 6 minutes. Turn the patties over and broil for 6 to 8 minutes more or till desired doneness.

■ While meat is broiling, seed and finely chop the cucumber. In a small saucepan combine the cucumber, tomato sauce, chives, and ¼ teaspoon oregano. Heat mixture till bubbly, stirring occasionally. Serve meat patties topped with the tomato mixture. Makes 4 servings.

PER SERVING

Calories	221
Protein	25 g
Carbohydrate	7 g
Fat	10 g
Cholesterol	80 mg
Sodium	418 mg
Potassium	429 mg

TIMETABLE

Preparation time:
10 minutes

Cooking time:
12 to 14 minutes

20 minutes or less

SPOON BURGERS

What's a Spoon Burger? It's a one-bun burger you spoon the meat on and eat with a fork.

1 pound lean ground beef
½ cup frozen chopped green pepper (see tip, page 39)
1 8-ounce can (1 cup) tomato sauce with chopped onion
1 tablespoon brown mustard *or* Dijon-style mustard
2 teaspoons Worcestershire sauce
3 hamburger buns

■ Break ground meat into large pieces while adding it to a medium skillet. Add frozen green pepper. Cook meat and green pepper over high heat till meat is brown and green pepper is tender. Drain off fat.

■ Stir in tomato sauce, mustard, and Worcestershire sauce. Bring mixture just to boiling; reduce the heat. Simmer, uncovered, about 5 minutes, or till mixture is heated through and flavors are well blended, stirring occasionally.

■ While meat is cooking, split hamburger buns and toast under the broiler. Divide meat mixture among toasted bun halves for an open-face sandwich. Makes 6 servings.

PER SERVING

Calories	205
Protein	18 g
Carbohydrate	15 g
Fat	8 g
Cholesterol	54 mg
Sodium	386 mg
Potassium	367 mg

TIMETABLE

Total preparation time:
15 minutes

SPROUT-TOPPED BURGERS

Be sure to put the cheese on the hot burger right away so it will melt.

1 egg white
¼ cup quick-cooking rolled oats
¼ cup frozen chopped onion (see tip, page 39)
½ teaspoon dried rosemary, crushed
¼ teaspoon salt
1 cup alfalfa sprouts
1 pound lean ground beef
1 1½-ounce slice low-fat mozzarella cheese

■ Preheat the broiler. Meanwhile, in a medium mixing bowl lightly beat the egg white. Stir in the oats, frozen onion, rosemary, and salt. Finely chop ½ *cup* of the sprouts and add to the mixture in the bowl. Add beef, then mix well. Shape meat mixture into four ¾-inch-thick patties.

■ Place patties on the unheated rack of a broiler pan. Broil patties 3 to 4 inches from the heat for 6 minutes. Turn the patties over and broil for 6 to 8 minutes more or till desired doneness.

■ While meat patties are broiling, cut the cheese slice into 8 crosswise strips. When the meat patties are done, immediately top *each* meat patty with *2* of the cheese strips. Garnish the tops of patties with the remaining sprouts. Makes 4 servings.

PER SERVING

Calories	246
Protein	28 g
Carbohydrate	5 g
Fat	12 g
Cholesterol	86 mg
Sodium	260 mg
Potassium	325 mg

TIMETABLE

Preparation time: 10 minutes

Cooking time: 12 to 14 minutes

CURRIED BEEF

Stir-frying the curry powder in hot oil mellows the flavor.

⅔ cup long grain rice
¾ pound boneless beef top round steak
   Nonstick spray coating
¾ cup frozen chopped green pepper (see tip, page 39)
½ cup frozen chopped onion (see tip, page 39)
1 teaspoon cooking oil
1 to 2 teaspoons curry powder
1 6-ounce can tomato juice
¼ cup raisins
1 teaspoon instant beef bouillon granules
½ cup cold water
1 tablespoon cornstarch

■ Prepare rice according to package directions, *except* omit the margarine or butter.

■ While the rice is cooking, trim fat from meat. Thinly slice the meat across the grain into bite-size strips. Spray a *cold* large skillet with nonstick coating. Preheat the skillet over medium-high heat.

■ Add pepper and onion to skillet and stir-fry for 2 minutes; remove vegetables from skillet and set aside. Add cooking oil to skillet. Add beef to skillet; stir-fry over high heat for 2 minutes or till nearly done. Add curry powder; stir-fry for 1 minute more.

■ Carefully stir in tomato juice, cooked onion and pepper, raisins, and bouillon granules. Stir together cold water and cornstarch. Stir into meat mixture. Cook and stir till thickened and bubbly, then cook and stir for 2 minutes more. Serve meat mixture over hot rice. Makes 4 servings.

PER SERVING

Calories	262
Protein	17 g
Carbohydrate	39 g
Fat	4 g
Cholesterol	39 mg
Sodium	636 mg
Potassium	453 mg

TIMETABLE

Total preparation time: 25 minutes

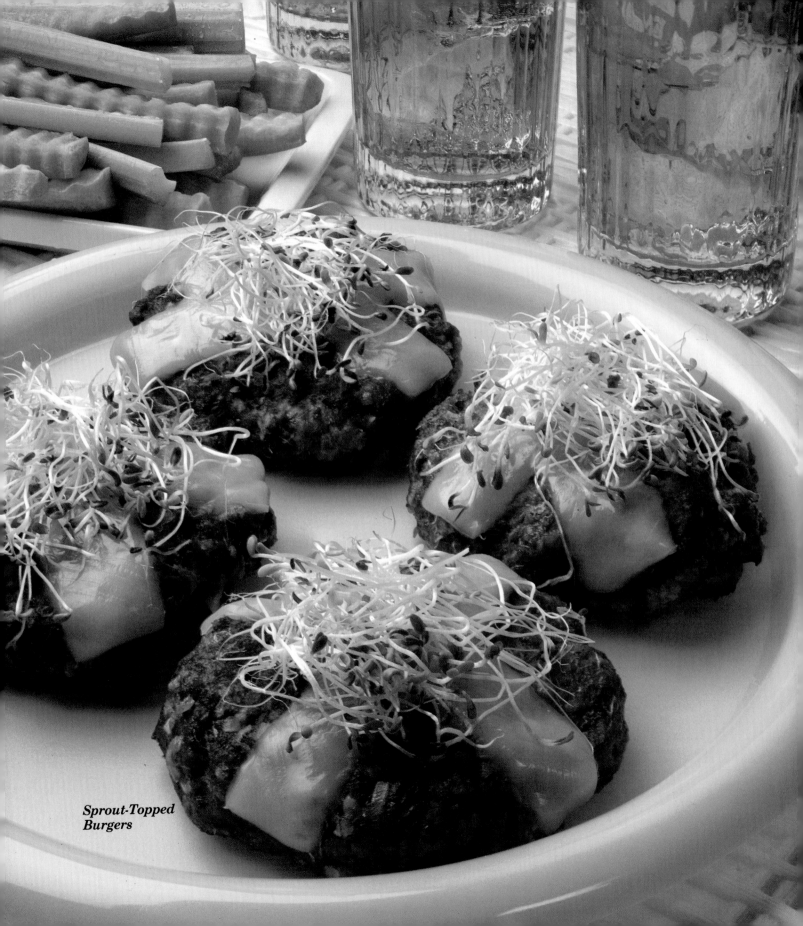

*Sprout-Topped
Burgers*

HAMBURGER HASH

Cracked wheat adds special flavor and extra nutrition to this old standby.

¾ pound lean ground beef
½ cup frozen chopped onion (see tip, page 39)
½ teaspoon bottled minced garlic *or* ⅛ teaspoon garlic powder
1 large potato
½ cup cracked wheat
½ cup frozen chopped green pepper (see tip, page 39)
2 teaspoons instant beef bouillon granules
¾ teaspoon dried thyme, crushed
¼ teaspoon pepper
1½ cups water
1 large tomato

■ Break ground meat into large pieces while adding it to a large skillet. Add frozen onion and garlic. Cook meat, onion, and garlic over high heat till meat is brown and onion is tender. Drain off fat.

■ While the meat is cooking, dice the *unpeeled* potato. Add potato to skillet, along with cracked wheat, frozen green pepper, bouillon granules, thyme, and pepper. Stir in water. Bring to boiling, then reduce heat. Cover and simmer for 15 minutes or till potatoes and cracked wheat are tender.

■ While meat mixture is cooking, cut the tomato into 8 wedges. Garnish meat mixture with tomato wedges. Makes 4 servings.

PER SERVING

Calories	270
Protein	22 g
Carbohydrate	28 g
Fat	8 g
Cholesterol	60 mg
Sodium	220 mg
Potassium	682 mg

TIMETABLE

Total preparation time: 25 minutes

SAUCY BEEF SKILLET

A top-of-the-range casserole with a from-the-oven full flavor.

1 16-ounce package loose-pack frozen cauliflower, broccoli, and carrots
1 pound lean ground beef
⅓ cup frozen chopped onion (see tip, page 39)
¼ teaspoon bottled minced garlic *or* dash garlic powder
1 tablespoon cornstarch
½ teaspoon salt
¼ teaspoon dried marjoram *or* dried basil, crushed
Dash pepper
1¼ cups skim milk
½ of an 8-ounce container reduced-calorie soft-style cream cheese

■ Cook frozen vegetables according to package directions; drain. Set aside and keep hot. Meanwhile, break ground meat into large pieces while adding it to a large skillet. Add frozen onion and garlic. Cook meat, onion, and garlic over high heat till meat is brown and onion is tender. Drain off fat.

■ Stir in cornstarch, salt, marjoram or basil, and pepper. Add milk. Cook and stir over medium-high heat till mixture is thickened and bubbly. Stir in cream cheese till melted. To serve, arrange vegetables on a plate. Spoon meat mixture over vegetables. Makes 4 servings.

PER SERVING

Calories	320
Protein	31 g
Carbohydrate	14 g
Fat	15 g
Cholesterol	98 mg
Sodium	570 mg
Potassium	747 mg

TIMETABLE

Total preparation time: 25 minutes

ORANGE FLANK STEAK

Slice flank steak across the grain to make it tender and succulent. (Pictured on pages 24 and 25.)

1 **pound beef flank steak**
½ **cup orange juice**
4 **teaspoons soy sauce**
1 **teaspoon cornstarch**
½ **teaspoon dried minced onion**
   Frozen snipped chives (optional)
   Orange wedges (optional)

■ Preheat the broiler. Meanwhile, trim fat from meat. Place meat on the unheated rack of a broiler pan. For sauce, in a small saucepan combine orange juice, soy sauce, cornstarch, and onion. Cook and stir till thickened and bubbly. Cook and stir for 2 minutes more; set aside.

■ Broil steak 3 to 4 inches from the heat for 4 to 5 minutes. Turn steak over. Brush with some of the sauce. Broil steak for 4 to 6 minutes more or till desired doneness. To serve, cut very thin slices diagonally across the grain. Spoon remaining sauce over meat. Sprinkle with chives and garnish with orange wedges, if desired. Makes 4 servings.

PER SERVING

Calories	185
Protein	25 g
Carbohydrate	5 g
Fat	7 g
Cholesterol	77 mg
Sodium	430 mg
Potassium	477 mg

TIMETABLE

Preparation time:
15 minutes

Cooking time:
8 to 11 minutes

QUICK SAUERBRATEN

The crumbled gingersnaps spice up and thicken the sauce of this traditional German dish.

¾ **pound boneless beef top round steak**
1 **tablespoon all-purpose flour**
½ **teaspoon dry mustard**
¼ **teaspoon salt**
¼ **teaspoon pepper**
   Nonstick spray coating
1 **medium onion**
1¼ **cups water**
¼ **cup vinegar**
1 **tablespoon brown sugar**
1 **bay leaf**
   Dash ground cloves
2 **cups medium noodles**
4 **gingersnaps**

■ Trim fat from meat. Cut meat into ½-inch pieces. Stir together flour, mustard, salt, and pepper; add meat and toss to coat well. Spray a *cold* medium skillet with nonstick coating. Quickly brown meat over medium-high heat.

■ While meat is browning, thinly slice onion. Carefully add the water, vinegar, onion slices, brown sugar, bay leaf, and cloves to skillet. Bring mixture to boiling, then reduce heat. Cover and simmer about 15 minutes or till meat is tender.

■ While meat is cooking, cook noodles according to package directions, *except* use a large saucepan and 4 cups *hot water*. Drain.

■ Crumble gingersnaps. Add to meat mixture. Cook and stir about 5 minutes or till mixture is slightly thickened. Remove and discard bay leaf. Serve mixture over hot cooked noodles. Makes 4 servings.

PER SERVING

Calories	242
Protein	20 g
Carbohydrate	29 g
Fat	5 g
Cholesterol	70 mg
Sodium	482 mg
Potassium	304 mg

TIMETABLE

Total preparation time:
about 40 minutes

20 minutes or less

VEAL-PEA POD STIR-FRY

Using precut frozen vegetables takes the work out of stir-fry preparation.

1   cup quick-cooking rice
1   6-ounce package frozen
       pea pods
1½   cups loose-pack frozen
       broccoli, green beans,
       mushrooms, and onions
12   ounces boneless veal
       Nonstick spray coating
½   cup cold water
2   tablespoons soy sauce
1   tablespoon cornstarch
¼   teaspoon ground ginger
1   teaspoon cooking oil

■ Cook rice according to package directions, *except* omit margarine or butter. Keep warm. Place frozen pea pods and frozen vegetables in a colander. Run *hot water* over vegetables just till thawed. Drain well.

■ While vegetables are draining, trim fat from meat. Thinly slice meat across the grain into bite-size strips, then set aside.

■ Spray a *cold* large skillet with nonstick coating. Preheat the skillet over high heat. For sauce, in a small bowl stir together cold water, soy sauce, cornstarch, and ginger. Set sauce aside.

■ Stir-fry pea pods and vegetables in the hot skillet about 2 minutes or just till crisp-tender. Remove vegetables from the skillet. Add cooking oil to the skillet. Stir-fry veal strips in skillet for 2 to 3 minutes or till brown. Push meat from center of skillet.

■ Stir sauce, then add it to center of the skillet. Cook and stir till thickened and bubbly. Return vegetables to the skillet and stir ingredients together. Cook and stir for 1 minute more. Serve mixture over hot cooked rice. Makes 4 servings.

PER SERVING

Calories	312
Protein	23 g
Carbohydrate	35 g
Fat	8 g
Cholesterol	61 mg
Sodium	783 mg
Potassium	514 mg

TIMETABLE

Total preparation time:
20 minutes

20 minutes or less

VEAL AND HAM BUNDLES

The low-calorie egg white is all you need to help the bread crumb coating stick.

2   slices thinly sliced ham
       (about 1½ ounces total)
2   tenderized veal cutlets
       (about 8 ounces total)
       Dash ground sage
1   egg white
2   tablespoons fine dry
       seasoned bread crumbs
1   teaspoon sesame seed
2   lemon wedges (optional)
       Parsley sprigs (optional)

■ Preheat the broiler. Center *1* ham slice atop *each* veal cutlet. Sprinkle lightly with sage. Fold cutlets in half, and seal around edges by pressing veal together. Beat egg white slightly. Brush veal bundles with egg white, then coat with a mixture of bread crumbs and sesame seed.

■ Broil veal bundles 4 to 5 inches from the heat for 5 minutes. Turn and broil for 5 minutes more or till meat is no longer pink and crumbs are golden brown. If desired, serve with lemon wedges to drizzle over meat, and garnish with parsley. Makes 2 servings.

PER SERVING

Calories	248
Protein	30 g
Carbohydrate	5 g
Fat	11 g
Cholesterol	92 mg
Sodium	406 mg
Potassium	457 mg

TIMETABLE

Preparation time:
10 minutes

Cooking time:
about 10 minutes

VEGETABLE-TOPPED PORK

Our food editors loved the taste of these tender burgers. We're sure you will, too.

8 ounces lean ground pork
2 teaspoons soy sauce
1 medium zucchini
1 medium carrot
⅔ cup orange juice
1 teaspoon frozen snipped chives (see tip, page 39)
2 teaspoons cornstarch
2 teaspoons soy sauce
½ teaspoon curry powder

■ Preheat a large skillet over medium heat. In a mixing bowl combine pork and 2 teaspoons soy sauce. Mix well. Shape meat mixture into two ½-inch-thick patties. Place patties in the preheated skillet. Cook patties over medium heat about 12 minutes or till no pink remains, turning once. (Partially cover skillet to prevent spattering.)

■ While the patties are cooking, slice zucchini and coarsely shred carrot. When patties are done, remove from skillet; drain fat. Place patties on a serving platter; cover and keep warm. Add zucchini, carrot, ⅓ *cup* of the orange juice, and chives to skillet. Cook, covered, for 3 to 5 minutes or just till vegetables are crisp-tender.

■ While vegetables are cooking, combine the remaining orange juice, cornstarch, 2 teaspoons soy sauce, and curry powder; add to skillet. Cook and stir till mixture is thickened and bubbly, then cook and stir for 2 minutes more. Serve vegetable mixture atop meat patties. Makes 2 servings.

PER SERVING

Calories	241
Protein	21 g
Carbohydrate	18 g
Fat	10 g
Cholesterol	58 mg
Sodium	744 mg
Potassium	758 mg

TIMETABLE

Total preparation time: 20 minutes

PIZZA-SAUCED PORK PATTIES

1 egg white
2 teaspoons dried minced onion
½ teaspoon dried oregano, crushed
¼ teaspoon salt
⅛ teaspoon pepper
1 pound lean ground pork
⅓ cup pizza sauce
¼ cup shredded mozzarella cheese (1 ounce)
¼ of a medium head lettuce

■ Preheat the broiler. Meanwhile, in a medium mixing bowl beat egg white slightly. Stir in onion, oregano, salt, and pepper. Add ground pork and mix well. Shape meat mixture into four ½-inch-thick patties.

■ Place patties on the unheated rack of a broiler pan. Broil 3 to 4 inches from the heat about 12 minutes or till no pink remains, turning once. Brush with some of the pizza sauce during the last few minutes of broiling. Sprinkle the cheese atop sauce and broil about 1 minute more or till cheese starts to melt.

■ While patties are cooking, shred lettuce and divide among 4 serving plates. To serve, place the meat patties atop shredded lettuce. Makes 4 servings.

PER SERVING

Calories	204
Protein	21 g
Carbohydrate	4 g
Fat	11 g
Cholesterol	62 mg
Sodium	341 mg
Potassium	360 mg

TIMETABLE

Preparation time: 15 minutes

Cooking time: 13 minutes

PORK CHOPS DIJON

Serve these juicy chops with crusty French or Italian bread slices, steamed green beans, and mugs of iced tea.

4 **pork loin chops, cut ½ to ¾ inch thick (1¼ to 1½ pounds total)**
2 **tablespoons reduced-calorie Italian salad dressing (not oil free)**
2 **tablespoons Dijon-style mustard**
¼ **teaspoon pepper**
1 **medium onion**
  Nonstick spray coating
4 **lettuce leaves**

■ Trim fat from pork chops. In a small bowl stir together the salad dressing, mustard, and pepper. Brush both sides of chops with the mustard mixture. Slice onion.

■ Spray a *cold* 12-inch skillet with nonstick coating. Cook chops and onion in skillet, covered, over medium-low heat for 20 minutes.

■ Turn the pork chops. Cook, covered, for 5 to 10 minutes more or till meat is tender and no pink remains. To serve, place chops on a platter lined with lettuce leaves. Top the pork chops with the cooked onions. Makes 4 servings.

PER SERVING

Calories	227
Protein	25 g
Carbohydrate	2 g
Fat	12 g
Cholesterol	71 mg
Sodium	261 mg
Potassium	424 mg

TIMETABLE

Preparation time:
10 minutes

Cooking time:
25 to 30 minutes

20 minutes or less

ORANGE-BASIL PORK

1½ **cups frozen crinkle-cut carrots**
12 **ounces pork tenderloin**
4 **stalks bok choy**
4 **green onions**
  Nonstick spray coating
½ **cup water**
¼ **cup frozen orange juice concentrate**
2 **teaspoons cornstarch**
1 **teaspoon instant chicken bouillon granules**
½ **teaspoon dried basil, crushed**
¼ **teaspoon bottled minced garlic**

■ Place frozen carrots in a colander. Run *hot water* over vegetables just till thawed. Drain thoroughly. Trim fat from pork. Thinly bias-slice pork into bite-size strips; set aside. Chop bok choy and cut green onions into 1-inch pieces; set aside.

■ Spray a *cold* large skillet with nonstick coating. Preheat the skillet over high heat. Meanwhile, for sauce, in a small bowl or custard cup stir together the water, orange juice concentrate, cornstarch, bouillon granules, and basil. Set sauce aside.

■ Stir-fry carrots, bok choy, green onions, and garlic in skillet over high heat for 2 minutes or just till vegetables are crisp-tender. Remove vegetables from skillet. Stir-fry pork strips for 3 to 4 minutes or till no pink remains. Push meat from center of skillet.

■ Stir sauce, then add it to center of skillet. Cook and stir till mixture is thickened and bubbly. Return vegetables to the skillet and stir to coat all ingredients well. Cook and stir for 1 minute more. Serve immediately. Makes 3 or 4 servings.

PER SERVING

Calories	184
Protein	20 g
Carbohydrate	19 g
Fat	3 g
Cholesterol	57 mg
Sodium	237 mg
Potassium	768 mg

TIMETABLE

Total preparation time:
20 minutes

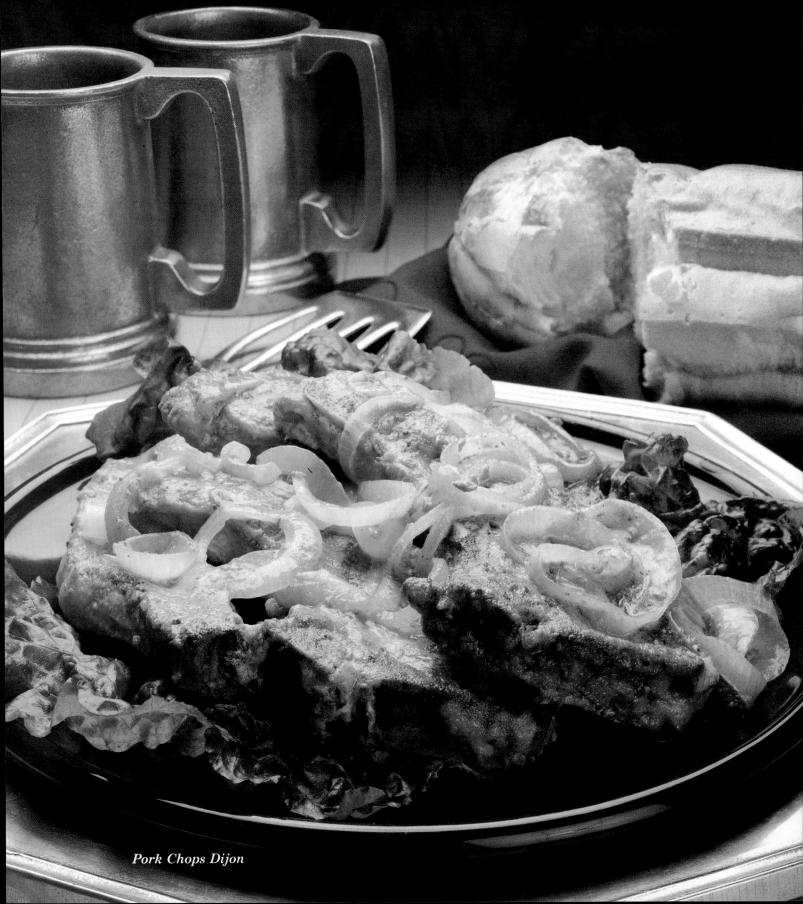
Pork Chops Dijon

20 minutes or less

SAUSAGE CHOWDER

Here's a quick cutting trick: Place the sausages side by side on the cutting board and cut crosswise into bite-size pieces all at once.

1½ cups water
½ of a 16-ounce package loose-pack frozen broccoli, cauliflower, and carrots
1 teaspoon dried Italian seasoning, crushed
6 brown-and-serve sausage links
1¾ cups skim milk
2 tablespoons cornstarch
2 ounces sliced process Swiss cheese

■ In a large saucepan bring the water to boiling. Add the frozen vegetables and Italian seasoning to saucepan. Return mixture to boiling, then reduce the heat. Cover and simmer for 5 minutes. *Do not drain.*

■ While the vegetables are cooking, cut the brown-and-serve sausage links into bite-size pieces. In a mixing bowl stir together the skim milk and cornstarch.

■ Stir the milk mixture and sausage links into vegetable mixture in saucepan. Cook and stir over medium-high heat till mixture is thickened and bubbly. Cook and stir for 2 minutes more.

■ Tear the cheese into pieces and stir it into the chowder till melted. Season chowder to taste with salt and pepper. Makes 3 servings.

PER SERVING

Calories	312
Protein	17 g
Carbohydrate	16 g
Fat	20 g
Cholesterol	45 mg
Sodium	753 mg
Potassium	568 mg

TIMETABLE

Total preparation time: 20 minutes

CITRUS SAMPLER

It's so easy to add a light, fresh flavor to foods with a bit of finely shredded citrus peel. Lemon, lime, orange—the possibilities are simply delicious. And keeping it on hand is no hassle either.

The next time a recipe calls for shredded citrus peel, shred more than you need. Place any extra shredded peel in a small airtight container, then label and freeze. It's ready to use another time. (Freshly shredded citrus peel also can be used in the recipes calling for frozen peel.)

SKILLET PORK CHOPS 'N' RICE

Choose Granny Smith, Jonathan, Winesap, or Rome Beauty apples.

1½ cups water
½ cup frozen chopped onion (see tip, page 39)
¼ cup frozen chopped green pepper (see tip, page 39)
1 teaspoon instant chicken bouillon granules
½ teaspoon ground cinnamon
⅔ cup long grain rice
2 small cooking apples
12 ounces fully cooked boneless smoked pork chops
2 tablespoons reduced-calorie orange marmalade

■ In a large skillet combine water, frozen onion, frozen green pepper, bouillon granules, and cinnamon. Stir in *uncooked* rice. Bring mixture to boiling, then reduce heat. Cover and simmer for 15 minutes.

■ While rice is cooking, core apples and cut into thin wedges. Stir apples into rice mixture in skillet. Place chops on top. Cover and simmer for 10 to 15 minutes more or till rice is tender and chops are heated through. Spread marmalade evenly over chops.

■ To serve, place the pork chops on individual serving plates and spoon rice in a mound beside chops. Makes 4 servings.

PER SERVING

Calories	298
Protein	20 g
Carbohydrate	41 g
Fat	5 g
Cholesterol	45 mg
Sodium	1,129 mg
Potassium	420 mg

TIMETABLE

Total preparation time:
30 minutes

PORK-VEGGIE POCKETS

2 pork cubed steaks (about 8 ounces total)
1 medium zucchini
1 small onion
Nonstick spray coating
½ cup tomato sauce with tomato tidbits
¼ teaspoon dried thyme, crushed
¼ teaspoon seasoned salt
¼ teaspoon pepper
2 large pita bread rounds
¾ cup shredded mozzarella cheese (3 ounces)

■ Cut the pork cubed steaks into bite-size pieces. Slice zucchini and onion; set aside. Spray a *cold* large skillet with nonstick coating. Preheat the skillet over high heat.

■ Cook the meat pieces in skillet for 4 to 5 minutes or till no pink remains. Drain off the fat. Add the zucchini, onion, tomato sauce, thyme, seasoned salt, and pepper to meat in skillet. Cook, covered, over medium heat for 6 to 8 minutes or just till the vegetables are crisp-tender, stirring occasionally. Remove the skillet from the heat.

■ While the vegetables are cooking, cut the pita bread rounds in half crosswise. Divide vegetable-meat mixture among pita halves. Top each pita half with some of the cheese. Makes 4 servings.

PER SERVING

Calories	274
Protein	21 g
Carbohydrate	26 g
Fat	9 g
Cholesterol	46 mg
Sodium	235 mg
Potassium	367 mg

TIMETABLE

Preparation time:
10 minutes

Cooking time:
10 to 13 minutes

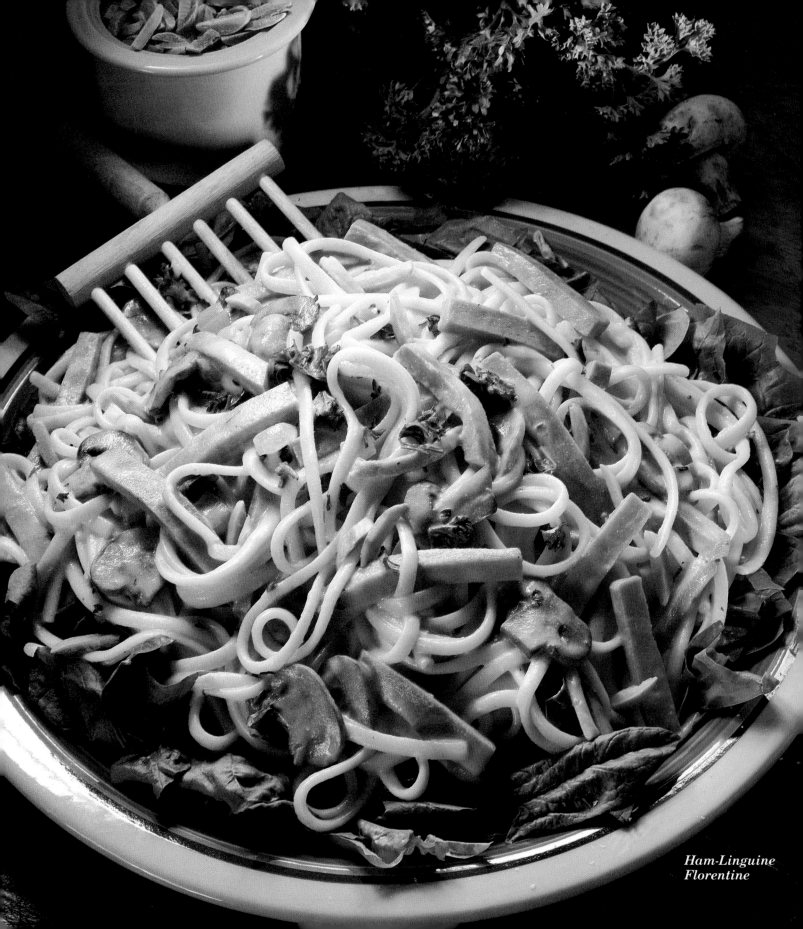

Ham-Linguine
Florentine

HAM-LINGUINE FLORENTINE

A pasta fork, like the one shown in the picture opposite, makes serving a snap.

3 ounces linguine
1 8-ounce fully cooked
   boneless ham slice
1 tablespoon slivered almonds
6 ounces fresh spinach
   (6 cups)
1 cup sliced fresh mushrooms
½ cup frozen chopped onion
   (see tip, page 39)
1 cup beef broth
½ cup skim milk
1 tablespoon cornstarch
½ teaspoon dried marjoram,
   crushed
2 tablespoons Dijon-style
   mustard
¼ cup frozen snipped parsley
   (see tip, page 39)

■ Cook the linguine according to package directions, *except* use a medium saucepan and 4 cups *hot water*. Let the linguine stand in hot water while finishing the recipe.

■ While pasta is cooking, cut ham into julienne strips; set aside. In a large saucepan cook almonds over medium heat about 1 to 2 minutes or till golden, stirring constantly. Remove almonds from saucepan; set aside. Coarsely chop the spinach and arrange it on a serving platter.

■ In the same saucepan, cook mushrooms and frozen onion in beef broth for 2 minutes or just till vegetables are tender. Meanwhile, in a screw-top jar combine milk and cornstarch. Cover and shake to mix well. Stir milk mixture and marjoram into saucepan. Cook and stir over medium-high heat till mixture is thickened and bubbly. Cook and stir for 1 minute more. Stir ham, mustard, and frozen parsley into saucepan; heat through. Drain the linguine and stir it into the ham mixture.

■ To serve, top spinach with hot linguine mixture. Sprinkle toasted almonds atop. Makes 3 servings.

PER SERVING

Calories	300
Protein	25 g
Carbohydrate	33 g
Fat	7 g
Cholesterol	41 mg
Sodium	1,895 mg
Potassium	887 mg

TIMETABLE

Total preparation time:
30 minutes

20 minutes or less

HAM AND BEAN SALAD

Put the garbanzo beans and ham in the refrigerator the night before or early in the morning—they'll be thoroughly chilled by mealtime.

½ of a 15-ounce can garbanzo
   beans, chilled
1 6¾-ounce can chunk-style
   ham *or* 1¼ cups diced
   fully cooked ham, chilled
½ of a medium head lettuce
1 stalk celery
¼ cup reduced-calorie
   mayonnaise *or* salad
   dressing
2 tablespoons chili sauce
1 tablespoon skim milk
¼ teaspoon dry mustard
⅛ teaspoon pepper

■ Drain beans and canned ham; set aside. Coarsely shred lettuce and slice celery; set aside. For dressing, in a small bowl stir together mayonnaise or salad dressing, chili sauce, milk, mustard, and pepper.

■ Divide shredded lettuce among 3 individual serving plates. Gently toss beans, ham, and celery together. Place one-third of the ham mixture in a mound atop lettuce on each plate. Drizzle dressing over salads. Sprinkle with paprika, if desired. Serve immediately. Makes 3 servings.

PER SERVING

Calories	225
Protein	17 g
Carbohydrate	17 g
Fat	10 g
Cholesterol	31 mg
Sodium	996 mg
Potassium	612 mg

TIMETABLE

Total preparation time:
15 minutes

20 minutes or less

LEMON-DILL LAMB CHOPS

Brush the lemon-dill sauce on the chops during the last few minutes of broiling.

4　lamb leg sirloin chops, cut 1 inch thick (1¼ pounds total)
3　tablespoons reduced-calorie mayonnaise *or* salad dressing
2　tablespoons Dijon-style mustard
2　teaspoons lemon juice
⅛　teaspoon dried dillweed *or* dried tarragon, crushed

■ Preheat the broiler. Meanwhile, trim fat from lamb chops. Place chops on the unheated rack of a broiler pan. Broil chops 3 inches from the heat for 6 minutes. Meanwhile, for sauce, in a small mixing bowl stir together mayonnaise or salad dressing, mustard, lemon juice, and dillweed or tarragon.

■ Turn chops over and broil for 3 minutes. Brush chops with some of the sauce. Broil for 1 to 3 minutes more or till desired doneness. Pass any remaining sauce. Makes 4 servings.

PER SERVING

Calories	170
Protein	20 g
Carbohydrate	1 g
Fat	9 g
Cholesterol	69 mg
Sodium	332 mg
Potassium	235 mg

TIMETABLE

Preparation time:
5 minutes

Cooking time:
10 to 12 minutes

20 minutes or less

GINGERED-PINEAPPLE LAMB CHOPS

4　lamb leg sirloin chops, cut 1 inch thick (1¼ pounds total)
1　tablespoon sugar
1　teaspoon cornstarch
½　cup unsweetened pineapple juice
2　tablespoons frozen chopped green pepper (see tip, page 39)
1　teaspoon soy sauce
¼　teaspoon ground ginger

■ Preheat the broiler. Meanwhile, trim fat from lamb chops. Place chops on the unheated rack of a broiler pan. Broil lamb chops 3 inches from the heat for 6 minutes. Turn chops over and broil for 4 to 6 minutes more or till desired doneness.

■ While chops are broiling, for sauce, in a small saucepan stir together sugar and cornstarch. Stir in pineapple juice, green pepper, soy sauce, and ginger. Cook and stir till mixture is thickened and bubbly. Then cook and stir for 2 minutes more. Serve sauce over the lamb chops. Makes 4 servings.

PER SERVING

Calories	162
Protein	20 g
Carbohydrate	8 g
Fat	5 g
Cholesterol	69 mg
Sodium	134 mg
Potassium	279 mg

TIMETABLE

Total preparation time:
20 minutes

SPICED-APRICOT LAMB BURGERS

Cooking the raisins with the rice makes them plump and juicy.

1 cup quick-cooking rice
¼ cup light raisins
1 egg
¼ cup fine dry bread crumbs
½ teaspoon onion salt
1 pound lean ground lamb
⅓ cup unsweetened pineapple juice
3 tablespoons reduced-calorie apricot preserves
⅛ teaspoon ground cinnamon
⅛ teaspoon ground cloves

■ Preheat the broiler. Prepare rice according to package directions, *except* add raisins with rice to the water. Meanwhile, in a medium mixing bowl stir together egg, bread crumbs, and onion salt. Add the lamb, then mix well.

■ Shape meat mixture into four ½-inch-thick patties. Place patties on the unheated rack of a broiler pan. Broil patties 3 to 4 inches from the heat for 5 minutes. Turn the patties over and broil for 4 to 5 minutes more for medium doneness.

■ While patties are cooking, for sauce, in a small bowl stir together pineapple juice, apricot preserves, cinnamon, and cloves. Brush some of the sauce mixture over lamb patties during the last 1 to 2 minutes of broiling. Serve lamb patties on a bed of the cooked rice-raisin mixture. Spoon remaining sauce atop. Serve immediately. Makes 4 servings.

PER SERVING

Calories	347
Protein	27 g
Carbohydrate	39 g
Fat	8 g
Cholesterol	148 mg
Sodium	546 mg
Potassium	506 mg

TIMETABLE

Total preparation time:
25 minutes

FINES-HERBES LAMB STEW

Fines herbes is a handy blend of dried thyme, oregano, sage, rosemary, marjoram, and basil leaves that complements many foods.

8 ounces lean boneless lamb
Nonstick spray coating
1 cup water
½ cup apple juice
1 teaspoon instant chicken bouillon granules
½ teaspoon dried fines herbes, crushed
¼ teaspoon salt
1 cup frozen mixed vegetables
½ cup frozen chopped green pepper (see tip, page 39)
1 tablespoon cornstarch
1 tablespoon cold water

■ Trim fat from lamb. Cut the lamb into bite-size strips. Spray a *cold* medium saucepan with nonstick coating. Preheat the saucepan over medium-high heat. Add lamb to saucepan. Cook lamb over medium-high heat till brown.

■ Remove saucepan from the heat. Carefully add the 1 cup water, apple juice, bouillon granules, fines herbes, and salt. Stir in the frozen mixed vegetables and green pepper. Bring mixture to boiling, then reduce heat. Cover and simmer about 10 minutes or till meat and vegetables are tender.

■ In a small bowl stir together cornstarch and 1 tablespoon cold water; stir into mixture in saucepan. Cook and stir till mixture is thickened and bubbly. Then cook and stir for 2 minutes more. To serve, ladle the stew into bowls. Makes 2 servings.

PER SERVING

Calories	281
Protein	28 g
Carbohydrate	25 g
Fat	7 g
Cholesterol	85 mg
Sodium	559 mg
Potassium	614 mg

TIMETABLE

Preparation time:
15 minutes

Cooking time:
12 minutes

20 minutes or less

BULGUR TACOS

When you bite into one of these super stuffed tacos, you'd never guess there isn't a bit of meat inside.

8　taco shells
1　cup hot water
⅓　cup bulgur
1　1⅛- to 1¼-ounce envelope taco seasoning mix
8　ounces tofu (fresh bean curd)
4　lettuce leaves
1　medium tomato
½　cup shredded cheddar cheese (2 ounces)
½　cup tomato sauce
　　Salsa (optional)

■ Heat taco shells according to package directions. Meanwhile, in a medium saucepan combine hot water, bulgur, and taco seasoning mix. Bring mixture to boiling, then reduce heat. Cover and simmer about 10 minutes or till water is absorbed and bulgur is tender.

■ While bulgur is cooking, drain and finely chop tofu; set aside. Roll lettuce leaves together; thinly slice to form shreds. Chop tomato. Place lettuce, tomato, and cheese in individual serving bowls.

■ When bulgur is done, stir in chopped tofu and tomato sauce. Simmer, uncovered, for 1 to 2 minutes or till of desired consistency.

■ To serve, fill taco shells with some of the bulgur mixture. Pass lettuce, tomatoes, cheese, and salsa, if desired. Makes 4 servings.

PER SERVING

Calories	258
Protein	12 g
Carbohydrate	29 g
Fat	12 g
Cholesterol	15 mg
Sodium	518 mg
Potassium	291 mg

TIMETABLE

Total preparation time: 20 minutes

BULGUR-CHEESE DINNER

2　14½-ounce cans tomato wedges *or* one 28-ounce can tomatoes
½　cup frozen mixed vegetables
½　cup bulgur
½　teaspoon sugar
½　teaspoon dried oregano, crushed
½　teaspoon ground cumin
½　teaspoon chili powder
½　teaspoon bottled minced garlic *or* ⅛ teaspoon garlic powder
¾　cup shredded mozzarella cheese (3 ounces)

■ Cut up whole canned tomatoes. In a medium saucepan combine *undrained* tomatoes, frozen vegetables, bulgur, sugar, oregano, cumin, chili powder, and garlic. Bring mixture to boiling, then reduce heat. Cover; simmer for 20 to 25 minutes or till liquid is absorbed and bulgur and vegetables are tender.

■ To serve, spoon mixture onto individual plates or into bowls; sprinkle with cheese. Makes 3 servings.

PER SERVING

Calories	246
Protein	14 g
Carbohydrate	37 g
Fat	6 g
Cholesterol	15 mg
Sodium	618 mg
Potassium	781 mg

TIMETABLE

Total preparation time: about 30 minutes

GREEK FRITTATA

This Italian-style scrambled egg dish will remind you of an open-faced omelet.

2 ounces tofu (fresh bean
  curd)
2 ounces feta cheese
1 small tomato
4 pitted ripe olives
4 eggs
¼ teaspoon dried Italian
  seasoning, crushed
⅛ teaspoon pepper
  Nonstick spray coating
1 tablespoon grated
  Parmesan cheese
1 teaspoon frozen snipped
  chives (see tip, page 39)

■ Cut up tofu (you should have about ⅓ cup). Crumble feta cheese (you should have about ⅓ cup). Set aside. Chop tomato and slice olives. Set aside.

■ In a blender container or food processor bowl combine eggs, tofu, feta cheese, Italian seasoning, and pepper. Cover and blend or process till smooth.

■ Spray a *cold* medium skillet with nonstick coating. Heat skillet till a drop of water sizzles. Pour in egg mixture. Cook over medium-low heat, lifting edges occasionally to allow uncooked portion of the egg mixture to flow underneath. Cook about 4 minutes or till top is almost set.

■ Top the egg mixture with the chopped tomato, olives, Parmesan cheese, and chives. Remove skillet from heat. Cover and let stand for 3 to 4 minutes or till set. To serve, use a wide spatula to lift individual servings from the skillet. Makes 3 servings.

PER SERVING

Calories	192
Protein	13 g
Carbohydrate	4 g
Fat	14 g
Cholesterol	385 mg
Sodium	389 mg
Potassium	177 mg

TIMETABLE

Preparation time:
10 minutes

Cooking time:
about 4 minutes

Standing time:
3 to 4 minutes

MEATLESS CHILI SOUP

Soup without crackers is no fun, so why not crunch on homemade tortilla chips (see recipe, page 30) as you savor this vegetable-packed soup.

1 15-ounce can garbanzo
  beans
1 12-ounce can whole kernel
  corn with sweet peppers
1 15½-ounce can red kidney
  beans
1 14½-ounce can beef broth
1 10-ounce can tomatoes with
  green chili peppers
½ cup frozen chopped onion
  (see tip, page 39)
2 teaspoons chili powder
½ teaspoon bottled minced
  garlic *or* ⅛ teaspoon
  garlic powder
¼ teaspoon crushed red
  pepper
⅛ teaspoon pepper
¼ cup plain low-fat yogurt

■ Drain the garbanzo beans and corn. Drain and rinse the kidney beans. In a large saucepan stir together the garbanzo beans, corn, kidney beans, broth, tomatoes, frozen onion, chili powder, garlic, red pepper, and pepper.

■ Bring the mixture to boiling, then reduce the heat. Cover and simmer for 20 minutes. To serve, ladle into bowls. Dollop each serving with *1 tablespoon* of the yogurt. Makes 4 servings.

PER SERVING

Calories	312
Protein	17 g
Carbohydrate	58 g
Fat	3 g
Cholesterol	1 mg
Sodium	1,300 mg
Potassium	867 mg

TIMETABLE

Preparation time:
15 minutes

Cooking time:
about 20 minutes

20 minutes or less

HERB OMELET

Savor this omelet plain or choose from three fabulous fillings. Any way you serve it, the omelet is sure to tickle your taste buds.

  Nonstick spray coating
2 **eggs**
2 **tablespoons water**
⅛ **teaspoon dried basil, oregano, thyme,**
    ***or* marjoram, crushed**
⅛ **teaspoon pepper**

■ Spray a *cold* medium skillet with nonstick coating. Preheat skillet over medium heat. Meanwhile, in a small mixing bowl use a fork to beat eggs; water; basil, oregano, thyme, or marjoram; and pepper together till well combined.

■ Pour egg mixture into the hot skillet. Cook eggs over medium heat. As eggs set, use a spatula to push cooked eggs toward center, tilting pan so uncooked eggs flow underneath to the pan surface (see photo 1). When eggs are set but still shiny (3 to 4 minutes), fold omelet in half and slide onto a serving plate (see photo 2). Makes 1 serving.

PER SERVING		TIMETABLE
Calories	**160**	Total preparation time: 10 minutes
Protein	12 g	
Carbohydrate	1 g	
Fat	11 g	
Cholesterol	550 mg	
Sodium	139 mg	
Potassium	140 mg	

Swiss-Sprout Omelet: Prepare Herb Omelet as directed above, *except* when eggs are set but still shiny, sprinkle ¼ cup shredded *Swiss cheese,* 1 tablespoon *alfalfa sprouts,* and 1 tablespoon *sunflower nuts* on *half* of the omelet. Fold unfilled half of the omelet over filling. Remove omelet from skillet as above. Top with 1 tablespoon *alfalfa sprouts* and 2 tablespoons chopped *tomato.*

Calories	**299**

Total preparation time: 15 minutes

Blue-Cheese-Tomato Omelet: Prepare Herb Omelet as directed above, *except* chop 1 small *tomato* and crumble 1 tablespoon *blue cheese.* When eggs are set but still shiny, sprinkle chopped tomato and cheese on *half* of the omelet. Fold unfilled half of the omelet over filling. Remove omelet from skillet as above.

Calories	**203**

Total preparation time: 15 minutes

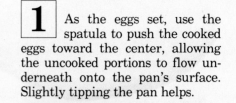

1 As the eggs set, use the spatula to push the cooked eggs toward the center, allowing the uncooked portions to flow underneath onto the pan's surface. Slightly tipping the pan helps.

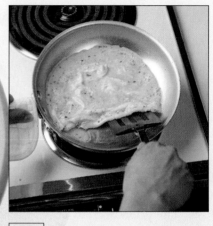

2 When the eggs are set but still shiny, sprinkle the filling ingredients on *half* of the omelet. Use the spatula to fold the unfilled half of the omelet over the filling, and carefully slide the omelet onto the serving plate.

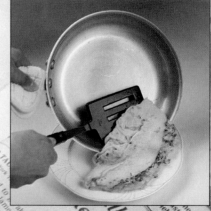

Omelet Olé: Prepare Herb Omelet as directed above left, *except* when eggs are set but still shiny, sprinkle ¼ cup shredded *Monterey Jack cheese* and 1 table-spoon chopped *pitted ripe olives* on *half* of the omelet. Fold unfilled half of the omelet over filling. Remove omelet from skillet. Sprinkle omelet with 2 table-spoons shredded *Monterey Jack cheese*, then spoon on 2 tablespoons *salsa.*

Calories	339

Total preparation time:
15 minutes

BARBECUE-STYLE CHICKEN

Freezing the chicken before placing it in the crockery cooker slows the cooking of the chicken. It will be tender, not overcooked, when the rest of the foods are done.

2 medium unpeeled potatoes
1 large green pepper
1 medium onion
1 tablespoon quick-cooking tapioca
2 pounds meaty chicken pieces, skin and fat removed, then frozen (see tip, below)
1 8-ounce can tomato sauce
2 tablespoons brown sugar
1 tablespoon Worcestershire sauce
2 teaspoons prepared mustard
½ teaspoon bottled minced garlic *or* ⅛ teaspoon garlic powder
¼ teaspoon salt

■ Cut potatoes into ½-inch pieces. Cut green pepper into thin strips and onion into thin slices.

■ In a 3½- or 4-quart electric crockery cooker place potatoes, green pepper, and onion. Sprinkle tapioca over vegetables. Place *frozen* chicken pieces on top.

■ In a small mixing bowl stir together tomato sauce, brown sugar, Worcestershire sauce, mustard, garlic, and salt. Pour mixture over chicken. Cover cooker. Cook on low-heat setting for 10 to 12 hours.

■ To serve, transfer chicken and vegetables to a serving bowl. Skim fat from sauce, then pour sauce over chicken and vegetables. Makes 5 servings.

PER SERVING

Calories	242
Protein	31 g
Carbohydrate	19 g
Fat	5 g
Cholesterol	95 mg
Sodium	549 mg
Potassium	752 mg

TIMETABLE

Preparation time:
15 minutes

Cooking time:
10 to 12 hours

FREEZING CHICKEN

With the help of your freezer, you can always have chicken on hand for our electric crockery cooker recipe above.

Before freezing the chicken, trim calories by removing all of the skin, as well as those hidden pockets of fat just beneath the skin. Then, arrange the chicken pieces in a single layer on a baking sheet. Cover and freeze the chicken till firm. Package the frozen pieces in moisture- and vaporproof wrap, label, and store in the freezer. When you're ready to cook, simply remove the number of pieces you need.

LAZY-DAY TURKEY

Feel like loafing? Then let your crockery cooker produce a succulent turkey dinner for you.

1 3- to 3½-pound frozen boneless turkey roast
2 stalks celery
1 small onion
1 medium carrot
½ cup water
½ teaspoon dried rosemary, crushed
1 tablespoon reduced-calorie orange marmalade

■ *About 12 hours before cooking,* place frozen turkey roast in the refrigerator to *partially* thaw.

■ Cut celery, onion, and carrot into large chunks. In a 3½- or 4-quart electric crockery cooker combine water and rosemary. Add the *partially thawed* turkey, then add celery, onion, and carrot chunks. Cover cooker. Cook on low-heat setting for 10 to 12 hours or until the internal temperature of the turkey roast is 180° to 185°.

■ To serve, in a small saucepan melt the orange marmalade. Discard liquid and vegetables from turkey in crockery cooker. Remove the net webbing from the turkey roast. Place turkey on a serving platter, then brush surface with marmalade. Serves 12 to 14.

PER SERVING

Calories	133
Protein	28 g
Carbohydrate	2 g
Fat	1 g
Cholesterol	70 mg
Sodium	69 mg
Potassium	389 mg

TIMETABLE

Preparation time:
10 minutes

Cooking time:
10 to 12 hours

PASTRY 'N' CHICKEN

We've tucked a tantalizing surprise inside this pastry-wrapped chicken: a superb mushroom filling.

4 boned skinless chicken breast halves (about 1 pound total)
1 2-ounce can mushroom stems and pieces
2 tablespoons reduced-calorie soft-style cream cheese
⅛ teaspoon dried fines herbes, crushed
1 tablespoon frozen sliced green onion (see tip, page 39)
1 4-ounce package (4) refrigerated crescent rolls

■ Preheat the oven to 350°. Meanwhile, place *1* piece of chicken, boned side up, between *2* pieces of clear plastic wrap. Working from the center to the edges, pound lightly with the flat side of a meat mallet to form a rectangle about ⅛ inch thick. Remove plastic wrap. Repeat with remaining chicken pieces.

■ Drain mushrooms. If necessary, cut up any large pieces. In a small mixing bowl stir together cream cheese and fines herbes. Then stir in mushrooms and onion. Spoon *one-fourth* of the mixture near the center of the top of *each* piece of chicken. Fold in sides of chicken, then roll up jelly-roll style. Place rolls, seam side down, in a shallow baking dish or pan.

■ Unroll crescent dough. Press perforations together to seal, forming *2* rectangles; roll or pat each into a 6x4-inch rectangle. Cut each rectangle in half crosswise, forming four 4x3-inch retangles. Place *1* rectangle over *each* roll, slightly pressing and stretching dough to shape over chicken. Cover loosely with foil. Bake in the 350° oven for 25 minutes. Remove foil. Bake for 10 to 15 minutes or till pastry is golden and chicken is tender and no longer pink. Serves 4.

PER SERVING

Calories	244
Protein	29 g
Carbohydrate	12 g
Fat	8 g
Cholesterol	73 mg
Sodium	398 mg
Potassium	386 mg

TIMETABLE

Preparation time:
15 minutes

Cooking time:
35 to 40 minutes

CHICKEN 'N' HAM ROLL-UPS

Tastes like classic chicken cordon bleu but with 347 fewer calories per serving.

4 boned skinless chicken
  breast halves (about
  1 pound total)
2 thin slices fully cooked
  ham (about 1½ ounces
  total)
2 thin slices mozzarella
  or Swiss cheese (about
  2 ounces total)
3 tablespoons fine dry bread
  crumbs
1 tablespoon grated
  Parmesan cheese
½ teaspoon dried basil,
  crushed
¼ teaspoon paprika

■ Preheat the oven to 350°. Meanwhile, place *1* piece of chicken, boned side up, between *2* pieces of clear plastic wrap. Working from the center to the edges, pound lightly with the flat side of a meat mallet to form a rectangle about ⅛ inch thick. Remove plastic wrap. Repeat with remaining chicken pieces.

■ Cut ham and cheese slices in half. Place *1* piece of ham and cheese on top of *each* piece of chicken. If necessary, trim ham and cheese to fit within ¼ inch of the edges. Fold in sides of chicken. Roll up jelly-roll style. If necessary, secure with wooden toothpicks.

■ In a shallow dish combine bread crumbs, Parmesan cheese, basil, and paprika. Brush chicken rolls with a little *water*, then roll the chicken in crumb mixture to coat. Place rolls in a shallow baking pan.

■ Bake in the 350° oven for 40 to 45 minutes or till chicken is tender and no longer pink. To serve, transfer chicken to a platter. Discard toothpicks. Serves 4.

PER SERVING

Calories	206
Protein	34 g
Carbohydrate	4 g
Fat	5 g
Cholesterol	81 mg
Sodium	340 mg
Potassium	352 mg

TIMETABLE

Preparation time:
15 minutes

Cooking time:
40 to 45 minutes

OVEN-FRIED CHICKEN

Every minute counts. Save yourself some time by using purchased cornflake crumbs instead of crushing cornflakes. (Pictured on page 25.)

   Nonstick spray coating
2 pounds meaty chicken
  pieces
⅔ cup cornflake crumbs
1½ teaspoons chili powder
½ teaspoon ground cumin
¼ teaspoon garlic salt
⅛ teaspoon ground red pepper

■ Preheat the oven to 375°. Meanwhile, spray a 13x9x2-inch baking pan with nonstick coating, then set aside. Remove skin and fat from chicken pieces. Set the chicken pieces aside.

■ In a shallow dish combine cornflake crumbs, chili powder, cumin, garlic salt, and red pepper. Rinse chicken pieces with *water*, then roll pieces in the crumb mixture to coat. Place chicken pieces in the prepared pan.

■ Bake chicken in the 375° oven for 45 to 50 minutes or till tender and no longer pink. To serve, transfer chicken to a serving platter. Makes 6 servings.

PER SERVING

Calories	165
Protein	20 g
Carbohydrate	9 g
Fat	5 g
Cholesterol	57 mg
Sodium	255 mg
Potassium	198 mg

TIMETABLE

Preparation time:
15 minutes

Cooking time:
45 to 50 minutes

ITALIAN SEASONED TURKEY BREAST HALF

1 teaspoon dried Italian
   seasoning, crushed
½ teaspoon salt
¼ teaspoon garlic powder
1 2- to 2½-pound fresh turkey
   breast half with bone
1 teaspoon cooking oil

■ Preheat the oven to 350°. Meanwhile, for seasoning mixture, in a small mixing bowl or custard cup combine Italian seasoning, salt, and garlic powder.

■ Remove and discard skin from turkey breast half. Using a sharp knife, cut *2* lengthwise slits about 1½ inches apart from the top to, *but not through,* the bottom of the turkey. Sprinkle seasoning mixture into the slits. Then rub oil over surface of turkey. Place turkey on a rack in a shallow roasting pan. Insert a meat thermometer near center of breast half. Cover loosely with foil.

■ Roast in the 350° oven for 1 to 1½ hours or till the thermometer registers 170°. Let stand for 10 minutes before slicing. Makes 8 to 10 servings.

PER SERVING

Calories	105
Protein	22 g
Carbohydrate	0 g
Fat	1 g
Cholesterol	56 mg
Sodium	177 mg
Potassium	267 mg

TIMETABLE

Preparation time:
5 minutes

Cooking time:
1 to 1½ hours

Standing time:
10 minutes

SPANISH CHICKEN BAKE

After working all day, mix up this easy dish, then put your feet up and read the paper while it bakes.

1⅓ cups water
1 4½-ounce package regular
   Spanish-style rice mix
1 2-ounce can mushroom
   stems and pieces
½ of a 4-ounce can diced
   green chili peppers
   (about ¼ cup)
4 boned skinless chicken
   breast halves (about
   1 pound total)
¼ cup finely shredded cheddar
   cheese (1 ounce)

■ Preheat the oven to 350°. Meanwhile, bring water to boiling. In a 10x6x2-inch baking dish combine the boiling water and rice mix. Drain mushrooms. Then stir mushrooms and chili peppers into rice mixture. Arrange chicken on top of the rice mixture. Cover tightly with foil.

■ Bake in the 350° oven for 35 to 40 minutes or till rice and chicken are tender and chicken is no longer pink. Sprinkle with cheese. Then bake, uncovered, for 2 to 3 minutes more or till cheese is melted. Makes 4 servings.

PER SERVING

Calories	234
Protein	30 g
Carbohydrate	16 g
Fat	4 g
Cholesterol	73 mg
Sodium	654 mg
Potassium	314 mg

TIMETABLE

Preparation time:
10 minutes

Cooking time:
37 to 43 minutes

SALMON 'N' SPINACH PUFF

Another way to thaw spinach is to place the frozen block in a microwave-safe casserole. Micro-cook, covered, on 30% power (medium-low) for 10 to 12 minutes.

Nonstick spray coating
1 6½-ounce can boneless, skinless pink salmon
1 10-ounce package frozen chopped spinach
2 tablespoons margarine *or* butter
2 cups low-fat cottage cheese
3 eggs
½ cup shredded Swiss cheese (2 ounces)
⅓ cup all-purpose flour
½ teaspoon dry mustard
¼ teaspoon frozen, finely shredded lemon peel (see tip, page 66)

■ Preheat the oven to 350°. Meanwhile, spray a 1½-quart soufflé dish *or* casserole with nonstick coating. Place dish in a 13x9x2-inch baking pan; set aside. Drain salmon, then flake it. Set salmon aside.

■ Place frozen spinach in a colander. Run *hot water* over spinach just till thawed. Then drain well, squeezing out excess water.

■ While thawing spinach, melt margarine or butter. In a blender container or food processor bowl place melted margarine or butter, cottage cheese, eggs, Swiss cheese, flour, mustard, and frozen lemon peel. Cover and blend or process till well combined. (When necessary, stop and scrape sides with a spatula.) Blend or process for 1 minute more.

■ Using a spoon, stir the salmon and drained spinach into the egg mixture. Pour mixture into the prepared soufflé dish or casserole. Pour *hot water* into pan around dish or casserole to a depth of 1 inch.

■ Bake in the 350° oven for 60 to 70 minutes or till a knife inserted near the center comes out clean. Serve immediately. Makes 6 servings.

PER SERVING

Calories	255
Protein	23 g
Carbohydrate	11 g
Fat	13 g
Cholesterol	161 mg
Sodium	571 mg
Potassium	361 mg

TIMETABLE

Preparation time: 20 minutes

Cooking time: 60 to 70 minutes

ONE-STEP SALMON BAKE

You don't need to cook the noodles separately—they cook during baking.

1 stalk celery
1 6½-ounce can boneless, skinless pink salmon
1 10¾-ounce can condensed cream of shrimp soup
1 cup skim milk
1 cup frozen cut broccoli
¼ teaspoon frozen, finely shredded lemon peel (see tip, page 66)
2½ ounces medium noodles (about 2 cups)
½ cup shredded mozzarella cheese (2 ounces)

■ Preheat the oven to 350°. Meanwhile, slice celery. Drain salmon, then break it into large chunks.

■ In a 1½-quart casserole combine celery, condensed soup, milk, frozen broccoli, frozen lemon peel, and ¼ teaspoon *pepper*. Add salmon and *uncooked* noodles, then toss lightly till mixed well.

■ Bake, covered, in the 350° oven about 50 minutes or till noodles are tender, stirring once after 25 minutes of cooking. Sprinkle salmon-noodle mixture with cheese. Then bake, uncovered, about 5 minutes more or till cheese is melted. Makes 4 servings.

PER SERVING

Calories	244
Protein	18 g
Carbohydrate	23 g
Fat	9 g
Cholesterol	48 mg
Sodium	730 mg
Potassium	397 mg

TIMETABLE

Preparation time: 10 minutes

Cooking time: about 55 minutes

SEAFOOD-STUFFED FISH

Save an extra minute by purchasing sliced mushrooms from the supermarket salad bar.

1 6-ounce package frozen
  crabmeat and shrimp
1 cup sliced fresh mushrooms
¼ cup frozen sliced green
  onion (see tip, page 39)
½ teaspoon bottled minced
  garlic *or* ⅛ teaspoon
  garlic powder
2 tablespoons water
¼ teaspoon salt
⅛ teaspoon chili powder
⅛ teaspoon pepper
¾ cup herb-seasoned stuffing
  mix
1 1½- to 2-pound fresh dressed
  redfish *or* red snapper
  Nonstick spray coating

■ Preheat the oven to 350°. Meanwhile, place crabmeat and shrimp in a colander. Run *cool water* over seafood just till thawed. Drain well. Chop; set aside.

■ While seafood is thawing, begin preparing the stuffing. In an uncovered medium saucepan cook the mushrooms, onion, and garlic in water till vegetables are tender, stirring frequently. Remove from heat. Stir in seafood, salt, chili powder, and pepper. Then stir in the stuffing mix.

■ To stuff fish, fill fish cavity with stuffing, lightly patting the stuffing to flatten evenly. (If all of the stuffing does not fit into the fish, place the remaining stuffing in a covered custard cup and bake for the last 10 minutes.) Tie or skewer fish closed.

■ Spray a large shallow baking pan with nonstick coating. Place stuffed fish in the pan. Cover loosely with foil. Bake in the 350° oven for 40 to 50 minutes or till fish flakes easily with a fork. Serves 5 or 6.

PER SERVING

Calories	266
Protein	37 g
Carbohydrate	17 g
Fat	5 g
Cholesterol	93 mg
Sodium	575 mg
Potassium	662 mg

TIMETABLE

Preparation time:
25 minutes

Cooking time:
40 to 50 minutes

COUSCOUS-STUFFED PIKE

Look for couscous (KOO-skoos), also known as Moroccan pasta, near the rice section in your supermarket.

1 medium apple
1 stalk celery
1¼ cups apple cider *or* apple
  juice
2 teaspoons Dijon-style
  mustard
½ teaspoon salt
¼ teaspoon onion powder
⅛ teaspoon pepper
¾ cup quick-cooking couscous
1 2- to 2½-pound fresh scaled,
  drawn pike, haddock, *or*
  lake trout
  Nonstick spray coating

■ Preheat the oven to 350°. Meanwhile, for stuffing, core and chop apple. Then chop celery. In a medium saucepan combine chopped apple, celery, apple cider or juice, mustard, salt, onion powder, and pepper. Bring to boiling, then reduce heat. Cover and simmer for 2 minutes. Remove saucepan from heat, then stir in couscous. Cover and let stand for 5 minutes.

■ To stuff fish, fill fish cavity with stuffing, lightly patting the stuffing to flatten evenly. (If all of the stuffing does not fit into the fish, place the remaining stuffing in a covered casserole and bake for the last 25 minutes.) Tie or skewer fish closed.

■ Spray a large shallow baking pan with nonstick coating. Place stuffed fish in the pan. Cover loosely with foil. Bake in the 350° oven for 45 to 55 minutes or till fish flakes easily with a fork. Serves 5 or 6.

PER SERVING

Calories	241
Protein	29 g
Carbohydrate	26 g
Fat	2 g
Cholesterol	75 mg
Sodium	353 mg
Potassium	573 mg

TIMETABLE

Preparation time:
20 minutes

Cooking time:
45 to 55 minutes

STUFFED HASH-BROWN LOAF

Calling all meat and potato lovers: Here's a slimming and satisfying meat-and-potato loaf.

1¼ cups frozen hash brown potatoes with onion and peppers
1 egg yolk
¼ teaspoon dried thyme, crushed
1 egg white
¼ cup quick-cooking rolled oats
3 tablespoons skim milk
1 tablespoon dried parsley flakes
½ teaspoon salt
⅛ teaspoon pepper
1½ pounds lean ground beef
½ cup pizza sauce *or* tomato sauce

■ Preheat the oven to 350°. Meanwhile, place the frozen potatoes in a colander. Run *hot water* over potatoes just till thawed. Drain well.

■ For stuffing, in a small mixing bowl slightly beat egg yolk. Stir in potatoes and thyme, then set aside. For meat mixture, in a medium mixing bowl slightly beat egg white. Stir in oats, milk, parsley, salt, and pepper. Add the beef, then mix well.

■ In a 9x9x2-inch baking pan pat *half* of the meat mixture into a 7-inch circle. On a sheet of waxed paper, pat the remaining meat into an 8-inch circle. Spread stuffing mixture on the smaller circle to within ½ inch of edges. Invert the 8-inch circle on top. Peel off paper. Press meat around edges to seal well.

■ Bake in the 350° oven for 1 hour. Spoon pizza or tomato sauce on top of loaf. Bake for 5 to 10 minutes more or till meat is well-done and no pink remains. Transfer meat loaf to a serving platter. Cut into wedges to serve. Makes 6 servings.

PER SERVING

Calories	263
Protein	26 g
Carbohydrate	13 g
Fat	11 g
Cholesterol	125 mg
Sodium	370 mg
Potassium	427 mg

TIMETABLE

Preparation time:
25 minutes

Cooking time:
65 to 70 minutes

BULGUR MEAT LOAF

Serve with baby carrots and a tossed salad for simple meal accompaniments.

1 egg white
⅓ cup skim milk
¼ cup quick-cooking rolled oats
3 tablespoons bulgur
½ teaspoon onion salt
¼ teaspoon ground sage
¼ teaspoon pepper
1 pound lean ground beef
1 tablespoon reduced-calorie apricot, peach, *or* cherry preserves, *or* orange marmalade

■ Preheat the oven to 350°. Meanwhile, in a medium mixing bowl slightly beat egg white. Stir in milk, oats, *uncooked* bulgur, onion salt, sage, and pepper. Add the beef, then mix well.

■ Shape meat mixture into a 6x3x2-inch loaf, then place it in an 8x8x2-inch baking pan.

■ Bake in the 350° oven for 50 to 55 minutes or till meat is well-done and no pink remains. Transfer meat loaf to a serving platter. Brush top of meat loaf with preserves or marmalade. Slice to serve. Serves 4.

PER SERVING

Calories	248
Protein	26 g
Carbohydrate	11 g
Fat	10 g
Cholesterol	80 mg
Sodium	290 mg
Potassium	351 mg

TIMETABLE

Preparation time:
10 minutes

Cooking time:
50 to 55 minutes

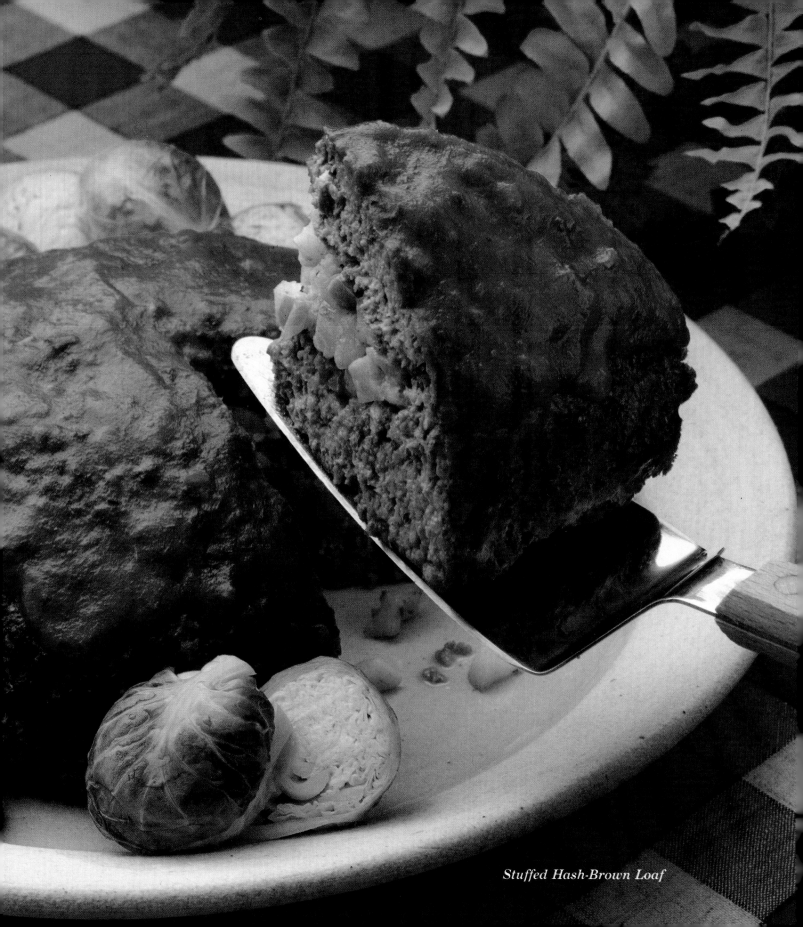

Stuffed Hash-Brown Loaf

SLIMMING BEEF BURGUNDY

Company coming? You'll spend less time in the kitchen cooking and more time with your guests when you serve this elegant classic.

½ cup cold water
2 tablespoons quick-cooking tapioca
1 pound boneless beef chuck pot roast *or* beef chuck steak
Nonstick spray coating
1 cup water
½ cup dry red wine
1 tablespoon instant beef bouillon granules
1 tablespoon tomato paste
1 bay leaf
⅛ teaspoon pepper
8 ounces fresh whole mushrooms
1 cup small frozen whole onions
2½ ounces medium noodles (about 2 cups)

■ Preheat the oven to 350°. Meanwhile, in a small mixing bowl combine ½ cup cold water and tapioca. Set tapioca mixture aside.

■ Trim fat from meat. Cut meat into ¾-inch cubes. Spray a *cold* large saucepan or Dutch oven with nonstick coating. Brown meat over medium-high heat.

■ While meat is browning, stir 1 cup water, wine, bouillon granules, tomato paste, bay leaf, and pepper into tapioca mixture. Add tapioca mixture to meat in saucepan or Dutch oven. Cook and stir just till boiling. Transfer meat mixture to a 1½-quart casserole.

■ Bake, covered, in the 350° oven for 1 hour. Add the mushrooms and onions. Then bake, covered, about 30 minutes more or till meat is tender. Meanwhile, cook noodles according to package directions, then drain. Remove bay leaf from meat mixture. Serve the meat mixture over noodles. Makes 4 servings.

PER SERVING

Calories	305
Protein	23 g
Carbohydrate	24 g
Fat	10 g
Cholesterol	77 mg
Sodium	600 mg
Potassium	538 mg

TIMETABLE

Preparation time: 25 minutes

Cooking time: about 1½ hours

DILLED ROUND STEAK

Long simmering tenderizes less expensive cuts of meats like round steak.

1 pound beef round steak, cut ¾ inch thick
Nonstick spray coating
1 small onion
¾ cup water
2 teaspoons lemon juice
½ teaspoon instant beef bouillon granules
¼ teaspoon garlic salt
¼ teaspoon dried dillweed
¼ teaspoon pepper
2 tablespoons cold water
1 tablespoon cornstarch

■ Trim fat from meat. Cut meat into 4 serving-size pieces. Spray a *cold* large skillet with nonstick coating. Add meat and brown over medium-high heat.

■ While the meat is browning, thinly slice onion. Carefully add water, onion, lemon juice, bouillon granules, garlic salt, dillweed, and pepper to skillet. Bring to boiling, then reduce heat. Cover and simmer about 45 minutes or till meat is tender. Meanwhile, stir together cold water and cornstarch.

■ To serve, transfer meat to a serving platter. Cover to keep warm. Spoon fat from juices. Stir cornstarch mixture into juices. Cook and stir over medium-high heat till thickened and bubbly. Cook and stir for 2 minutes more. Serve with meat. Makes 4 servings.

PER SERVING

Calories	136
Protein	21 g
Carbohydrate	3 g
Fat	4 g
Cholesterol	59 mg
Sodium	206 mg
Potassium	252 mg

TIMETABLE

Preparation time: 10 minutes

Cooking time: about 50 minutes

ALL-DAY POT ROAST

Spend only 15 minutes starting dinner in the morning and come home to a hot, hearty main dish that's ready and waiting.

1   1½-pound boneless beef
     chuck eye roast, eye of
     round roast, *or* round
     rump roast
     Nonstick spray coating
4   medium potatoes
1   4-ounce can mushroom
     stems and pieces
1   10-ounce package frozen
     tiny whole carrots
½   teaspoon dried tarragon *or*
     basil, crushed
¼   teaspoon salt
1   10¾-ounce can condensed
     golden mushroom soup

■ Trim fat from meat. Spray a *cold* large skillet with nonstick coating, then add meat and brown over high heat on all sides. Meanwhile, scrub and quarter potatoes. Drain mushrooms.

■ In a 3½- to 4-quart electric crockery cooker place potatoes, mushrooms, frozen carrots, and tarragon or basil. Place browned meat on top of vegetables. Sprinkle with salt. Pour condensed soup over meat. Cover and cook on low-heat setting for 10 to 12 hours.

■ To serve, transfer meat and vegetables to a serving platter. Serve the sauce over meat and vegetables. Makes 5 servings.

PER SERVING

Calories	345
Protein	23 g
Carbohydrate	33 g
Fat	14 g
Cholesterol	58 mg
Sodium	747 mg
Potassium	1,057 mg

TIMETABLE

Preparation time:
15 minutes

Cooking time:
10 to 12 hours

VEAL STEW

8   ounces veal stew meat
     Nonstick spray coating
¼   cup frozen chopped onion
     (see tip, page 39)
1   10-ounce package frozen
     succotash
1¼   cups water
2   tablespoons frozen chopped
     green pepper (see tip,
     page 39)
1   tablespoon quick-cooking
     tapioca
1½   teaspoons instant chicken
     bouillon granules
¼   teaspoon dried dillweed
¼   teaspoon pepper

■ Trim fat from meat. Cut meat into 1-inch cubes. Spray a *cold* large saucepan with nonstick coating. Add all of the meat and frozen onion. Brown meat over medium-high heat, stirring occasionally. Then drain off fat.

■ Add the frozen succotash, water, green pepper, tapioca, bouillon granules, dillweed, and pepper to meat in saucepan.

■ Bring mixture to boiling, then reduce heat. Cover and simmer about 1 hour or till meat is tender. Stir before serving. Makes 2 servings.

PER SERVING

Calories	261
Protein	22 g
Carbohydrate	33 g
Fat	6 g
Cholesterol	53 mg
Sodium	730 mg
Potassium	677 mg

TIMETABLE

Preparation time:
25 minutes

Cooking time:
about 1 hour

APPLE-RAISIN PORK LOAF

We added applesauce and raisins for a pleasant hint of sweetness.

1 egg white
¼ cup quick-cooking rolled oats
2 tablespoons raisins
1 tablespoon dried minced onion
1 teaspoon prepared mustard
¾ teaspoon salt
¼ teaspoon pepper
1 8½-ounce can applesauce
1 pound lean ground pork
⅛ teaspoon ground cinnamon

■ Preheat the oven to 350°. Meanwhile, in a medium mixing bowl slightly beat egg white. Stir in rolled oats, raisins, onion, mustard, salt, pepper, and ¼ *cup* of the applesauce. Add the pork, then mix well. Shape meat mixture into a 6x4-inch loaf, then place it in an 8x8x2-inch baking pan.

■ Bake in the 350° oven about 55 minutes or till meat is well-done and no pink remains.

■ In a small saucepan combine remaining applesauce and cinnamon. Cook till heated through. To serve, transfer meat loaf to a serving platter. Slice loaf and serve with heated applesauce. Serves 4.

PER SERVING

Calories	249
Protein	20 g
Carbohydrate	21 g
Fat	10 g
Cholesterol	58 mg
Sodium	487 mg
Potassium	392 mg

TIMETABLE

Preparation time:
10 minutes

Cooking time:
about 55 minutes

PORK 'N' LENTIL CHILI

For low-calorie chili toppings, try alfalfa sprouts, shredded lettuce, or chopped carrot or tomato.

8 ounces lean boneless pork
Nonstick spray coating
1 16-ounce can tomatoes
3 stalks celery
1 cup dry lentils
1 cup water
1 6-ounce can hot-style tomato juice
½ cup frozen chopped onion (see tip, page 39)
2 teaspoons chili powder
1 teaspoon sugar
¼ teaspoon garlic powder
¼ teaspoon ground cumin

■ Trim fat from meat. Cut the meat into ½-inch cubes. Spray a *cold* large saucepan with nonstick coating. Quickly brown meat over medium-high heat, then drain off fat.

■ While meat is browning, cut up tomatoes and slice celery. Stir the *undrained* tomatoes, celery, lentils, water, tomato juice, frozen onion, chili powder, sugar, garlic, and cumin into meat in saucepan.

■ Bring mixture to boiling, then reduce heat. Cover and simmer about 1 hour or till lentils and meat are tender. Spoon fat from chili. To serve, ladle chili into individual bowls. Makes 3 servings.

PER SERVING

Calories	394
Protein	30 g
Carbohydrate	54 g
Fat	8 g
Cholesterol	39 mg
Sodium	571 mg
Potassium	1,376 mg

TIMETABLE

Preparation time:
10 minutes

Cooking time:
about 1 hour

FRUITED PORK STEW

Dried fruit, sage, and cloves combine for a wonderfully unique flavor.

1 pound lean boneless pork
  Nonstick spray coating
2 medium carrots
1 medium onion
2 cups water
½ of an 8-ounce package mixed
  dried fruit
½ cup orange juice
2 tablespoons quick-cooking
  tapioca
2 teaspoons instant chicken
  bouillon granules
¼ teaspoon ground sage
⅛ teaspoon ground cloves
⅔ cup long grain rice
  (optional)

■ Trim fat from meat. Cut the meat into 1-inch cubes. Spray a *cold* large saucepan with nonstick coating. Quickly brown meat over medium-high heat, then drain off fat.

■ While meat is browning, cut carrots into 1-inch pieces and slice onion. Stir the carrots, onion, water, dried fruit, orange juice, tapioca, bouillon granules, sage, and cloves into meat in saucepan.

■ Bring mixture to boiling, then reduce heat. Cover and simmer about 1 hour or till the meat is tender. Meanwhile, if desired, cook rice according to package directions.

■ To serve, spoon fat from stew. If desired, serve over hot cooked rice in individual bowls. Makes 4 servings.

PER SERVING

Calories	274
Protein	19 g
Carbohydrate	28 g
Fat	9 g
Cholesterol	58 mg
Sodium	246 mg
Potassium	716 mg

TIMETABLE

Preparation time:
10 minutes

Cooking time:
about 1 hour

HAM 'N' KRAUT CASSEROLE

Many meat departments sell ham that's already cubed.

1 14-ounce can sauerkraut
  with caraway seed
2 cups cubed fully cooked
  ham (about 10 ounces)
1 cup frozen hash brown
  potatoes with onion
  and peppers
½ cup reduced-calorie
  Thousand Island salad
  dressing
1 cup plain croutons
¼ cup shredded cheddar
  cheese (1 ounce)

■ Preheat the oven to 350°. Meanwhile, rinse and drain sauerkraut. Using kitchen shears, snip sauerkraut. In a large mixing bowl combine sauerkraut, ham, and frozen hash brown potatoes. Add salad dressing, then stir till well mixed. Transfer the mixture to a 1½-quart casserole.

■ Bake, covered, in the 350° oven about 45 minutes or till heated through. Remove casserole from oven, then sprinkle with croutons and cheese. Cover and let stand about 5 minutes or till cheese melts. Serves 4.

PER SERVING

Calories	273
Protein	20 g
Carbohydrate	22 g
Fat	12 g
Cholesterol	45 mg
Sodium	1,752 mg
Potassium	472 mg

TIMETABLE

Preparation time:
15 minutes

Cooking time:
about 45 minutes

Standing time:
about 5 minutes

FRUIT-FILLED BUNDLES

Tender pork, fruit, honey, and spices—yummy!

½ cup mixed dried fruit bits (about 2 ounces)
⅓ cup water
1 teaspoon dried minced onion
¼ teaspoon ground ginger
4 pork cubed steaks (about 1 pound total)
⅛ teaspoon salt
    Dash pepper
2 teaspoons honey

■ Preheat the oven to 350°. Meanwhile, for filling, in a small saucepan combine fruit bits, water, onion, and ginger. Bring to boiling, then reduce heat. Cover and simmer for 3 minutes. Drain the fruit mixture, reserving liquid.

■ Sprinkle cubed steaks with the salt and pepper. Place *one-fourth* of the fruit mixture on the center of *each* cubed steak. Fold 1 side over filling. Then fold in the 2 opposite sides. Fold bundle over the remaining side to enclose the filling. Place bundles, seam side down, in an 11x7x1½-inch baking pan. Brush bundles with the reserved fruit liquid.

■ Bake in the 350° oven for 55 to 60 minutes or till no pink remains. Just before serving, brush bundles with honey. Makes 4 servings.

PER SERVING

Calories	199
Protein	16 g
Carbohydrate	13 g
Fat	9 g
Cholesterol	59 mg
Sodium	117 mg
Potassium	358 mg

TIMETABLE

Preparation time:
10 minutes

Cooking time:
55 to 60 minutes

PORK CHOP-BULGUR BAKE

A hearty one-dish meal for two.

½ medium carrot
½ stalk celery
½ cup water
¼ cup bulgur
1 teaspoon instant chicken bouillon granules
½ teaspoon dried minced onion
¼ teaspoon dried tarragon, crushed
2 pork loin rib chops, cut ½ inch thick (about 8 ounces total)
1½ cups frozen cut broccoli
2 tablespoons catsup
1 tablespoon dry red wine *or* water

■ Preheat the oven to 375°. Meanwhile, coarsely shred carrot and slice celery. In a small saucepan combine carrot, celery, ½ cup water, bulgur, bouillon granules, onion, and tarragon. Bring to boiling. Remove saucepan from heat.

■ Spoon bulgur mixture into a 9-inch pie plate or divide mixture between 2 individual baking dishes. Trim fat from pork chops. Place chops atop bulgur mixture in dish. Arrange broccoli around edge of dish. Cover dish tightly with foil.

■ Bake, covered, in the 375° oven for 45 minutes or till meat is tender and no pink remains. Meanwhile, in a small bowl combine catsup and wine or water. Spoon catsup mixture over pork chops. Bake, uncovered, for 5 minutes more. Makes 2 servings.

PER SERVING

Calories	244
Protein	18 g
Carbohydrate	24 g
Fat	8 g
Cholesterol	46 mg
Sodium	432 mg
Potassium	579 mg

TIMETABLE

Preparation time:
15 minutes

Cooking time:
50 minutes

FETA LAMB BURGERS

For fast cleanup, shape the burgers on waxed paper.

2 tablespoons fine dry bread crumbs
2 tablespoons plain low-fat yogurt
1 teaspoon dried oregano, crushed
¼ teaspoon ground nutmeg
⅛ teaspoon garlic powder
1 pound lean ground lamb
¼ cup crumbled feta cheese
2½ cups fresh spinach
¼ of a small cucumber
⅓ cup plain low-fat yogurt

■ Preheat the oven to 350°. Meanwhile, in a medium mixing bowl combine bread crumbs, 2 tablespoons yogurt, oregano, nutmeg, and garlic powder. Add the lamb, then mix well.

■ Shape meat mixture into eight ¼-inch-thick oval patties. Place *1 tablespoon* feta cheese on top of *each* of *4* patties. Place remaining patties on top. Press meat around edges to seal well. Place patties on a rack in a shallow baking pan.

■ Bake in the 350° oven about 40 minutes or till done. Meanwhile, clean and tear spinach, then set spinach aside. Chop cucumber. In a small mixing bowl stir together cucumber and ⅓ cup yogurt.

■ To serve, place spinach on individual plates. Place lamb burgers on spinach. Spoon yogurt-cucumber mixture on top of burgers. Makes 4 servings.

PER SERVING

Calories	170
Protein	21 g
Carbohydrate	6 g
Fat	7 g
Cholesterol	67 mg
Sodium	190 mg
Potassium	477 mg

TIMETABLE

Preparation time: 20 minutes

Cooking time: about 40 minutes

CURRIED LAMB CHOPS

Smother your lamb chops in a rich, creamy sauce—and to think you won't be cheating on your diet!

4 lamb leg sirloin *or* shoulder chops, cut ¾ inch thick (about 1¼ pounds total)
Nonstick spray coating
2 tablespoons chutney
½ of a 10¾-ounce can condensed cream of celery soup
¼ cup water
2 teaspoons curry powder
1 teaspoon dried minced onion
⅔ cup long grain rice

■ Preheat the oven to 350°. Meanwhile, trim fat from lamb chops. Spray a *cold* large skillet with nonstick coating, then add chops and brown over medium-high heat.

■ For the sauce, cut up chutney. In a small mixing bowl combine chutney, condensed soup, water, curry powder, and onion.

■ Place browned chops in a 10x6x2-inch baking dish. Pour sauce over chops. Cover with foil.

■ Bake in the 350° oven for 45 to 60 minutes or till chops are tender. Meanwhile, cook rice according to package directions, *except* omit the margarine or butter. Serve chops and sauce with hot cooked rice. Makes 4 servings.

PER SERVING

Calories	260
Protein	18 g
Carbohydrate	32 g
Fat	6 g
Cholesterol	58 mg
Sodium	690 mg
Potassium	272 mg

TIMETABLE

Preparation time: 10 minutes

Cooking time: 45 to 60 minutes

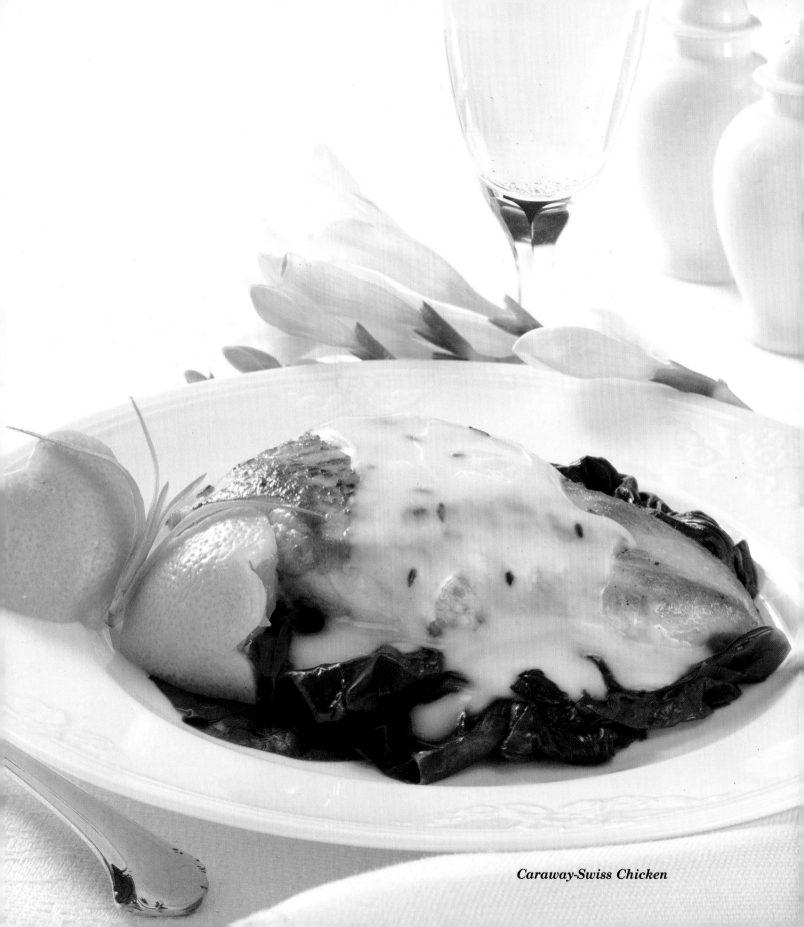

Caraway-Swiss Chicken

CARAWAY-SWISS CHICKEN

Add a colorful garnish like the butterfly trim in the photo. It's made of lemon wedges and chives or slivers of green onion tops.

1 10-ounce package
   frozen spinach
   Nonstick spray coating
4 boned skinless chicken
   breast halves (about
   1 pound total)
¾ cup skim milk
2 teaspoons cornstarch
1½ teaspoons instant chicken
   bouillon granules
¼ teaspoon caraway seed
⅛ teaspoon pepper
2 ounces process Swiss
   cheese, torn into pieces

■ Cook spinach according to package directions; drain well. Divide among 4 au gratin baking dishes. Meanwhile, spray a *cold* large skillet with nonstick coating. Add chicken. Cook over medium heat for 8 to 10 minutes or till tender and no longer pink, turning pieces occasionally. Place chicken atop spinach.

■ For sauce, combine milk, cornstarch, bouillon, caraway, and pepper. Cook and stir till thickened and bubbly. Add cheese; stir till melted. Pour atop chicken. Cover with foil; seal, label, and freeze. Serves 4.

Conventional oven: Bake frozen casserole, covered, in a 375° oven for 45 to 50 minutes or till hot.

Microwave oven: Remove foil from frozen casserole (use a microwave-safe baking dish); cover with vented microwave-safe plastic wrap. Micro-cook 1 serving on 70% power (medium-high) for 6 to 7 minutes or till heated through, turning dish once.

PER SERVING

Calories	208
Protein	33 g
Carbohydrate	6 g
Fat	5 g
Cholesterol	79 mg
Sodium	470 mg
Potassium	658 mg

TIMETABLE

Advance preparation time: 30 minutes

Final preparation time: 45 to 50 minutes

LAYERED TURKEY SALAD

6 ounces sliced fully cooked
   smoked turkey breast
1 medium tomato
2 stalks celery
1 cup low-fat cottage cheese
3 tablespoons skim milk
2 tablespoons crumbled
   blue cheese
1 teaspoon lemon juice
¼ teaspoon Worcestershire
   sauce
   Dash garlic powder
3 cups torn mixed salad
   greens
1 10-ounce package frozen
   peas
¼ cup frozen chopped onion
¼ cup shredded cheddar
   cheese (1 ounce)

■ Cut stack of sliced turkey into bite-size pieces. Seed and chop tomato. Wrap chopped tomato in a clear plastic bag; chill till serving time. Chop celery. Set turkey and celery aside.

■ For dressing, in a blender container or food processor bowl place cottage cheese, milk, blue cheese, lemon juice, Worcestershire sauce, and garlic powder. Cover; blend or process for 30 seconds or till smooth.

■ To assemble salad, in a medium clear glass salad bowl layer torn mixed greens, turkey, frozen peas, celery, and onion. Spread dressing atop salad. Cover and chill for 6 to 24 hours.

■ To serve, sprinkle salad with cheddar cheese and chopped tomato; toss. Makes 4 or 5 servings.

PER SERVING

Calories	214
Protein	25 g
Carbohydrate	16 g
Fat	6 g
Cholesterol	29 mg
Sodium	929 mg
Potassium	558 mg

TIMETABLE

Advance preparation time: 15 minutes

Chilling time: 6 to 24 hours

PEPPER-TURKEY KABOBS

Leave a little space between the ingredients on the skewer—the kabob will cook more quickly and evenly.

1 pound turkey breast tenderloin steaks *or* boned skinless chicken breast halves
2 small onions
1 medium green pepper
1 medium sweet red *or* green
   pepper
¼ cup white wine vinegar
3 tablespoons soy sauce
2 tablespoons water
1 teaspoon ground ginger
1 teaspoon bottled minced
   garlic *or* ¼ teaspoon
   garlic powder
   Nonstick spray coating

■ Cut poultry into 1-inch pieces. Cut onions into wedges. Cut green and sweet red peppers into 1-inch pieces. For the marinade, in a 13x9x2-inch baking dish combine the vinegar, soy sauce, water, ginger, and garlic. Set aside.

■ For kabobs, use five 12-inch-long skewers. Alternately thread poultry, onion, and peppers, leaving a ¼-inch space between pieces. Place kabobs in the baking dish; turn to coat with marinade. Cover and marinate kabobs in the refrigerator for 8 to 24 hours.

■ To serve, preheat the broiler. Meanwhile, spray the unheated rack of a broiler pan with nonstick coating. Drain kabobs, reserving marinade; place on rack. Broil kabobs 4 inches from the heat for 3 minutes. Brush with marinade; turn. Broil for 3 to 5 minutes more or till poultry is tender and no longer pink and vegetables are crisp-tender. Serves 5.

PER SERVING

Calories	129
Protein	24 g
Carbohydrate	6 g
Fat	1 g
Cholesterol	56 mg
Sodium	664 mg
Potassium	433 mg

TIMETABLE

Advance preparation time:
25 minutes

Chilling time:
8 to 24 hours

Final preparation time:
6 to 8 minutes

PARTS AREN'T JUST PARTS!

Have you noticed the number of new poultry parts and products available lately? It can be mind-boggling if you're not sure what's what. So, to help you make the most of these wonderfully convenient and versatile products, here's a rundown on some of the items:

Turkey breast tenderloins are the whole muscle on the inside of the breast.

Turkey breast tenderloin steaks are ½-inch-thick, lengthwise cuts from the tenderloin. *Turkey breast steaks* are ½- to 1-inch-thick crosswise cuts from the whole or half breast. Steaks that are ½ inch thick can be used interchangeably with boned skinless chicken breast halves of the same weight.

The turkey breast also can be sliced crosswise into ¼- to ⅜-inch-thick, boneless pieces, called *turkey breast slices or cutlets.* Slices or cutlets can be used interchangeably with skinless, boneless chicken breast halves that have been pounded to the same thickness.

WINE-SAUCED CHICKEN

3½ ounces fine noodles
   (1¾ cups)
1 pound boned skinless
   chicken breast halves *or*
   turkey breast tenderloin
   steaks
   Nonstick spray coating
1 7½-ounce can tomatoes
1 4-ounce can sliced
   mushrooms
⅓ cup tomato sauce
¼ cup dry red wine
1 tablespoon cornstarch
1½ teaspoons instant chicken
   bouillon granules
½ teaspoon bottled minced
   garlic *or* ⅛ teaspoon
   garlic powder
¼ teaspoon dried basil,
   crushed
¾ cup small frozen whole
   onions

■ Cook pasta according to package directions, *except* use a large saucepan and 4 cups *hot water;* drain. Rinse with cold water; drain.

■ While pasta is cooking, slice poultry into ¾-inch-wide strips. Spray a *cold* large skillet with nonstick coating. Add poultry. Cook over medium-high heat about 4 minutes or till tender and no longer pink, turning pieces over occasionally.

■ While poultry is cooking, cut up tomatoes and drain mushrooms. In a saucepan combine *undrained* tomatoes, mushrooms, tomato sauce, wine, cornstarch, bouillon granules, garlic, and basil. Cook and stir over medium-high heat till mixture is thickened and bubbly. Then cook and stir for 2 minutes more; remove from heat. Stir in poultry and onions.

■ Spoon the pasta to 1 side of 4 individual shallow baking dishes. Then spoon the poultry-tomato mixture on the other sides of the dishes. Cover with clear plastic wrap and then foil; seal, label, and freeze. Makes 4 single-serving entrées.

Conventional oven: Remove plastic wrap. Cover with foil. Bake frozen casserole, covered, in a 375° oven for 1 hour or till heated through.

Microwave oven: Remove foil from frozen casserole (use a microwave-safe baking dish); cover with vented microwave-safe plastic wrap or waxed paper. Micro-cook 1 serving on 70% power (medium-high) for 9 minutes or till heated through, turning dish once. Or, micro-cook 2 servings on medium-high for 16 to 18 minutes or till heated through, turning dishes once.

PER SERVING

Calories	277
Protein	31 g
Carbohydrate	28 g
Fat	3 g
Cholesterol	89 mg
Sodium	802 mg
Potassium	627 mg

TIMETABLE

Advance preparation time:
30 minutes

Final preparation time:
1 hour

NIÇOISE SUPPER SALAD

Halve two pitted ripe olives as a flavorful garnish for each serving.

½　cup water
½　teaspoon salt
8　ounces fresh skinless cod *or* haddock fillets (about ½ inch thick)
½　of a 9-ounce package (about 1 cup) frozen whole *or* cut green beans
1　8½-ounce can whole white potatoes
2　small tomatoes
½　of a small red onion
⅔　cup reduced-calorie Italian salad dressing
1　tablespoon snipped parsley
　　Lettuce leaves

■ In a large skillet combine water and salt; bring just to boiling. Meanwhile, cut fish into 4 equal portions. Carefully add fish to boiling water. Return just to boiling; reduce heat. Cover and simmer gently for 4 to 6 minutes or till fish flakes easily with a fork. Use a slotted spatula to transfer fish to a shallow baking dish; strain and reserve ¼ *cup* of the fish liquid.

■ While fish is cooking, run frozen green beans under *cool water* to separate; drain. Cover beans; chill. Cut potatoes into cubes, tomatoes into thin wedges, and onion into slices; place in small plastic bags or bowls. For marinade, combine reserved fish liquid, salad dressing, and parsley. Pour some of the marinade over the fish and vegetables in the bags or bowls. Seal or cover; marinate in the refrigerator for 8 to 24 hours, occasionally turning the bags.

■ To serve, line a plate with lettuce leaves. With a slotted spoon transfer fish and vegetables to plate, reserving marinade. Arrange beans on salad; drizzle each serving with 1 tablespoon marinade. Serves 2.

PER SERVING	
Calories	258
Protein	23 g
Carbohydrate	23 g
Fat	9 g
Cholesterol	47 mg
Sodium	838 mg
Potassium	944 mg

TIMETABLE

Advance preparation time: 30 minutes

Chilling time: 8 to 24 hours

Final preparation time: 5 minutes

LEMON-ORANGE ROUGHY

Planning a special dinner for two? This elegant lemony fish and couscous recipe halves easily (use ¼ teaspoon onion salt).

1　small carrot
1　cup quick-cooking couscous
¾　teaspoon onion salt
⅛　teaspoon lemon-pepper seasoning
　　Dash ground nutmeg
1　cup water
　　Nonstick spray coating
1　pound fresh skinless orange roughy, flounder, red snapper, *or* salmon fillets (about ½ inch thick)
½　of a lemon
1　tomato (optional)

■ Finely shred carrot. In a mixing bowl combine carrot, couscous, onion salt, lemon-pepper seasoning, and nutmeg. Add water; stir.

■ Spray 4 individual au gratin baking dishes with nonstick coating. Divide couscous mixture among dishes. Cut fish into 4 equal portions. Place *1* fish portion atop couscous mixture in each au gratin dish, tucking under any thin edges to make fish an even thickness. Cut lemon half into 4 slices. Place *1* slice atop each piece of fish. Cover with foil. Refrigerate for 3 to 24 hours.

■ To serve, bake fish, covered, in a 450° oven for 18 to 20 minutes or till fish flakes easily with a fork. Meanwhile, if desired, cut tomato into wedges; serve with fish. Makes 4 servings.

PER SERVING	
Calories	208
Protein	21 g
Carbohydrate	26 g
Fat	0 g
Cholesterol	54 mg
Sodium	449 mg
Potassium	445 mg

TIMETABLE

Advance preparation time: 10 minutes

Chilling time: 3 to 24 hours

Final preparation time: 18 to 20 minutes

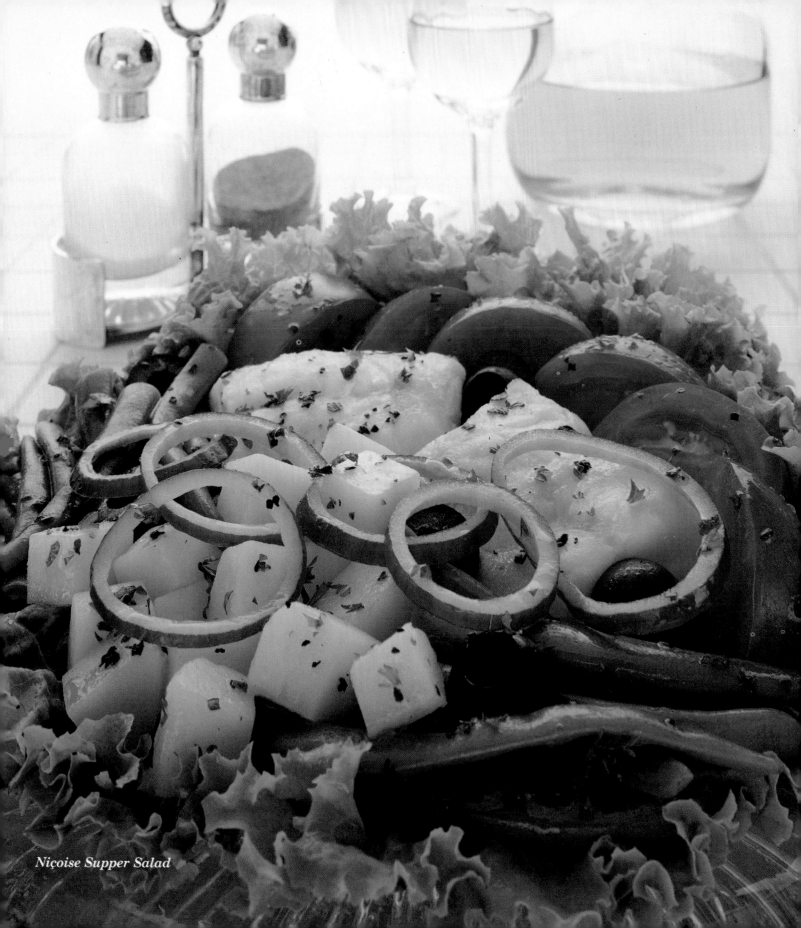

Niçoise Supper Salad

SWISS STEAKLETS

Here's a slick trick for cutting up the tomatoes quickly: do it right in the can with a pair of kitchen shears.

Nonstick spray coating
4 beef cubed steaks (about 1 pound total)
1 7½-ounce can tomatoes
1 stalk celery
½ cup frozen chopped onion (see tip, page 39)
¼ cup water
1 tablespoon steak sauce
¼ teaspoon dried basil, crushed
¼ teaspoon garlic salt
½ of a small green pepper
1 tablespoon cornstarch
1 tablespoon cold water

■ Spray a *cold* 12-inch skillet with nonstick coating. Preheat the skillet. Brown the meat on both sides in the hot skillet. Drain off the fat. Return the meat to the skillet.

■ While the meat is browning, cut up tomatoes; slice celery. Add *undrained* tomatoes, celery, onion, the ¼ cup water, steak sauce, and basil to skillet with the meat. Cover and simmer about 10 minutes.

■ With a slotted spatula transfer meat to 4 individual baking dishes, reserving sauce. Sprinkle the meat with garlic salt. Slice green pepper into 4 rings. Place *1* ring atop each piece of meat.

■ For sauce, stir together the cornstarch and 1 tablespoon cold water; add to mixture in skillet. Cook and stir till mixture is thickened and bubbly. Pour sauce atop meat in individual baking dishes. Cover with clear plastic wrap and then foil; seal, label, and freeze. Makes 4 single-serving entrées.

Conventional oven: Remove plastic wrap. Cover with foil. Bake frozen casserole, covered, in a 375° oven for 45 to 50 minutes or till heated through.

Microwave oven: Remove foil from frozen casserole (use a microwave-safe baking dish); cover with vented microwave-safe plastic wrap or waxed paper. Micro-cook 1 serving on 70% power (medium-high) for 6 to 7 minutes or till heated through, turning dish once. Or, micro-cook 2 servings on medium-high for 12 to 14 minutes or till heated through, turning and rearranging dishes every 4 minutes.

PER SERVING

Calories	171
Protein	20 g
Carbohydrate	8 g
Fat	6 g
Cholesterol	59 mg
Sodium	397 mg
Potassium	451 mg

TIMETABLE

Advance preparation time: 25 minutes

Final preparation time: 45 to 50 minutes

VEGETABLE-BEEF ORIENTAL

Before serving, top with ½ cup chow mein noodles (we've included them in the calorie count and nutrition analysis).

12 ounces lean ground beef
1 stalk celery
½ cup frozen chopped green pepper (see tip, page 39)
½ cup frozen chopped onion
¼ teaspoon bottled minced garlic
1 10¾-ounce can condensed golden mushroom soup
1 tablespoon dry sherry
1 tablespoon soy sauce
¼ teaspoon five-spice powder
¼ teaspoon ground ginger
1 8-ounce can sliced water chestnuts
1 4-ounce can sliced mushrooms

■ Break beef into large pieces while adding it to a large skillet. Slice celery. Cook meat, celery, green pepper, onion, and garlic over high heat till meat is brown and vegetables are tender. Drain off fat. Stir in soup, sherry, soy sauce, five-spice powder, and ginger. Drain water chestnuts and mushrooms; stir into skillet. Transfer mixture to a 1½-quart casserole. Cover. Seal, label, and freeze. Makes 4 servings.

Conventional oven: Bake frozen casserole, covered, in a 400° oven for 1 to 1¼ hours or till heated through. Top with chow mein noodles.

Microwave oven: Micro-cook frozen casserole (use a microwave-safe baking dish), covered, on 70% power (medium-high) for 23 to 27 minutes or till hot, stirring occasionally. Top with chow mein noodles.

PER SERVING

Calories	250
Protein	20 g
Carbohydrate	15 g
Fat	12 g
Cholesterol	61 mg
Sodium	781 mg
Potassium	433 mg

TIMETABLE

Advance preparation time: 15 minutes

Final preparation time: 1 to 1¼ hours

ITALIAN BEEF PATTIES

Moisten the custard cup with water before you use it to flatten the meat patties. Then it won't stick to the meat mixture.

1 egg
¼ cup fine dry bread crumbs
1 teaspoon dried Italian seasoning, crushed
¼ teaspoon onion powder
¼ teaspoon salt
1 pound lean ground beef
½ cup pizza sauce
1 tablespoon grated Parmesan cheese
¼ cup frozen chopped green pepper (see tip, page 39) *or* ¼ cup sliced fresh mushrooms
¼ cup shredded mozzarella cheese (1 ounce)

■ Preheat the oven to 425°. Slightly beat egg. Add crumbs, Italian seasoning, onion powder, and salt. Add beef; mix well. Shape meat into four ½-inch-thick patties; place in a shallow ungreased baking pan. With a 6-ounce custard cup flatten centers to about ¼ inch in center, forming ½-inch-wide rims.

■ Bake patties in the 425° oven for 8 to 10 minutes or till no longer pink. Drain. Combine pizza sauce and Parmesan cheese; spoon into centers of patties. Top with green pepper and mozzarella cheese. Cool completely; place in a single layer in an airtight freezer container. Seal, label, and freeze. Serves 4.

Conventional oven: Place frozen patties in a shallow baking pan. Cover with foil. Bake in a 350° oven about 45 minutes or till heated through.

Microwave oven: Place frozen patty in a shallow microwave-safe baking dish. Cover with waxed paper. Micro-cook 1 patty on 70% power (medium-high) about 5 minutes or till hot, rotating dish once.

PER SERVING

Calories	278
Protein	29 g
Carbohydrate	9 g
Fat	13 g
Cholesterol	154 mg
Sodium	489 mg
Potassium	316 mg

TIMETABLE

Advance preparation time: 25 minutes

Final preparation time: 45 to 50 minutes

BEEF-STUFFED PEPPERS

The green pepper shells will be just a bit crisper when cooked in the microwave.

8 ounces lean ground beef
¼ cup frozen chopped onion
(see tip, page 39)
1 7½-ounce can tomatoes
⅓ cup quick-cooking rice
2 tablespoons raisins
2 tablespoons water
1 to 2 teaspoons curry powder
¼ teaspoon salt
2 medium green peppers
1 tablespoon chopped
peanuts

■ Break ground meat into large pieces while adding it to a medium skillet. Cook meat and frozen onion over high heat till meat is brown and onion is tender. Drain. Cut up tomatoes; add *undrained* tomatoes to meat in skillet. Stir in *uncooked* rice, raisins, water, curry powder, and salt.

■ While meat is cooking, cut peppers in half lengthwise. Remove seeds and membranes. Spoon meat mixture into peppers. Place *2* pepper halves in 2 individual baking dishes. Cover with clear plastic wrap and then foil; seal, label, and freeze. Serves 2.

Conventional oven: Remove plastic wrap. Add 2 tablespoons water to each dish. Cover with foil. Bake frozen casserole, covered, in a 375° oven about 1 hour or till hot. Sprinkle with peanuts.

Microwave oven: Remove foil from frozen casserole (use a microwave-safe baking dish); cover with vented microwave-safe plastic wrap or waxed paper. Micro-cook 1 serving on 70% power (medium-high) for 7 to 8 minutes or till heated through, turning dish once.

PER SERVING

Calories	395
Protein	29 g
Carbohydrate	43 g
Fat	13 g
Cholesterol	80 mg
Sodium	526 mg
Potassium	1,004 mg

TIMETABLE

Advance preparation time:
15 minutes

Final preparation time:
about 1 hour

GARLIC FLANK STEAK

Marinated in a garlic-Worcestershire sauce mixture, this recipe certainly lives up to its name!

1 pound beef flank steak
2 tablespoons vinegar
2 tablespoons water
1 tablespoon Worcestershire
sauce
1 tablespoon cooking oil
1 teaspoon bottled minced
garlic *or* ¼ teaspoon
garlic powder
¼ teaspoon crushed red
pepper

■ Score flank steak on both sides. Place meat in a plastic bag; set in a bowl. For marinade, in a bowl combine vinegar, water, Worcestershire sauce, cooking oil, garlic, and red pepper. Pour marinade over meat in bag. Close bag. Marinate in the refrigerator for 4 to 24 hours, turning bag occasionally.

■ Preheat the broiler. Meanwhile, remove meat from marinade; reserve marinade. Place meat on the unheated rack of a broiler pan. Broil meat 3 to 4 inches from the heat for 5 minutes; brush with marinade. Turn meat over and brush with marinade. Broil for 3 to 5 minutes more or to desired doneness. Transfer meat to a platter. Thinly slice meat diagonally across the grain. Makes 4 servings.

PER SERVING

Calories	185
Protein	23 g
Carbohydrate	1 g
Fat	9 g
Cholesterol	72 mg
Sodium	82 mg
Potassium	201 mg

TIMETABLE

Advance preparation time:
5 minutes

Chilling time:
4 to 24 hours

Final preparation time:
8 to 10 minutes

MUSHROOM FREEZER PIZZA

Put away the knife and fork. This is a pick-it-up pizza!

1 6½-ounce package pizza
   crust mix
8 ounces lean ground beef
¼ cup frozen chopped onion
   (see tip, page 39)
¼ cup frozen chopped green
   pepper (see tip, page 39)
1 8-ounce can pizza sauce
¼ to ½ teaspoon crushed red
   pepper
1 3-ounce can sliced
   mushrooms
½ cup shredded mozzarella
   cheese (2 ounces)

■ Preheat the oven to 425°. Meanwhile, prepare pizza crust mix according to package directions. Spread dough on a greased 12-inch pizza pan. Prick crust; bake for 10 minutes in the 425° oven. Meanwhile, break meat into large pieces while adding it to a saucepan. Cook meat, onion, and green pepper over high heat till meat is brown and vegetables are tender. Drain. Stir in pizza sauce and red pepper.

■ Spread meat mixture over crust. Drain mushrooms; place atop meat mixture. Top with mozzarella cheese. Cover with clear plastic wrap and then foil; seal, label, and freeze.

■ To serve, remove foil. Bake frozen pizza, uncovered, in a 425° oven for 20 to 25 minutes or till crust is brown and topping is hot. Cut into 8 wedges. Serves 4.

PER SERVING

Calories	344
Protein	22 g
Carbohydrate	43 g
Fat	9 g
Cholesterol	48 mg
Sodium	846 mg
Potassium	267 mg

TIMETABLE

Advance preparation time:
20 minutes

Final preparation time:
20 to 25 minutes

BEEFY MACARONI AND CHEESE

⅔ cup elbow macaroni *or*
   corkscrew macaroni
12 ounces lean ground beef
½ cup frozen chopped onion
   (see tip, page 39)
1 10¾-ounce can condensed
   golden mushroom soup
¼ cup water
½ teaspoon dried basil,
   crushed
¼ teaspoon garlic powder
1 9-ounce package frozen cut
   green beans
¼ cup shredded cheddar
   cheese (1 ounce)

■ Cook pasta according to package directions, *except* use a medium saucepan and 3 cups *hot water*. Drain well. Return pasta to saucepan. Meanwhile, break ground meat into large pieces while adding it to a medium skillet. Cook meat and onion over high heat till meat is brown and onion is tender. Drain.

■ Stir soup, water, basil, and garlic powder into pasta. Place frozen beans in a colander; run *hot water* over to separate. Drain well. Stir beans and meat into soup mixture; spoon into a 10x6x2-inch baking dish. Cover with foil; seal, label, and freeze. Serves 4.

Conventional oven: Bake frozen casserole, covered, in a 375° oven for 1 to 1¼ hours or till heated through, stirring after 45 minutes. Top with cheese.

Microwave oven: Remove foil from frozen casserole (use a microwave-safe baking dish); cover with vented microwave-safe plastic wrap or waxed paper. Microcook on 70% power (medium-high) for 18 to 22 minutes or till hot, stirring twice. Top with cheese.

PER SERVING

Calories	355
Protein	25 g
Carbohydrate	28 g
Fat	16 g
Cholesterol	68 mg
Sodium	974 mg
Potassium	456 mg

TIMETABLE

Advance preparation time:
25 minutes

Final preparation time:
1 to 1¼ hours

CURRIED PORK WITH RICE

12 ounces pork tenderloin
1 large apple
  Nonstick spray coating
¼ cup frozen chopped onion
  (see tip, page 39)
1½ teaspoons curry powder
½ teaspoon salt
⅛ teaspoon ground ginger
1 tablespoon cornstarch
2 cups skim milk
¾ cup quick-cooking rice
¼ cup raisins

■ Trim fat from pork and thinly slice meat into bite-size strips. Peel, core, and chop apple. Spray a *cold* large skillet with nonstick coating. Preheat the skillet. Cook pork strips about 3 minutes or till no longer pink; remove from skillet. Set aside.

■ Add apple, onion, curry powder, salt, and ginger to the drippings in the skillet. Cook and stir till apple and onion are tender.

■ Stir together cornstarch and ¼ *cup* of the milk; add to apple mixture in the skillet with remaining milk. Cook and stir till mixture is thickened and bubbly. Then cook and stir for 2 minutes more. Stir in pork, *uncooked* rice, and raisins.

■ Divide pork mixture among 4 individual baking dishes. Cover with foil; seal, label, and freeze. Makes 4 single-serving entrées.

Conventional oven: Bake frozen casseroles, covered, in a 375° oven for 55 to 60 minutes or till heated through. Stir before serving.

Microwave oven: Remove the foil from frozen casserole (use a microwave-safe baking dish); cover casserole with vented microwave-safe plastic wrap or waxed paper. Micro-cook 1 serving on 70% power (medium-high) for 5 to 7 minutes or till casserole is heated through, turning dish once and stirring once during cooking.

PER SERVING

Calories	250
Protein	19 g
Carbohydrate	37 g
Fat	3 g
Cholesterol	45 mg
Sodium	362 mg
Potassium	594 mg

TIMETABLE

Advance preparation time: 25 minutes

Final preparation time: 55 to 60 minutes

TANGERINE CHOPS

4 pork loin chops, cut ½ inch thick (about 1 to 1¼ pounds total)
¼ cup frozen tangerine *or* orange juice concentrate
2 tablespoons water
1 tablespoon soy sauce
1 tablespoon molasses
½ teaspoon bottled minced garlic *or* ⅛ teaspoon garlic powder
¼ teaspoon ground ginger

■ Trim fat from chops. Pierce chops with a fork. Place in a single layer in an 8x8x2-inch baking dish.

■ For marinade, in a small mixing bowl stir together tangerine or orange juice concentrate, water, soy sauce, molasses, garlic, and ginger. Pour marinade over chops. Turn chops over to coat them with the marinade. Cover with clear plastic wrap and marinate chops in the refrigerator for 8 to 24 hours.

■ Before serving, preheat the broiler. Drain chops, reserving marinade. Place chops on the unheated rack of a broiler pan. Brush chops with some of the marinade. Broil chops 3 inches from the heat for 4 minutes. Turn chops over and brush with additional marinade. Broil about 3 to 4 minutes more or till meat is tender and no pink remains. Serves 4.

PER SERVING

Calories	283
Protein	27 g
Carbohydrate	10 g
Fat	14 g
Cholesterol	87 mg
Sodium	322 mg
Potassium	599 mg

TIMETABLE

Advance preparation time:
10 minutes

Chilling time:
8 to 24 hours

Final preparation time:
7 to 8 minutes

HAM AND PASTA SALAD

Lettuce cups are a quick and attractive way to serve a salad. For each cup, use a firm, curved inner leaf from a head of lettuce.

½ of a 7-ounce package (1 cup) corkscrew macaroni
1 small zucchini
1 small green pepper
1 small carrot
8 ounces fully cooked ham
2 tablespoons frozen chopped onion (see tip, page 39)
⅓ cup reduced-calorie blue cheese salad dressing
2 tablespoons skim milk
1 large tomato *or* 8 cherry tomatoes
4 lettuce leaves

■ Cook pasta according to package directions, *except* use a medium saucepan and 4 cups unsalted *hot water*. Drain; rinse with cold water. Drain. Meanwhile, slice zucchini. Cut green pepper into bite-size strips. Shred carrot. Cut ham into cubes.

■ In a mixing bowl combine macaroni, zucchini, green pepper, carrot, ham, and onion. For dressing, combine salad dressing and skim milk. Pour dressing over pasta mixture and toss lightly to coat. Cover and chill for 6 to 24 hours.

■ To serve, cut large tomato into 8 wedges (or, halve cherry tomatoes). Place lettuce leaves on individual plates. Divide pasta salad among plates, and garnish each serving with tomato wedges or cherry tomato halves. Makes 4 servings.

PER SERVING

Calories	232
Protein	16 g
Carbohydrate	26 g
Fat	7 g
Cholesterol	30 mg
Sodium	859 mg
Potassium	433 mg

TIMETABLE

Advance preparation time:
20 minutes

Chilling time:
6 to 24 hours

Final preparation time:
10 minutes

HAM SANDWICH STRATA

This cheesy ham 'n' egg dish is perfect for a brunch or light supper.

Nonstick spray coating
1 medium carrot
1 6-ounce package sliced fully cooked ham
8 very thin slices firm-texture rye *or* wheat bread
1 cup shredded mozzarella cheese (4 ounces)
3 eggs
1½ cups skim milk
1 tablespoon frozen snipped chives (see tip, page 39)
1 teaspoon dry mustard
¼ teaspoon garlic powder
¼ teaspoon bottled hot pepper sauce
Apple slices and grapes (optional)

■ Spray an 8x8x2-inch baking dish with nonstick coating. Shred carrot.

■ Place *2* slices of the ham atop *each* of 4 bread slices. Top with remaining bread slices, making 4 sandwiches. Arrange sandwiches in the prepared baking dish. Sprinkle mozzarella cheese and carrot atop.

■ In a medium mixing bowl beat eggs; stir in milk, chives, mustard, garlic powder, and hot pepper sauce. Pour egg mixture over cheese-topped sandwiches. Cover and chill for 4 to 24 hours.

■ Preheat the oven to 325°. Bake the strata, uncovered, for 40 to 45 minutes or till a knife inserted near the center comes out clean. Let the strata stand for 5 minutes before serving. While the strata is baking, if desired, prepare fruit for garnish. Cut the strata into squares to serve. Makes 4 to 6 servings.

PER SERVING

Calories	303
Protein	27 g
Carbohydrate	22 g
Fat	12 g
Cholesterol	246 mg
Sodium	907 mg
Potassium	450 mg

TIMETABLE

Advance preparation time: 10 minutes

Chilling time: 4 to 24 hours

Final preparation time: 40 to 45 minutes

PORK ROAST ON TAP

Succulent beer-marinated pork calls for a baked potato accompaniment. Use medium baking potatoes—they'll cook in the same amount of time as the roast.

1 2-pound boneless pork loin roast
1 12-ounce can beer
2 tablespoons honey
1 teaspoon bottled minced garlic *or* ¼ teaspoon garlic powder
¼ teaspoon ground cloves
½ teaspoon pepper

■ Trim fat from roast. Pierce roast several times with a long-tined fork. Place roast in a plastic bag; set in a large bowl. For marinade, combine beer, honey, garlic, and cloves. Pour marinade over meat in bag.

■ Close bag. Marinate roast in the refrigerator for 8 to 24 hours, turning bag occasionally.

■ Preheat the oven to 325°. Meanwhile, remove the roast from the marinade. Place roast on a rack in a shallow roasting pan. Insert a meat thermometer, placing bulb so it rests in the center of the roast. Sprinkle roast with pepper. Roast, uncovered, for 1½ to 1¾ hours or till the thermometer registers 170°. Slice to serve. Makes 6 to 8 servings.

PER SERVING

Calories	259
Protein	24 g
Carbohydrate	8 g
Fat	12 g
Cholesterol	77 mg
Sodium	60 mg
Potassium	384 mg

TIMETABLE

Advance preparation time: 10 minutes

Chilling time: 8 to 24 hours

Final preparation time: 1½ to 2 hours

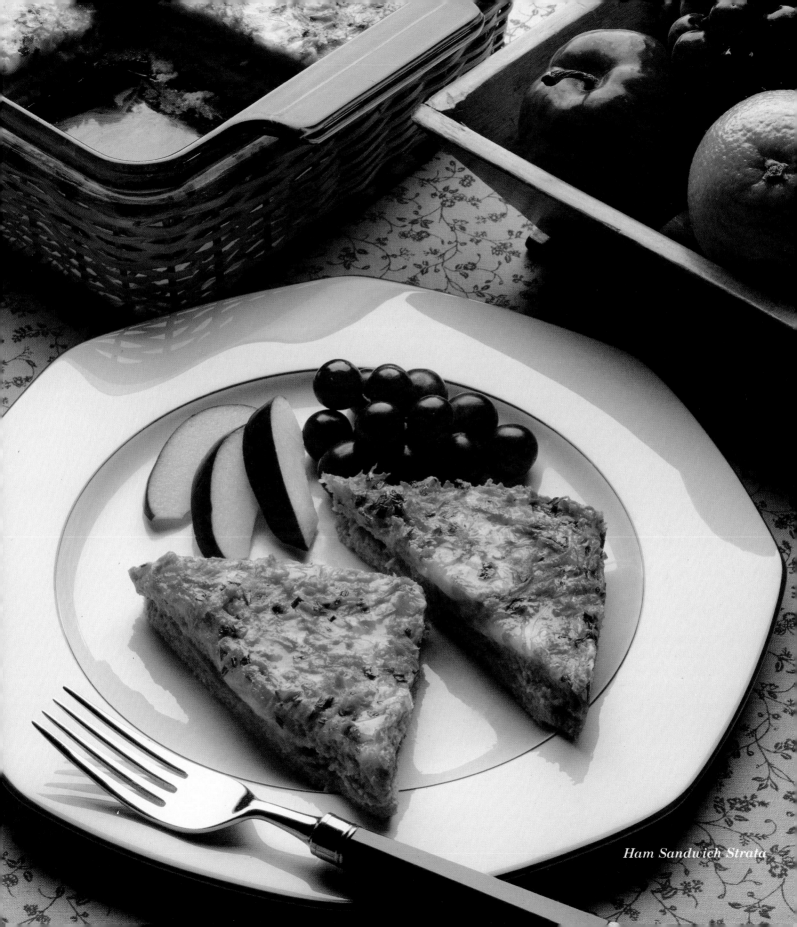

Ham Sandwich Strata

CHEESE 'N' SPINACH SHELLS

Conchiglioni are large, seashell-shaped pasta shells.

12 conchiglioni (about 5 ounces)
1 10-ounce package frozen chopped spinach
1 cup low-fat cottage cheese
1 egg
½ cup grated Parmesan cheese
½ cup shredded mozzarella cheese (2 ounces)
1 tablespoon dried parsley flakes
¼ teaspoon dried oregano, crushed
   Dash ground red pepper
1 8-ounce can tomato sauce

■ Cook pasta according to package directions, *except* use a large saucepan and 5 cups *hot water*. Drain. Meanwhile, cook spinach in a small amount of boiling water about 2 minutes or just till thawed. Drain well, pressing out excess liquid. Drain cottage cheese. In a mixing bowl combine egg, spinach, cottage cheese, Parmesan cheese, mozzarella cheese, parsley, oregano, and red pepper.

■ Spoon about ¼ *cup* of the cheese mixture into *each* shell. Place *3* shells in *each* of 4 shallow baking dishes. Spoon tomato sauce atop. Cover with clear plastic wrap and then foil; seal, label, and freeze. Serves 4.

Conventional oven: Remove plastic wrap. Cover with foil. Bake frozen casseroles, covered, in a 375° oven for 45 to 50 minutes or till heated through.

Microwave oven: Remove foil from frozen casserole (use a microwave-safe baking dish); cover with vented microwave-safe plastic wrap or waxed paper. Micro-cook 1 serving on 70% power (medium-high) for 6 to 8 minutes, giving dish a half-turn every 3 minutes.

PER SERVING

Calories	329
Protein	25 g
Carbohydrate	36 g
Fat	9 g
Cholesterol	91 mg
Sodium	1,208 mg
Potassium	645 mg

TIMETABLE

Advance preparation time: 30 minutes

Final preparation time: 45 to 50 minutes

VEGETABLE-SWISS STRATA

1 cup frozen mixed vegetables
¼ cup frozen chopped onion
¼ cup water
1 4-ounce can mushroom stems and pieces
4 slices firm-texture white bread
3 ounces sliced process Swiss cheese
3 eggs
1½ cups skim milk
½ teaspoon dried basil, crushed
¼ teaspoon salt
¼ teaspoon pepper

■ In a saucepan combine frozen mixed vegetables, onion, and water. Bring to boiling; reduce heat. Cover and simmer for 5 minutes or till vegetables are nearly tender. Drain well. Meanwhile, drain mushrooms.

■ Arrange the bread slices in an 8x8x2-inch baking dish. Top bread with cooked vegetables and drained mushrooms. Tear cheese slices and arrange pieces on top of vegetables. In a bowl beat eggs; stir in milk, basil, salt, and pepper. Pour egg mixture over bread and cheese mixture. Cover and chill for 4 to 24 hours.

■ Preheat the oven to 325°. Bake the strata, uncovered, for 50 to 55 minutes or till a knife inserted near the center comes out clean. Let the strata stand for 5 minutes before serving. Makes 4 servings.

PER SERVING

Calories	272
Protein	17 g
Carbohydrate	26 g
Fat	11 g
Cholesterol	227 mg
Sodium	780 mg
Potassium	425 mg

TIMETABLE

Advance preparation time: 15 minutes

Chilling time: 4 to 24 hours

Final preparation time: 50 to 55 minutes

ZUCCHINI LASAGNA

If you'd rather eat the lasagna right away, simply bake it, covered, in a 375° oven for 40 to 45 minutes or till heated through.

Nonstick spray coating
½ cup frozen chopped onion
  (see tip, page 39)
½ teaspoon bottled minced
  garlic *or* ⅛ teaspoon
  garlic powder
2 medium zucchini
1 15-ounce can tomato sauce
2 tablespoons tomato paste
¾ teaspoon dried Italian
  seasoning, crushed
1 cup low-fat ricotta cheese
2 tablespoons grated
  Parmesan cheese
2 tablespoons skim milk
1 tablespoon dried parsley
  flakes
4 no-boil lasagna noodles
1 4-ounce package shredded
  mozzarella cheese (1 cup)

■ Spray a *cold* large skillet with nonstick coating; preheat skillet. Cook onion and garlic in skillet just till onion is tender. Meanwhile, shred the zucchini (you should have about 3 cups). Stir zucchini, tomato sauce, tomato paste, and Italian seasoning into skillet. Simmer the mixture, uncovered, for 5 minutes, stirring occasionally.

■ While the tomato mixture is simmering, in a mixing bowl combine ricotta cheese, Parmesan cheese, milk, and parsley flakes. Set aside.

■ Run lasagna noodles under *warm* water *(do not boil noodles)*. Place *2* noodles in a 10x6x2-inch baking dish (if necessary, trim to fit). Spread *half* of the tomato mixture over noodles. Layer remaining noodles on top. Spread ricotta mixture atop noodles, and top with remaining tomato mixture. Sprinkle mozzarella cheese atop. Cover with clear plastic wrap and then foil; seal, label, and freeze.

■ To serve, thaw lasagna overnight in the refrigerator. Remove plastic wrap. Cover with foil. Bake, covered, in a 375° oven for 1 to 1¼ hours or till lasagna is heated through. Let stand for 5 minutes before serving. Makes 6 servings.

For individual casseroles: Assemble the lasagna in the 10x6x2-inch baking dish and freeze for 1½ to 2 hours or till lasagna is nearly firm. Cut the lasagna into 6 portions. Transfer each portion to a lightly greased 10-ounce casserole. Cover with clear plastic wrap and then foil; seal, label, and freeze.

Conventional oven (individual casseroles): Remove plastic wrap. Cover with foil. Bake frozen individual casseroles in a 375° oven for 50 minutes. Uncover; bake about 10 minutes more or till heated through. Let stand for 5 minutes before serving.

Microwave oven (individual casserole): Remove plastic wrap and foil from frozen casserole (use a microwave-safe baking dish). Loosely cover with waxed paper. Micro-cook 1 casserole on 70% power (medium-high) for 5 to 7 minutes, giving the dish a half-turn once. Let stand 5 minutes before serving.

PER SERVING

Calories	209
Protein	14 g
Carbohydrate	22 g
Fat	8 g
Cholesterol	25 mg
Sodium	667 mg
Potassium	560 mg

TIMETABLE

Advance preparation time:
20 minutes

Thawing time:
overnight

Final preparation time:
1 to 1¼ hours

Microwave Basics

Learn more about your microwave oven for successful micro-cooking. It's all here—information on microwave safety, oven wattage, and cookware, as well as cooking techniques.

Micro-cooking is an ideal way to prepare foods when you're on a diet, because micro-cooking requires little or no added fat. Micro-cooking also is a way to get in and out of the kitchen quickly, so you have less time to nibble.

Microwave Safety

Your microwave oven is one of the safest appliances in your kitchen. To make sure you are operating, cleaning, and maintaining your microwave oven properly, read the manufacturer's suggestions given in your oven manual.

Oven Wattage and Power Levels

The higher the output wattage of your microwave oven, the faster it cooks on high power. Most larger models provide between 600 and 700 watts of cooking power. They cook faster than the models that provide only 400 to 550 watts. Look in your owner's manual or on your oven to find the power output. (The time ranges within our recipes are based on timings for ovens providing 600 to 700 watts of cooking power. If your oven differs, use the owner's manual as a guide.)

Variable power means that a microwave oven has more than one power setting. Manufacturers name power levels differently, but most of their terms mean about the same thing. Some use numbers (10, 9, 8, and so forth), with 10 equal to 100%. Others rely on words (high, medium, and so forth), with high equal to 100%. Still others use cooking terms (cook, roast, bake, defrost), with cook comparable to 100%. In our recipes, we refer to the percentage and to the word description of the power level you should use—for example, 100% power (high).

If your owner's manual doesn't mention the percentage of power assigned to each power level, here's a test to roughly determine what it is: Fill each of two identical cups with 1 cup of water. Make sure the water is the same temperature in both cups. Cook one cup of water on 100% power and record the time it takes to boil. Cook the other cup of water on the power level you want to test. If the water takes twice as long to boil as on 100%, you have 50% power. If it takes 10 times as long, you have 10% power.

Microwave Cookware

An advantage of cooking in a microwave oven is that often you can mix, cook, and serve in one container.

Microwave-safe materials include glass, ceramics, certain plastics, paper, wood, and straw. Glass is ideal for microwave cooking because it lets you see through it to check the food for doneness. Use glass that's heat resistant or oven tempered.

Some plastics also work well in the microwave oven. Follow the container manufacturer's directions regarding which plastics can be used.

Paper products generally work well in the microwave. Waxed paper is handy because it prevents spattering without trapping the steam. Paper plates, napkins, and towels offer easy cleanup. To be safe, use paper products in your microwave for no more than 10 minutes. Don't use paper towels made from recycled paper because the paper can catch fire. Select undyed paper products because the dyes on colored paper can leak onto the food. Look for products labeled "microwave safe," then follow the manufacturer's instructions.

Use wood and straw products only to heat foods for a short period of time. Your owner's manual will tell you whether you can use metal in your oven.

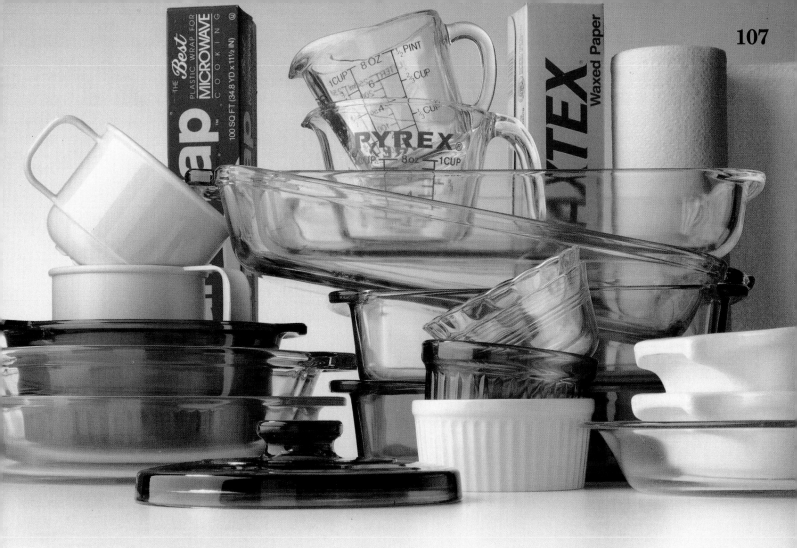

Dish Test

If you can't find the manufacturer's "microwave-safe" notice on the dish label, use this easy test:

Pour ½ cup cold water into a 1-cup glass measure. Set the cup of water in the microwave oven either inside or beside the dish to be tested. Cook on 100% power (high) for 1 minute. Remove the dish from the oven. If the dish is cool and the water in the measure is warm, you can cook with the dish. If the dish is warm and the water in the measure also is warm, you can reheat in the dish, but don't cook with it. If the dish is hot and the water in the measure is cool, don't use the dish in the microwave oven. Also, do not use containers with metallic trim or markings. Metal in the trim may blacken or overheat and crack the dish.

Cooking Techniques

Often a recipe calls for covering the food as it cooks. Casserole lids or vented microwave-safe clear plastic wrap hold the steam inside. Vent the wrap by turning back one corner. This cuts steam pressure but still allows some steam to build. (If your microwave oven has a browning unit, don't use plastic wrap with the unit.) Because steam builds even with venting, remove coverings carefully, making sure the steam escapes away from you. When your recipe says to loosely cover, placed waxed paper atop the food.

Stirring, turning, and rearranging are other micro-cooking techniques. Moving foods during cooking helps ensure that all parts cook evenly. To do this, you can stir mixtures, rearrange small pieces, turn large pieces over, or turn the dish.

SPEEDY LASAGNA

No-boil lasagna noodles—what a great time-saver! Look for them in the dry pasta section of the supermarket.

8 ounces ground turkey sausage
1½ cups low-fat cottage cheese (small curd)
1 4½-ounce jar sliced mushrooms
1 15½-ounce jar chunky spaghetti sauce
¼ cup frozen chopped onion (see tip, page 39)
¼ cup frozen chopped green pepper (see tip, page 39)
1 egg white
½ cup shredded mozzarella cheese (2 ounces)
1 teaspoon dried parsley flakes
Nonstick spray coating
6 no-boil lasagna noodles
2 tablespoons grated Parmesan cheese

■ In a 1½-quart microwave-safe casserole break turkey sausage into pieces. Cover. Micro-cook on 100% power (high) for 3 to 4 minutes or till no longer pink, stirring after 2 minutes; drain. Meanwhile, place cottage cheese in a colander to drain. Drain mushrooms.

■ Stir mushrooms, spaghetti sauce, onion, and green pepper into turkey in casserole, then set aside. In a medium mixing bowl, slightly beat egg white. Then stir in cottage cheese, mozzarella, and parsley.

■ Spray an 8x8x2-inch microwave-safe baking dish with nonstick coating. Run noodles under *warm* water (*do not boil noodles*). Place 2 noodles in dish (if necessary, break to fit). Spread with *half* of the cheese mixture and *one-third* of the sauce. Repeat layers, ending with sauce. Sprinkle with Parmesan cheese.

■ Cover dish with vented microwave-safe plastic wrap. Cook on 70% power (medium-high) for 15 to 18 minutes or till heated through, rotating dish a quarter-turn after 8 minutes. Let stand for 5 minutes before cutting. Makes 6 servings.

PER SERVING	
Calories	305
Protein	23 g
Carbohydrate	30 g
Fat	10 g
Cholesterol	42 mg
Sodium	1,114 mg
Potassium	263 mg

TIMETABLE

Preparation time: 20 minutes

Cooking time: 18 to 22 minutes

Standing time: 5 minutes

20 minutes or less

CHICKEN CHILI

Ready to eat in about 18 minutes.

1 6¾-ounce can chunk-style chicken *or* 1 cup chopped cooked chicken (see tip, opposite)
1 7½-ounce can tomatoes
1 8-ounce can red kidney beans
¼ cup frozen chopped green pepper (see tip, page 39)
¼ cup frozen chopped onion (see tip, page 39)
2 teaspoons chili powder
½ teaspoon bottled minced garlic *or* ⅛ teaspoon garlic powder
¼ teaspoon ground cumin

■ Cut large pieces of canned chicken into bite-size pieces. Set chicken aside. Cut up tomatoes. Drain kidney beans. In a 1½-quart microwave-safe casserole combine *undrained* tomatoes, drained kidney beans, frozen green pepper, onion, chili powder, garlic, cumin, and ¼ cup *water*.

■ Micro-cook, covered, on 100% power (high) for 4 minutes. Stir in the *undrained* chicken. Then cook, covered, on high for 3 to 4 minutes more or till heated. To serve, ladle chili into bowls. Makes 2 servings.

PER SERVING	
Calories	256
Protein	27 g
Carbohydrate	23 g
Fat	6 g
Cholesterol	62 mg
Sodium	266 mg
Potassium	814 mg

TIMETABLE

Preparation time: 10 minutes

Cooking time: 7 to 8 minutes

20 minutes or less

MEXICALI CHUNKS

When it's party time, serve this scrumptious entrée as an appetizer. It makes eight 109-calorie servings.

1 **pound boned skinless chicken breast halves** *or* **turkey breast tenderloin steaks**
¼ **cup cornmeal**
1 **teaspoon chili powder**
½ **teaspoon paprika**
¼ **to** ½ **teaspoon ground red pepper**
¼ **teaspoon salt**
2 **tablespoons margarine** *or* **butter**
Iceberg lettuce (optional)
½ **cup mild salsa** *or* **plain low-fat yogurt**

■ In a 12x7½x2-inch microwave-safe baking dish place poultry. Cover dish with vented microwave-safe plastic wrap. Micro-cook on 100% power (high) for 3 minutes. Turn poultry pieces over, then rearrange by moving the outside pieces to the center of dish. Cook, covered, on high for 3 to 4 minutes more or till poultry is tender and no longer pink.

■ While poultry is cooking, in a plastic bag combine cornmeal, chili powder, paprika, red pepper, and salt.

■ Cut cooked poultry into 1-inch pieces. Put pieces into the bag. Close bag and shake to coat poultry.

■ In a microwave-safe pie plate cook margarine or butter, uncovered, on high for 30 to 45 seconds or till melted. Add coated poultry pieces. Toss lightly till poultry is coated with margarine. Cook, uncovered, on high about 1 minute or till heated through. Meanwhile, if desired, shred some lettuce. If desired, serve the chicken on shredded lettuce. Serve salsa or yogurt as a dipping sauce. Makes 4 servings.

PER SERVING

Calories	217
Protein	27 g
Carbohydrate	8 g
Fat	8 g
Cholesterol	66 g
Sodium	483 mg
Potassium	398 mg

TIMETABLE

Total preparation time: 15 minutes

MICRO-COOKING POULTRY

What do you do when your recipe calls for cooked chicken or turkey and you don't have any leftover roasted poultry on hand? Our quick solution is to cook some poultry in the microwave oven.

To micro-cook the poultry, place 8 ounces boned skinless chicken breast halves or turkey breast tenderloin steaks in a 10x6x2-inch microwave-safe baking dish. Or, place 1 pound of the poultry in a 12x7½x2-inch baking dish. Cover with vented microwave-safe plastic wrap. Micro-cook on 100% power (high) for 1½ minutes for 8 ounces of poultry, 3 minutes for 1 pound. Turn pieces over, then rearrange by moving the outside pieces to center of dish. Cook, covered, on high for 1 to 2 minutes more for 8 ounces, 3 to 4 minutes more for 1 pound, or till tender and no longer pink. Then cut up poultry and use as directed in your recipe.

STUFFED PEPPERS

Here's a nifty tip from our Test Kitchen: For even cooking, move the center pepper halves to the ends of the dish halfway through cooking.

4   medium green *or* sweet red peppers *or* a combination of sweet peppers
2   6¾-ounce cans chunk-style chicken *or* 2 cups chopped cooked chicken (see tip, page 109)
1   7-ounce can whole kernel corn
1   15-ounce can Spanish rice
¼   cup frozen sliced green onion (see tip, page 39)
     Few dashes bottled hot pepper sauce
¼   cup finely shredded cheddar cheese (1 ounce)

■ Cut peppers in half lengthwise. Remove seeds and membranes. Place peppers, cut side down, in a 12x7½x2-inch microwave-safe baking dish. Cover with vented microwave-safe plastic wrap. Micro-cook on 100% power (high) for 6 to 8 minutes or till nearly tender, rearranging peppers after 3 minutes. Drain.

■ While peppers are cooking, drain canned chicken and corn. Break canned chicken into chunks. In a 1½-quart microwave-safe casserole combine chicken, corn, Spanish rice, frozen onion, and pepper sauce. Stir lightly till mixed. Cook, uncovered, on high about 6 minutes or till heated, stirring after 3 minutes.

■ Turn peppers cut side up. Mound chicken mixture into pepper shells. Cook, covered, on high for 2 minutes or till heated and peppers are tender. Sprinkle with cheese; cover and let stand about 2 minutes or till cheese melts. Makes 4 servings.

PER SERVING

Calories	352
Protein	27 g
Carbohydrate	34 g
Fat	13g
Cholesterol	67 mg
Sodium	1,024 mg
Potassium	729 mg

TIMETABLE

Preparation time:
10 minutes

Cooking time:
14 to 16 minutes

Standing time:
about 2 minutes

ORIENTAL TURKEY LOAF

Soy sauce, ginger, and water chestnuts add a savory hint of the Orient.

½   of an 8-ounce can sliced water chestnuts
1   egg
¼   cup quick-cooking rolled oats
⅓   cup frozen chopped green pepper (see tip, page 39)
1   tablespoon dried minced onion
1   tablespoon soy sauce
½   teaspoon ground ginger
1   pound ground raw turkey
¼   cup reduced-calorie apricot preserves *or* orange marmalade
1   teaspoon soy sauce
¼   teaspoon dry mustard

■ Drain, then chop, water chestnuts. In a medium mixing bowl slightly beat egg. Stir in water chestnuts, oats, frozen green pepper, onion, 1 tablespoon soy sauce, and ginger. Add turkey, then mix well.

■ In a 9-inch microwave-safe pie plate shape turkey into a ring with a 6-inch diameter, leaving a 2-inch-round hole in the center. Cover with waxed paper.

■ Micro-cook turkey loaf on 100% power (high) for 8 to 10 minutes or till turkey is no longer pink, rotating dish a quarter-turn every 3 minutes.

■ While turkey loaf is cooking, prepare glaze. For glaze, in a small mixing bowl stir together apricot preserves or orange marmalade, 1 teaspoon soy sauce, and dry mustard. Brush glaze over top of the cooked turkey loaf, then let stand for 5 minutes. To serve, cut into wedges. Makes 4 servings.

PER SERVING

Calories	220
Protein	28 g
Carbohydrate	14 g
Fat	5 g
Cholesterol	142 mg
Sodium	468 mg
Potassium	487 mg

TIMETABLE

Preparation time:
15 minutes

Cooking time:
8 to 10 minutes

Standing time:
5 minutes

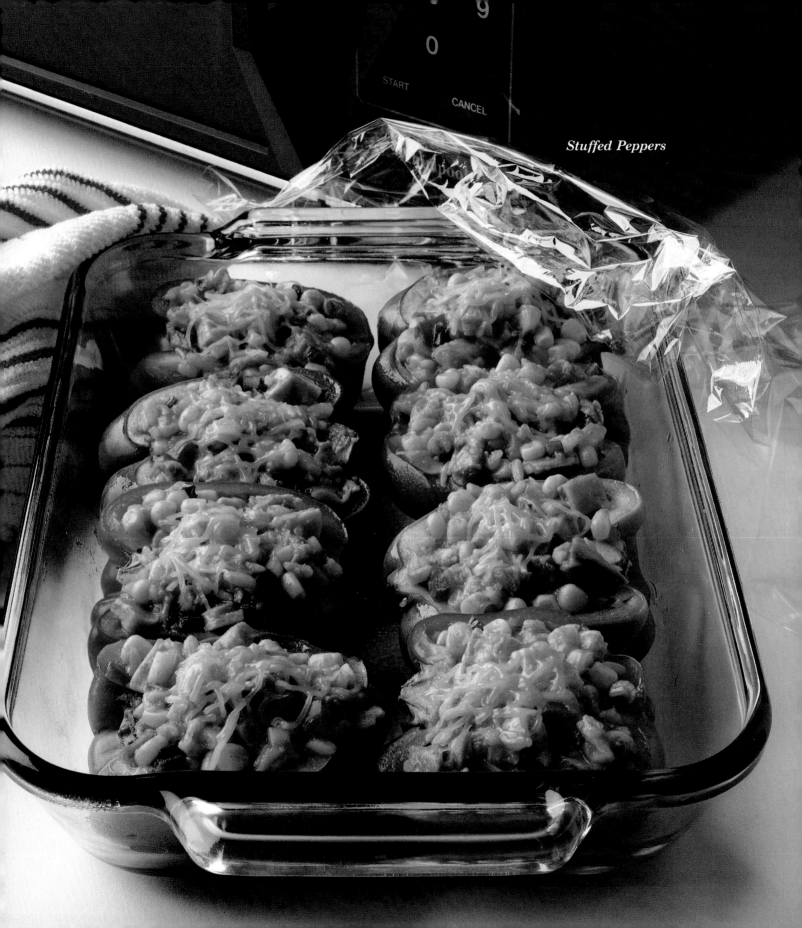

Stuffed Peppers

HALIBUT VÉRONIQUE

In order to get four small fish steaks that weigh a total of about a pound, have the steaks cut from the smaller, tail end of the fish.

1 cup sliced fresh mushrooms
2 tablespoons frozen
   sliced green onion
   (see tip, page 39)
1 tablespoon margarine
   or butter
4 small fresh halibut *or* other
   fish steaks, cut 1 inch
   thick (about 1 pound total)
½ cup seedless red *or*
   green grapes
¼ cup cold water
1½ teaspoons cornstarch
½ teaspoon instant chicken
   bouillon granules
3 tablespoons dry white
   wine

■ In a 12x7½x2-inch microwave-safe baking dish combine the mushrooms, frozen onion, and margarine or butter. Cover with vented microwave-safe plastic wrap. Micro-cook on 100% power (high) for 5 to 6 minutes or till tender, stirring after 3 minutes. Remove vegetables from dish. Set vegetables aside.

■ In the same dish arrange fish in a single layer. Cook, covered, on high for 5 to 6 minutes or till fish flakes easily with a fork, rearranging steaks and turning steaks over after 3 minutes. Using a wide slotted spatula, transfer fish to a serving platter. Cover fish to keep warm.

■ While fish is cooking, cut grapes in half. For sauce, in a small microwave-safe bowl or a 2-cup measure stir together cold water, cornstarch, and bouillon granules. Cook, uncovered, on high for 1 to 1½ minutes, till mixture is thickened and bubbly, stirring every 30 seconds. Then stir in vegetables, grapes, and wine. Cook, uncovered, on high for 1 minute. Spoon sauce over fish to serve. Makes 4 servings.

PER SERVING

Calories	177
Protein	23 g
Carbohydrate	6 g
Fat	6 g
Cholesterol	36 mg
Sodium	148 mg
Potassium	606 mg

TIMETABLE

Preparation time:
10 minutes

Cooking time:
12 to 15 minutes

20 minutes or less

SESAME-TOPPED FILLETS

Fillets cook more evenly if you turn under the thinner ends so the fillet is about the same thickness overall.

1 pound fresh skinless
   flounder, lake trout,
   or orange roughy fillets
   (about ½ inch thick)
3 tablespoons fine dry
   seasoned bread crumbs
1 tablespoon liquid margarine
1 tablespoon sesame seed
¼ teaspoon dried dillweed

■ Place the fillets in a single layer in a 10x6x2-inch microwave-safe baking dish, tucking under any thin edges. Cover dish with vented microwave-safe plastic wrap. Micro-cook fish on 100% power (high) for 3 minutes. Drain well.

■ While fish is cooking, prepare crumb mixture. For crumb mixture, in a small mixing bowl combine bread crumbs, margarine, sesame seed, and dillweed. Stir till well mixed.

■ Sprinkle crumb mixture on top of fish. Then cook, uncovered, on high for 1 to 3 minutes or till fish flakes easily with a fork, rotating dish a half-turn once. Makes 4 servings.

PER SERVING

Calories	145
Protein	20 g
Carbohydrate	4 g
Fat	5 g
Cholesterol	57 mg
Sodium	152 mg
Potassium	409 mg

TIMETABLE

Preparation time:
5 minutes

Cooking time:
4 to 6 minutes

20 minutes or less

SALMON-SHRIMP CHOWDER

Salmon, shrimp, and mushrooms in a rich-tasting creamy broth.

½ cup sliced fresh mushrooms
¼ cup frozen sliced green
    onion (see tip, page 39)
2 tablespoons dry white wine
    or water
1½ teaspoons instant chicken
    bouillon granules
    Dash pepper
1 6½-ounce can boneless,
    skinless pink salmon
2¼ cups skim milk
3 tablespoons all-purpose
    flour
2 tablespoons nonfat dry
    milk powder
¾ cup frozen cooked shrimp
    (about 3 ounces)

■ In a 1½-quart microwave-safe casserole combine mushrooms, frozen green onion, wine or water, bouillon granules, and pepper. Micro-cook, covered, on 100% power (high) for 2 to 3 minutes or till tender. Meanwhile, drain the salmon. Set salmon aside.

■ In a small mixing bowl stir together skim milk, flour, and dry milk powder. Then stir milk mixture into cooked vegetables. Cook, uncovered, on high for 5 to 8 minutes or till thickened and bubbly, stirring after every minute. Gently stir in salmon and frozen shrimp. Cook, uncovered, about 2 minutes more or till heated through. Makes 3 servings.

PER SERVING

Calories	239
Protein	28 g
Carbohydrate	19 g
Fat	4 g
Cholesterol	61 mg
Sodium	380 mg
Potassium	732 mg

TIMETABLE

Preparation time:
5 minutes

Cooking time:
9 to 13 minutes

FISHING FOR FLAVORS

Hooked on the idea of fixing fish, but unsure you'll like the flavor of a particular type of fish? Follow this handy guide when selecting from the variety of fish available.
• Cod, flounder, haddock, halibut, orange roughy, sea bass, and sole are popular because of their very delicate flavor.
• Pike, pollack, and red snapper are mild in flavor.
• Catfish can take on the flavor of the water they're grown in. Farm-raised catfish have a delicate flavor, and lake catfish have a slightly richer flavor.

MUSHROOM-STUFFED FISH ROLLS

½ of a small head romaine
1 cup sliced fresh mushrooms
2 teaspoons margarine *or* butter
½ teaspoon dried marjoram, crushed
4 4-ounce fresh skinless flounder *or* sole fillets
1½ teaspoons cornstarch
¼ teaspoon instant chicken bouillon granules
1 egg yolk
1 tablespoon lemon juice
Paprika

■ Cut center ribs from romaine leaves. Then chop romaine (you should have about 3 cups). Set aside.

■ In a 1-quart microwave-safe casserole combine mushrooms and margarine. Micro-cook, covered, on 100% power (high) for 2 minutes. Add romaine. Cook, covered, on high for 1 minute. Drain. Stir in marjoram, ¼ teaspoon *salt*, and ⅛ teaspoon *pepper*. Spoon ¼ *cup* mixture near center of *each* fillet. Roll fillets around filling (see photo 1). If necessary, secure with wooden toothpicks. Place rolls, seam side down, in a 10x6x2-inch microwave-safe baking dish. Cover with vented microwave-safe plastic wrap (see photo 2).

■ Cook on high for 3 minutes. Rearrange fish rolls by moving outside rolls to center of dish, then rotate dish a half-turn. Cook, covered, on high for 2 to 4 minutes or till fish flakes easily with a fork.

■ In a 2-cup microwave-safe measure combine cornstarch and bouillon granules. Stir in ½ cup *water* and egg yolk. Cook, uncovered, on high for 1½ to 2 minutes or till thickened and bubbly, stirring every 30 seconds. Stir in lemon juice. Discard toothpicks, then transfer rolls to a platter. Spoon on sauce. Sprinkle with paprika. Makes 4 servings.

PER SERVING		TIMETABLE
Calories	150	Total preparation time: 25 minutes
Protein	22 g	
Carbohydrate	3 g	
Fat	5 g	
Cholesterol	117 mg	
Sodium	277 mg	
Potassium	710 mg	

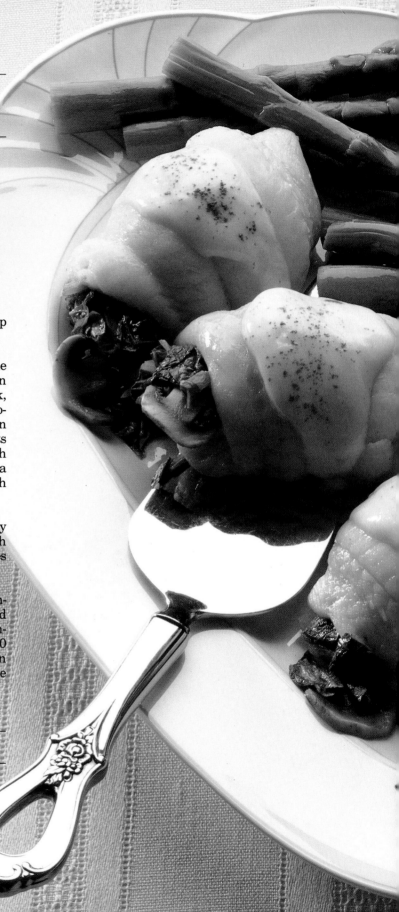

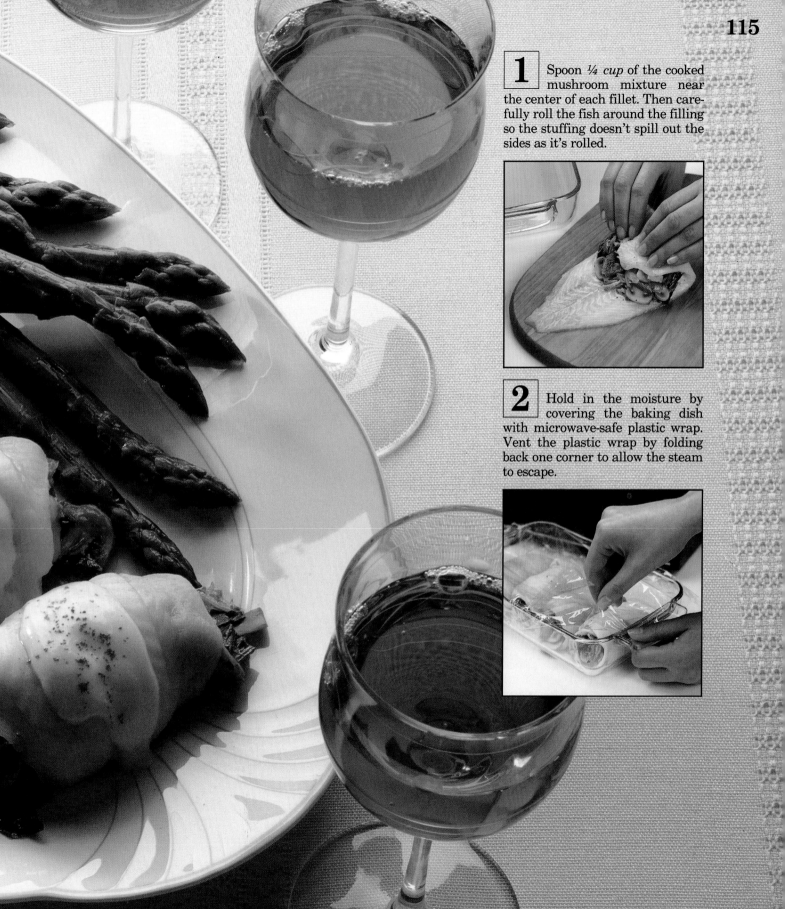

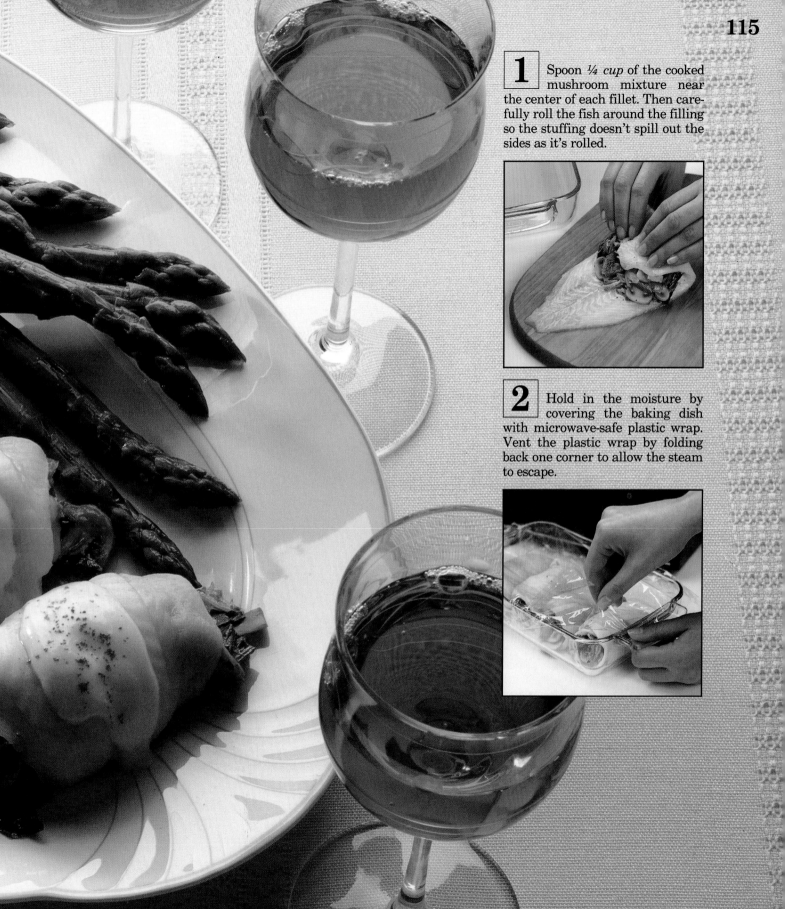

1 Spoon ¼ *cup* of the cooked mushroom mixture near the center of each fillet. Then carefully roll the fish around the filling so the stuffing doesn't spill out the sides as it's rolled.

2 Hold in the moisture by covering the baking dish with microwave-safe plastic wrap. Vent the plastic wrap by folding back one corner to allow the steam to escape.

GERMAN BEEF SALAD

A new twist to an old-time favorite: We added beef and spinach to this German potato salad.

¾ **pound beef top round steak**
½ **cup frozen chopped onion (see tip, page 39)**
2 **tablespoons cooking oil**
1 **tablespoon sugar**
1 **tablespoon cornstarch**
1 **teaspoon instant beef bouillon granules**
¼ **teaspoon celery seed**
½ **cup water**
¼ **cup vinegar**
1 **16-ounce can sliced potatoes**
6 **ounces fresh spinach**

■ Trim fat from meat. Thinly slice meat across the grain into bite-size strips. In a 2-quart microwave-safe casserole combine meat and frozen onion. Micro-cook, covered, on 100% power (high) for 3 to 5 minutes or till meat is done, stirring every 2 minutes. Drain off liquid. Set meat aside.

■ For dressing, in the same casserole stir together cooking oil, sugar, cornstarch, bouillon granules, and celery seed. Then stir in water and vinegar. Cook, uncovered, on high for 3 to 4 minutes or till thickened and bubbly, stirring after every minute.

■ Drain potatoes. Add potatoes and meat to dressing. Then cook, covered, on high for 1 to 2 minutes or till heated through. Meanwhile, clean and tear spinach to make about 5 cups. Place in a large salad bowl.

■ Add hot meat-potato mixture to spinach, and toss lightly till coated. Serve immediately. Serves 4.

PER SERVING

Calories	254
Protein	21 g
Carbohydrate	19 g
Fat	11 g
Cholesterol	54 mg
Sodium	357 mg
Potassium	658 mg

TIMETABLE

Preparation time:
10 minutes

Cooking time:
7 to 11 minutes

20 minutes or less

DILLY MEAT RING

Shaping the meat into a ring helps it cook more evenly in the microwave oven.

1 **small carrot**
1 **egg white**
¼ **cup skim milk**
2 **tablespoons fine dry bread crumbs**
1 **tablespoon frozen snipped chives (see tip, page 39)**
1 **teaspoon Worcestershire sauce**
½ **teaspoon garlic salt**
¼ **teaspoon pepper**
1 **pound lean ground beef**
½ **cup plain low-fat yogurt**
⅛ **teaspoon dried dillweed**

■ Coarsely shred carrot. In a medium mixing bowl slightly beat egg white. Stir in carrot, skim milk, bread crumbs, frozen chives, Worcestershire sauce, garlic salt, and pepper. Add beef, then mix well.

■ In a 9-inch microwave-safe pie plate shape the meat mixture into a ring with a 6-inch diameter, leaving a 2-inch-round hole in the center of the ring. Loosely cover with waxed paper.

■ Micro-cook meat loaf on 100% power (high) for 7 to 9 minutes or till meat is well-done and no pink remains, rotating dish a quarter-turn every 3 minutes. Meanwhile, for sauce, in a small mixing bowl stir together the yogurt and dillweed.

■ To serve, transfer meat loaf to a platter. Cut into wedges and serve with yogurt sauce. Serves 4.

PER SERVING

Calories	234
Protein	27 g
Carbohydrate	7 g
Fat	10 g
Cholesterol	82 mg
Sodium	371 mg
Potassium	419 mg

TIMETABLE

Preparation time:
10 minutes

Cooking time:
7 to 9 minutes

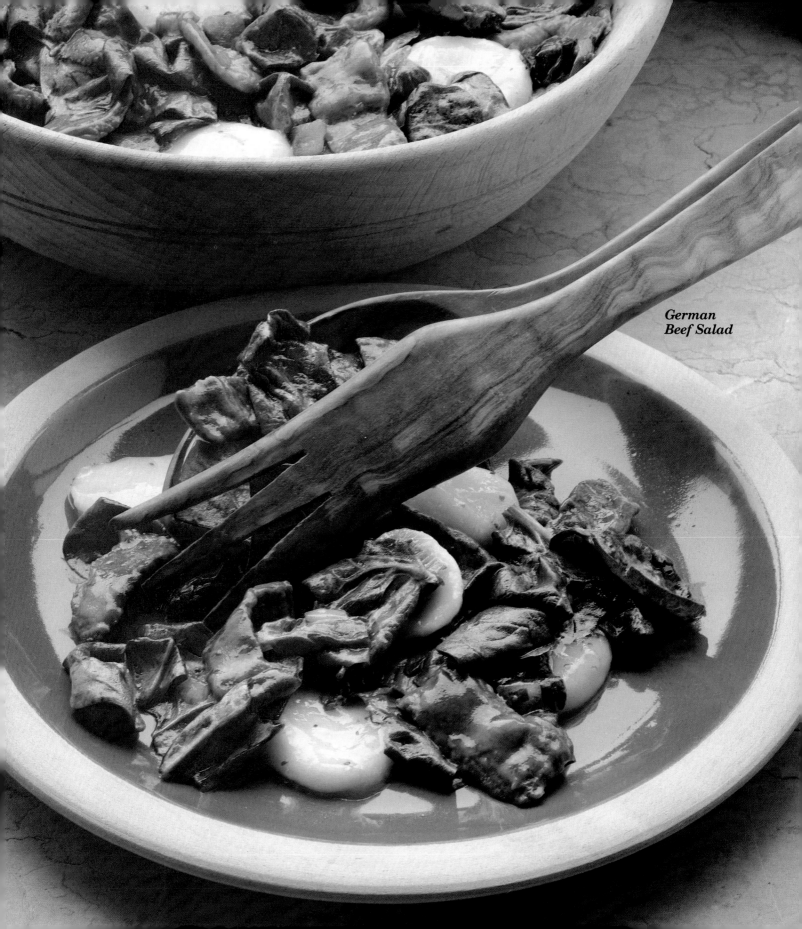

*German
Beef Salad*

STROGANOFF POTATOES

Ladle our tantalizing low-calorie beef stroganoff over piping hot potatoes, and you'll never miss oodles of noodles.

2   medium baking potatoes
      (6 to 8 ounces each)
1   2½-ounce package very
      thinly sliced smoked beef
½   of a small tomato
½   cup skim milk
1   tablespoon all-purpose flour
1   teaspoon frozen snipped
      chives (see tip, page 39)
⅛   teaspoon garlic powder
⅛   teaspoon pepper
1   2-ounce can chopped
      mushrooms
¼   cup plain low-fat yogurt

■ Scrub potatoes, then use a fork to prick potatoes several times. Place potatoes on a microwave-safe plate in the microwave oven, evenly spacing the potatoes. Micro-cook, uncovered, on 100% power (high) for 8 to 10 minutes or till tender, rearranging and turning potatoes over after 4 minutes. Meanwhile, cut beef into strips. Seed and chop tomato.

■ In a 1-quart microwave-safe casserole combine milk, flour, chives, garlic, and pepper. Cook, uncovered, on high for 2 to 3 minutes or till thickened and bubbly, stirring after every minute. Drain mushrooms. Stir mushrooms and beef into sauce. Cook on high for 1 to 2 minutes or till *very* hot. Stir in yogurt.

■ To serve, use a hot pad to gently roll the potatoes under your hand to loosen pulp. Cut a lengthwise slit in each potato, then press ends and push up. Place the potatoes on dinner plates. Spoon beef mixture on top. Sprinkle with tomato. Makes 2 servings.

PER SERVING

Calories	269
Protein	16 g
Carbohydrate	47 g
Fat	2 g
Cholesterol	19 mg
Sodium	618 mg
Potassium	1,463 mg

TIMETABLE

Preparation time:
10 minutes

Cooking time:
11 to 15 minutes

20 minutes or less

BORSCHT-STYLE STEW

Traditionally borscht is served dolloped with sour cream. We use plain yogurt as a low-calorie alternative.

8   ounces lean ground beef
¼   cup frozen chopped onion
      (see tip, page 39)
½   teaspoon instant beef
      bouillon granules
½   teaspoon Worcestershire
      sauce
⅛   teaspoon pepper
1   cup shredded cabbage
1   8¼-ounce can diced beets
1   8-ounce can stewed
      tomatoes
⅓   cup cold water
1   tablespoon cornstarch
2   tablespoons plain low-fat
      yogurt

■ In a 1½-quart microwave-safe casserole break ground beef into pieces. Add frozen onion. Micro-cook, covered, on 100% power (high) for 3 to 4 minutes or till meat is no longer pink and onion is tender, stirring after 2 minutes. Drain off fat.

■ Stir bouillon granules, Worcestershire sauce, and pepper into meat mixture. Then stir in the cabbage, *undrained* beets, and *undrained* tomatoes. Cook, covered, on high for 5 minutes, stirring after 2 minutes.

■ In a small bowl combine water and cornstarch, then stir it into meat mixture. Cook, uncovered, on high for 3 to 5 minutes or till thickened and bubbly, stirring every minute. To serve, ladle the stew into individual bowls. Top with yogurt. Makes 2 servings.

PER SERVING

Calories	292
Protein	27 g
Carbohydrate	24 g
Fat	10 g
Cholesterol	81 mg
Sodium	769 mg
Potassium	857 mg

TIMETABLE

Preparation time:
5 minutes

Cooking time:
11 to 14 minutes

BEEF 'N' POTATO CASSEROLE

Mashed potatoes on top, with saucy meat and vegetables underneath, create a hearty one-dish meal.

⅔ cup skim milk
¼ teaspoon salt
1 cup packaged instant mashed potato flakes
1 teaspoon frozen snipped chives (see tip, page 39)
2 cups loose-pack frozen broccoli, French-style green beans, onions, and red pepper
8 ounces cooked boneless beef *or* pork
1 10½-ounce can turkey gravy
½ teaspoon dried thyme, crushed
½ teaspoon bottled minced garlic *or* ⅛ teaspoon garlic powder
¼ teaspoon pepper

■ In a medium microwave-safe bowl combine milk, salt, and ⅔ cup *hot water*. Stir in potato flakes and frozen chives. Cover with vented microwave-safe plastic wrap. Micro-cook on 100% power (high) for 2½ minutes. Let stand covered.

■ While potatoes are cooking, place the frozen vegetables in a colander. Run *hot water* over vegetables till thawed, then drain well. Trim fat from meat. Slice meat into bite-size strips.

■ In a 1½-quart microwave-safe casserole combine gravy, thyme, garlic, and pepper. Stir in vegetables and meat. Cook, uncovered, on high for 3 to 4 minutes or till heated. Stir potatoes, then spoon potatoes into 4 mounds on top of the meat-vegetable mixture. Cook, uncovered, on high for 3 to 4 minutes or till sauce is bubbly and potatoes are heated, rotating casserole a half-turn after 2 minutes. Makes 4 servings.

PER SERVING

Calories	192
Protein	17 g
Carbohydrate	19 g
Fat	5 g
Cholesterol	37 mg
Sodium	626 mg
Potassium	427 mg

TIMETABLE

Preparation time:
10 minutes

Cooking time:
8 to 11 minutes

TOMATO-SAUCED VEAL

Can't find orzo? Then serve the vegetable-sauced veal over spaghetti.

¾ pound boneless veal *or* 1 pound pork sirloin chops
1 7½-ounce can tomatoes
½ of a 6-ounce can (⅓ cup) tomato paste
2 tablespoons frozen sliced green onion (see tip, page 39)
2 tablespoons dry white wine *or* water
½ teaspoon sugar
1 small zucchini
⅔ cup orzo (4 ounces)
2 tablespoons crumbled feta cheese

■ Trim fat from meat (discard bone from pork). Cut meat into ¾-inch cubes. Cut up tomatoes.

■ In a 1½-quart microwave-safe casserole combine meat, *undrained* tomatoes, tomato paste, onion, wine or water, and sugar. Micro-cook, covered, on 100% power (high) for 5 to 6 minutes or till mixture boils. Stir, then cook, covered, on 50% power (medium) for 10 to 12 minutes more or till meat is nearly tender.

■ While meat is cooking, cut zucchini in half lengthwise, then slice and set aside. On the range top in a medium saucepan heat 3½ cups *hot water* to boiling. Add orzo. Return to boiling. Boil gently for 5 to 8 minutes or till tender. Drain well. Keep warm.

■ Stir zucchini into meat mixture. Cook, covered, on medium for 4 to 5 minutes or till zucchini is tender. Sprinkle cheese over meat mixture. Then serve meat with hot cooked orzo. Makes 4 servings.

PER SERVING

Calories	295
Protein	21 g
Carbohydrate	30 g
Fat	9 g
Cholesterol	63 mg
Sodium	341 mg
Potassium	617 mg

TIMETABLE

Preparation time:
15 minutes

Cooking time:
19 to 23 minutes

SOUFFLÉED ASPARAGUS

Look for tofu, a soybean curd, in the produce department of the supermarket.

1   10-ounce package frozen asparagus *or* broccoli spears
1   tablespoon water
8   ounces tofu (fresh bean curd)
2   ounces American cheese
⅔   cup reduced-calorie mayonnaise *or* salad dressing
½   teaspoon frozen, finely shredded lemon peel (see tip, page 66)
2   egg whites
⅛   teaspoon cream of tartar
2   tablespoons sliced almonds (toasted, if desired)

■ In an 8x8x2-inch microwave-safe baking dish place frozen vegetables. Sprinkle with water. Cover with vented microwave-safe plastic wrap. Micro-cook on 100% power (high) for 5 to 7 minutes, separating and rearranging vegetables after 3 minutes. Drain, then arrange vegetables evenly in the baking dish.

■ While vegetables are cooking, drain and finely chop tofu. Shred cheese. In a small bowl stir together cheese, mayonnaise or salad dressing, and lemon peel. In another mixing bowl beat the egg whites and cream of tartar together till stiff peaks form (tips stand straight). Fold *half* of the mayonnaise mixture into egg whites. Fold tofu into the remaining mayonnaise mixture. Spoon tofu mixture on top of vegetables in baking dish. Then spoon egg white mixture on top of tofu mixture. Sprinkle with almonds.

■ Cook, uncovered, on 50% power (medium) for 8 to 10 minutes or till a knife inserted near the center comes out clean, rotating dish a quarter-turn every 3 minutes. Makes 4 servings.

PER SERVING

Calories	250
Protein	12 g
Carbohydrate	7 g
Fat	20 g
Cholesterol	13 mg
Sodium	458 mg
Potassium	274 mg

TIMETABLE

Preparation time:
15 minutes

Cooking time:
13 to 17 minutes

SPAGHETTI-STYLE SQUASH

Swap pasta for lower-calorie spaghetti squash.

½   of a 2½- to 3-pound spaghetti squash (halve squash lengthwise)
2   tablespoons water
1   15-ounce can garbanzo beans
1   15½-ounce jar extra-thick spaghetti sauce
¼   cup frozen snipped parsley (see tip, page 39)
¼   cup grated Parmesan cheese

■ Scoop out and discard seeds from squash. In a shallow microwave-safe baking dish place squash, cut side down. Add water. Cover with vented microwave-safe plastic wrap. Micro-cook on 100% power (high) for 8 to 12 minutes or till pulp can just be pierced with a fork, rotating dish a half-turn after 5 minutes. Let stand, covered, for 5 minutes.

■ Drain beans. In a 1½-quart microwave-safe casserole stir together beans, spaghetti sauce, and parsley. Cook, covered, on high for 4 to 6 minutes or till hot, stirring every 2 minutes. Keep covered; set aside.

■ Using a fork, shred and separate squash pulp into strands (see photo 2, page 155). Pile squash on a serving platter. Spoon on spaghetti sauce mixture. Sprinkle with cheese. Makes 3 servings.

PER SERVING

Calories	310
Protein	16 g
Carbohydrate	47 g
Fat	7 g
Cholesterol	7 mg
Sodium	1,159 mg
Potassium	793 mg

TIMETABLE

Preparation time:
10 minutes

Cooking time:
12 to 18 minutes

20 minutes or less

RICE 'N' BEAN STUFFED PEPPERS

½ cup frozen whole kernel
   corn
¼ cup frozen chopped onion
   (see tip, page 39)
1 tablespoon water
½ cup herbed tomato sauce
⅓ cup quick-cooking rice
¼ teaspoon sugar
⅛ teaspoon pepper
1 8-ounce can red kidney
   beans
1 large green or sweet red
   pepper
2 tablespoons shredded
   mozzarella cheese
   (½ ounce)

■ In a 1-quart microwave-safe casserole combine frozen corn, onion, and water. Micro-cook, covered, on 100% power (high) for 2 minutes. Then stir in tomato sauce, *uncooked* rice, sugar, and pepper. Cook, covered, on high for 2 to 3 minutes or till bubbly, stirring after 1 minute. Drain beans, then stir them into rice mixture. Cover and set aside.

■ Cut pepper in half lengthwise. Remove seeds and membranes. Place pepper halves, cut side down, in a microwave-safe pie plate. Cover with vented microwave-safe plastic wrap. Cook on high about 3 minutes or till nearly tender. Drain.

■ Turn pepper halves cut side up. Mound rice mixture into pepper shells. Cook, covered, on high about 2 minutes or till rice mixture is heated and peppers are tender, rotating dish a half-turn after 1 minute. Sprinkle with cheese. Makes 2 servings.

PER SERVING

Calories	257
Protein	12 g
Carbohydrate	48 g
Fat	3 g
Cholesterol	4 mg
Sodium	370 mg
Potassium	764 mg

TIMETABLE

Preparation time:
5 minutes

Cooking time:
9 to 10 minutes

MEXICALI SPUDS

If you need only two servings, halve this recipe. Micro-cook the two potatoes for 8 to 10 minutes and the salsa mixture about 1 minute.

4 medium baking potatoes
   (6 to 8 ounces each)
1 8-ounce can red kidney
   beans
½ cup salsa
1 cup low-fat cottage cheese
½ cup shredded cheddar
   cheese (2 ounces)

■ Scrub potatoes, then use a fork to prick potatoes several times. Place potatoes on a microwave-safe plate in the microwave oven, evenly spacing the potatoes. Micro-cook, uncovered, on 100% power (high) for 14 to 17 minutes or till tender, rearranging and turning potatoes over after 7 minutes.

■ Drain kidney beans. In a small microwave-safe bowl stir together beans and salsa. Cover with vented microwave-safe plastic wrap. Cook on 100% power (high) for 2 to 4 minutes or till heated through, stirring after 1½ minutes. Meanwhile, use a hot pad to gently roll potatoes under your hand to loosen pulp. Cut a crisscross slit in each potato. Place potatoes on a microwave-safe plate. Press potato ends to separate.

■ To serve, spoon cottage cheese into potatoes. Then pour salsa mixture over potatoes. Sprinkle with cheese. Cook, uncovered, on high about 1 minute or till cheese begins to melt. Makes 4 servings.

PER SERVING

Calories	292
Protein	17 g
Carbohydrate	42 g
Fat	6 g
Cholesterol	20 mg
Sodium	531 mg
Potassium	1,197 mg

TIMETABLE

Preparation time:
5 minutes

Cooking time:
17 to 22 minutes

Slimming Side Dishes

Dilled Corn and Pea Pods
(see recipe, page 133)

iets, like wardrobes, need color and variety to make them excitingly different. So, dress up your meals with timesaving side dishes. Check the medley of ideas on the following pages—from crisp, cool salads to steamy, hot vegetables. They're packed with flavor and texture but light on calories.

Parsley-Pesto-Style Toss
(see recipe, page 141)

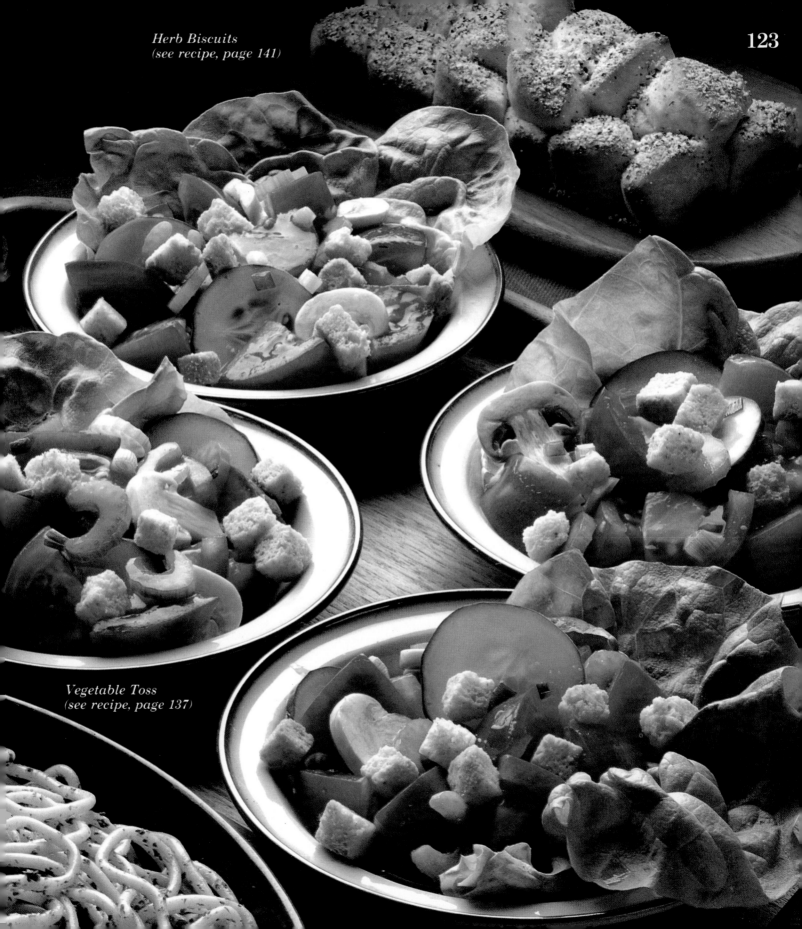

Herb Biscuits
(see recipe, page 141)

Vegetable Toss
(see recipe, page 137)

20 minutes or less

LEEKS WITH PEA PODS

8   **ounces leeks**
¼   **teaspoon bottled minced**
garlic *or* **dash garlic**
powder
2   **teaspoons margarine** *or*
butter
¼   **cup dry white wine**
⅛   **teaspoon salt**
Dash pepper
1   **6-ounce package frozen**
pea pods

■ Trim, then slice, leeks (you should have about 2 cups). In a large skillet cook the leeks and garlic in margarine or butter over medium heat for 2 minutes.

■ Add wine, salt, and pepper to leeks in the skillet. Bring to boiling. Reduce heat. Cover and simmer for 3 to 4 minutes or till tender, stirring occasionally.

■ Stir frozen pea pods into leek mixture. Return to boiling, then reduce heat. Simmer, uncovered, about 2 minutes or till vegetables are heated through and liquid is nearly evaporated. Makes 4 servings.

PER SERVING

Calories	80
Protein	2 g
Carbohydrate	12 g
Fat	2 g
Cholesterol	0 mg
Sodium	104 mg
Potassium	158 mg

TIMETABLE

Total preparation time:
15 minutes

20 minutes or less

GARLIC SUMMER SQUASH

Enjoying a bumper crop of summer squash? Here's a dandy way to use it.

2   **medium yellow summer**
squash *or* **zucchini**
(about 12 ounces total)
3   **medium green onions**
2   **teaspoons margarine** *or*
butter
½   **teaspoon bottled minced**
garlic *or* **⅛ teaspoon**
garlic powder
⅛   **teaspoon salt**
⅛   **teaspoon lemon-pepper**
seasoning

■ Cut the yellow squash or zucchini into bite-size chunks. Bias-slice green onions into 1-inch pieces.

■ In a medium skillet melt margarine or butter. Then add the squash, green onions, garlic, salt, and lemon-pepper seasoning. Toss gently to coat. Cover and cook over medium heat about 5 minutes or just till tender, stirring once. Makes 4 servings.

PER SERVING

Calories	38
Protein	1 g
Carbohydrate	4 g
Fat	2 g
Cholesterol	0 mg
Sodium	91 mg
Potassium	201 mg

TIMETABLE

Total preparation time:
10 minutes

SAUCY BROCCOLI AND ONIONS

1 **10-ounce package frozen cut broccoli**
½ **cup small frozen whole onions**
2 **ounces Neufchâtel cheese** *or* **2 ounces (¼ cup) reduced-calorie soft-style cream cheese**
½ **cup skim milk**
1 **teaspoon cornstarch**
⅛ **teaspoon dried thyme, crushed**
⅛ **teaspoon pepper**
1 **tablespoon grated Parmesan cheese**

■ In a medium saucepan cook broccoli and onions together according to package directions for broccoli. Then drain the vegetables, reserving ¼ *cup* of the cooking liquid. Set vegetables aside. Meanwhile, if using Neufchâtel cheese, cut it into cubes.

■ In the saucepan stir together milk, cornstarch, thyme, and pepper. Stir in the reserved liquid. Cook and stir till mixture is thickened and bubbly.

■ Stir Neufchâtel cheese or soft-style cream cheese into the mixture in the saucepan. Cook and stir till melted. Then add broccoli and onions. Toss lightly till mixed. Cook just till heated through.

■ To serve, transfer broccoli mixture to a serving bowl. Sprinkle with Parmesan cheese. Serves 4.

PER SERVING

Calories	85
Protein	6 g
Carbohydrate	8 g
Fat	4 g
Cholesterol	13 mg
Sodium	119 mg
Potassium	233 mg

TIMETABLE

Total preparation time: 20 minutes

CHEESY CELERIAC

Celeriac, also know as celery root, has a strong celery flavor that complements the pleasant hint of blue cheese in the sauce.

12 **ounces celeriac**
½ **cup skim milk**
1 **teaspoon cornstarch**
1 **tablespoon crumbled blue cheese**
1 **tablespoon frozen snipped parsley (see tip, page 39)**
1 **tablespoon chopped walnuts**

■ Peel celeriac, then cut into julienne sticks (you should have about 2 cups). Meanwhile, in a medium saucepan bring about 1 inch of *water* to boiling, then reduce heat to a simmer. Place celeriac in a steamer basket. Carefully place basket over the simmering water. Cover and steam about 5 minutes or till celeriac is crisp-tender.

■ For sauce, in a small saucepan stir together milk and cornstarch. Cook and stir till thickened and bubbly. Then cook and stir for 1 minute more. Stir in cheese and parsley. Cook and stir till cheese melts.

■ To serve, transfer celeriac to a serving bowl. Pour sauce over celeriac, then sprinkle with nuts. Serves 4.

PER SERVING

Calories	60
Protein	3 g
Carbohydrate	9 g
Fat	2 g
Cholesterol	2 mg
Sodium	114 mg
Potassium	289 mg

TIMETABLE

Total preparation time: 20 minutes

CHEESE-SAUCED KOHLRABI

Kohlrabies look like green tennis balls with tops of oval, dark green leaves. Choose those less than 3 inches in diameter for less woody texture.

3　medium kohlrabies (about 12 ounces total)
4　wheat crackers
1　ounce American cheese
2　tablespoons frozen chopped onion (see tip, page 39)
1　teaspoon margarine *or* butter
1½　teaspoons cornstarch
½　cup skim milk

■ Peel kohlrabies, then cut into cubes (you should have about 2 cups). Meanwhile, in a medium saucepan bring about 1 inch *water* to boiling. Reduce heat to a simmer. Place kohlrabies in a steamer basket. Carefully place basket over the simmering water. Cover and steam for 12 to 13 minutes or till tender.

■ While kohlrabies are steaming, crush crackers. Set crushed crackers aside. Shred cheese (you should have ¼ cup). In a small saucepan cook onion in margarine or butter till tender. Then stir in cornstarch. Add milk. Cook and stir till thickened and bubbly. Then cook and stir for 2 minutes more. Stir in cheese. Cook and stir till cheese melts.

■ To serve, add kohlrabies to sauce in saucepan. Toss lightly till coated. Transfer kohlrabies to a serving bowl. Sprinkle with crushed crackers. Serves 4.

PER SERVING

Calories	90
Protein	4 g
Carbohydrate	11 g
Fat	4 g
Cholesterol	7 mg
Sodium	166 mg
Potassium	373 mg

TIMETABLE

Preparation time: 15 minutes

Cooking time: 12 to 13 minutes

SWISS VEGGIE SOUP

Pair this side-dish soup with a half-sandwich for a filling lunch. Or, make the soup into two main-dish servings by adding small pieces of leftover cooked meat.

2½　cups loose-pack frozen broccoli, cauliflower, and carrots
½　cup frozen chopped onion (see tip, page 39)
½　cup water
½　teaspoon instant chicken bouillon granules
3　slices process Swiss cheese (3 ounces total)
1　cup skim milk

■ In a medium saucepan combine frozen vegetables, onion, water, and bouillon granules. Bring to boiling, then reduce heat. Cover and simmer about 10 minutes or till vegetables are tender. *Do not drain.* Meanwhile, tear the cheese slices into bite-size pieces and set aside.

■ Transfer all of the vegetables and cooking liquid to a blender container or food processor bowl. Add milk. Cover and blend or process till smooth.

■ Return mixture to saucepan. Stir in cheese. Cook and stir till cheese melts. To serve, ladle the soup into individual bowls. Makes 4 servings.

PER SERVING

Calories	118
Protein	9 g
Carbohydrate	9 g
Fat	6 g
Cholesterol	19 mg
Sodium	390 mg
Potassium	295 mg

TIMETABLE

Total preparation time: 25 minutes

LEMONY BEANS

Perk up frozen green beans with a splash of lemon juice.

1 **9-ounce package frozen cut
    green beans**
¼ **cup frozen chopped onion
    (see tip, page 39)**
½ **of an 8-ounce can sliced
    water chestnuts**
1 **tablespoon lemon juice
    Dash pepper**

◼ In a medium saucepan cook beans according to package directions, *except* add frozen onion. Drain beans and onion and transfer to a serving bowl.

◼ While beans and onion are cooking, drain water chestnuts. Add water chestnuts to cooked beans and onion, then sprinkle with lemon juice and pepper. Toss lightly till coated. Makes 4 servings.

PER SERVING

Calories	46
Protein	2 g
Carbohydrate	11 g
Fat	0 g
Cholesterol	0 mg
Sodium	5 mg
Potassium	195 mg

TIMETABLE

Total preparation time:
10 minutes

WHAT'S GRAZING ALL ABOUT?

The term *grazing* simply refers to nibbling on smaller amounts of food throughout the day.

If you choose to be among the grazers, beware! Calories from all those snacks can easily get out of control. And, keeping track of the calories may be more difficult than tallying calories for three meals. It's easy to forget small bites of food.

If you decide to graze, be sure to eat a variety of foods that will contribute to good nutrition. It's essential not to shortchange yourself on important nutrients that your body needs.

VEGETABLE SOUP

Carrots, spinach, turnips, and the heavenly aroma of soy sauce make this a colorful, side-dish soup.

2½ **cups water**
 1 **medium onion**
 2 **small turnips *or* potatoes**
 1 **cup frozen crinkle-cut carrots**
 4 **teaspoons soy sauce**
 2 **teaspoons instant chicken bouillon granules**
2½ **ounces fresh spinach (2 cups loosely packed)**
 2 **tablespoons miso (soybean paste) (optional)**

■ In a medium saucepan bring water to boiling. Meanwhile, slice onion, then separate onion into rings. Peel turnips or potatoes (see photo 1); cut into julienne sticks.

■ Add onion, turnips or potatoes, frozen carrots, soy sauce, and instant bouillon granules to water in the saucepan. Bring to boiling, then reduce heat. Cover and simmer for 8 to 10 minutes or till the vegetables are tender.

■ While soup is simmering, wash and remove stems from spinach (see photo 2). Tear spinach into bite-size pieces. If desired, stir miso into soup mixture. Stir in spinach and heat through. To serve, ladle soup into individual bowls. Makes 6 to 8 servings.

PER SERVING		TIMETABLE
Calories	**28**	Total preparation time: 30 minutes
Protein	1 g	
Carbohydrate	6 g	
Fat	0 g	
Cholesterol	0 mg	
Sodium	388 mg	
Potassium	222 mg	

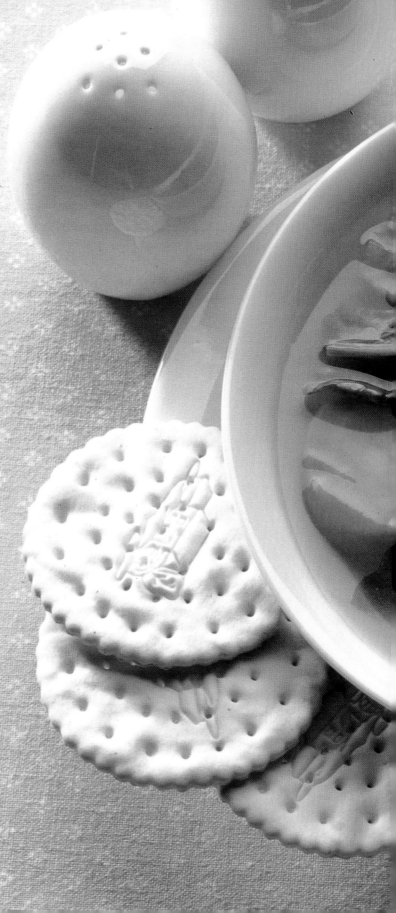

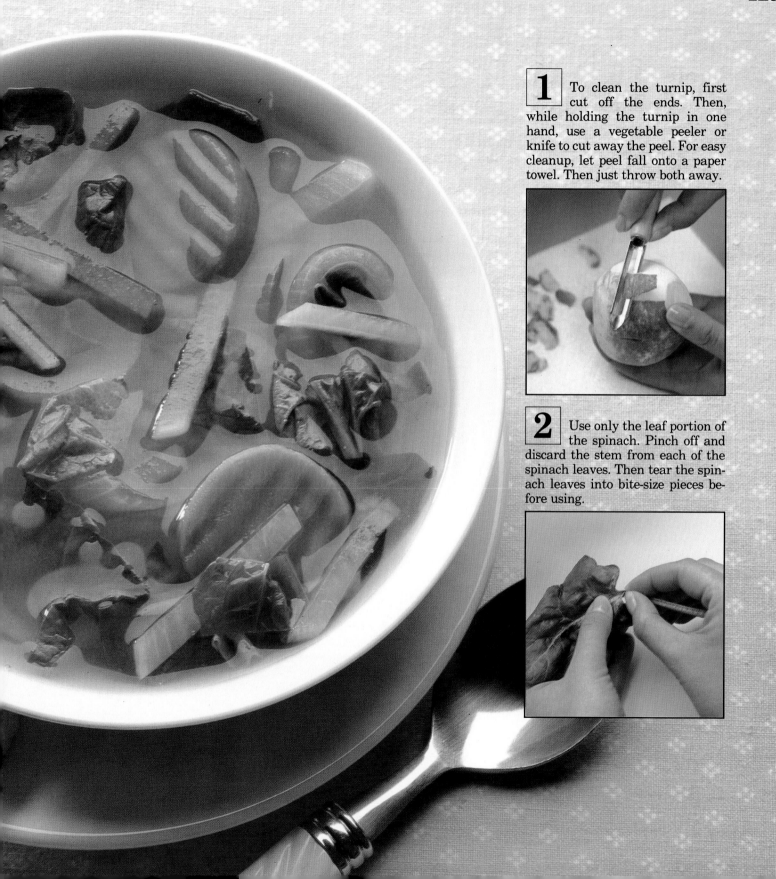

1 To clean the turnip, first cut off the ends. Then, while holding the turnip in one hand, use a vegetable peeler or knife to cut away the peel. For easy cleanup, let peel fall onto a paper towel. Then just throw both away.

2 Use only the leaf portion of the spinach. Pinch off and discard the stem from each of the spinach leaves. Then tear the spinach leaves into bite-size pieces before using.

20 minutes or less

BEANS 'N' MUSHROOMS

Transform frozen beans into a quick, festive vegetable combo.

1	9-ounce package frozen French-style green beans
2	teaspoons margarine *or* butter
1½	cups sliced fresh mushrooms (4 ounces)
½	teaspoon frozen, finely shredded lemon peel (see tip, page 66)
1	tablespoon chopped pimiento
	Dash pepper
1	teaspoon lemon juice

■ Place frozen beans in a colander. Run *hot water* over beans just till thawed. Drain well.

■ While beans are draining, preheat a large skillet over medium-high heat. Add margarine or butter to hot skillet. Then add the drained beans and stir-fry for 1 minute. Add mushrooms and lemon peel, then stir-fry for 2 minutes more. Stir in pimiento and pepper. Sprinkle with lemon juice. Serve immediately. Makes 3 or 4 servings.

PER SERVING

Calories	62
Protein	2 g
Carbohydrate	9 g
Fat	3 g
Cholesterol	0 mg
Sodium	35 mg
Potassium	312 mg

TIMETABLE

Total preparation time: 10 minutes

---

20 minutes or less

CHINESE CABBAGE STIR-FRY

¼	of a small head Chinese cabbage
1	cup fresh bean sprouts
	Nonstick spray coating
1	tablespoon cold water
1	tablespoon teriyaki sauce *or* soy sauce
¼	teaspoon cornstarch
¼	teaspoon bottled minced garlic *or* dash garlic powder
¼	cup frozen sliced green onion (see tip, page 39)

■ Coarsely chop Chinese cabbage (you should have about 2 cups). Remove the root portions from bean sprouts. Set cabbage and sprouts aside.

■ Spray a *cold* wok or large skillet with nonstick coating. Preheat the wok or skillet over high heat. Meanwhile, for sauce, in a custard cup stir together cold water, teriyaki sauce or soy sauce, cornstarch, and garlic.

■ Add cabbage, bean sprouts, and frozen onion to hot wok or skillet, then stir-fry for 2 to 3 minutes or till vegetables are nearly tender. Push vegetables from center of wok or skillet.

■ Stir sauce, then add to center of wok or skillet. Cook and stir till thickened and bubbly. Cook and stir for 30 seconds more. Stir in vegetables to coat with sauce. Serve immediately. Makes 2 servings.

PER SERVING

Calories	36
Protein	3 g
Carbohydrate	7 g
Fat	0 g
Cholesterol	0 mg
Sodium	547 mg
Potassium	256 mg

TIMETABLE

Preparation time: 15 minutes

Cooking time: 4 to 5 minutes

JICAMA STIR-FRY

Jicamas (HEE-kuh-muhs) resemble turnips in shape but have a delicate water-chestnutlike flavor.

8 ounces jicama
2½ ounces fresh spinach (2 cups loosely packed)
4 cherry tomatoes
2 green onions
½ cup cold water
1 teaspoon cornstarch
1 teaspoon soy sauce
½ teaspoon instant chicken *or* beef bouillon granules
½ teaspoon grated gingerroot *or* ⅛ teaspoon ground ginger
Nonstick spray coating
¼ teaspoon bottled minced garlic *or* dash garlic powder

■ Prepare vegetables by peeling jicama, then cutting into ½-inch-thick sticks (you should have about 1½ cups). Wash and remove stems from spinach. Tear spinach into bite-size pieces. Cut cherry tomatoes in half. Bias-slice green onions into 1-inch pieces. Set vegetables aside.

■ For the sauce, in a small bowl or custard cup stir together cold water, cornstarch, soy sauce, bouillon granules, and ginger. Set sauce aside.

■ Spray a *cold* wok or large skillet with nonstick coating. Preheat wok or skillet over high heat. Add the jicama, then stir-fry for 3 minutes. Add onions and garlic, then stir-fry vegetables about 1 minute more or till jicama is nearly tender. Push vegetables from center of the wok or skillet.

■ Stir sauce, then add to center of the wok or skillet. Cook and stir till thickened and bubbly. Cook and stir for 1 minute more. Add spinach and tomatoes. Cook and stir just till spinach is wilted. Serve immediately. Makes 4 servings.

PER SERVING

Calories	39
Protein	2 g
Carbohydrate	9 g
Fat	0 g
Cholesterol	0 mg
Sodium	147 mg
Potassium	141 mg

TIMETABLE

Preparation time: 15 minutes

Cooking time: about 8 minutes

20 minutes or less

PAN-FRIED JERUSALEM ARTICHOKES

8 ounces Jerusalem artichokes
1 tablespoon margarine *or* butter
¼ cup frozen sliced green onion (see tip, page 39)
¼ teaspoon bottled minced garlic *or* dash garlic powder
1 tablespoon frozen snipped parsley (see tip, page 39)

■ Peel artichokes, then thinly slice. Meanwhile, in a medium skillet melt margarine or butter.

■ Add artichokes, frozen onion, and garlic to skillet. Cook and stir vegetables over medium-high heat about 3 minutes or till artichoke slices are golden brown, then reduce heat. Cover and cook for 3 to 4 minutes or till vegetables are tender. Add parsley, then cook and stir for 30 seconds more. Serves 4.

PER SERVING

Calories	73
Protein	1 g
Carbohydrate	11 g
Fat	3 g
Cholesterol	0 mg
Sodium	37 mg
Potassium	269 mg

TIMETABLE

Total preparation time: 15 minutes

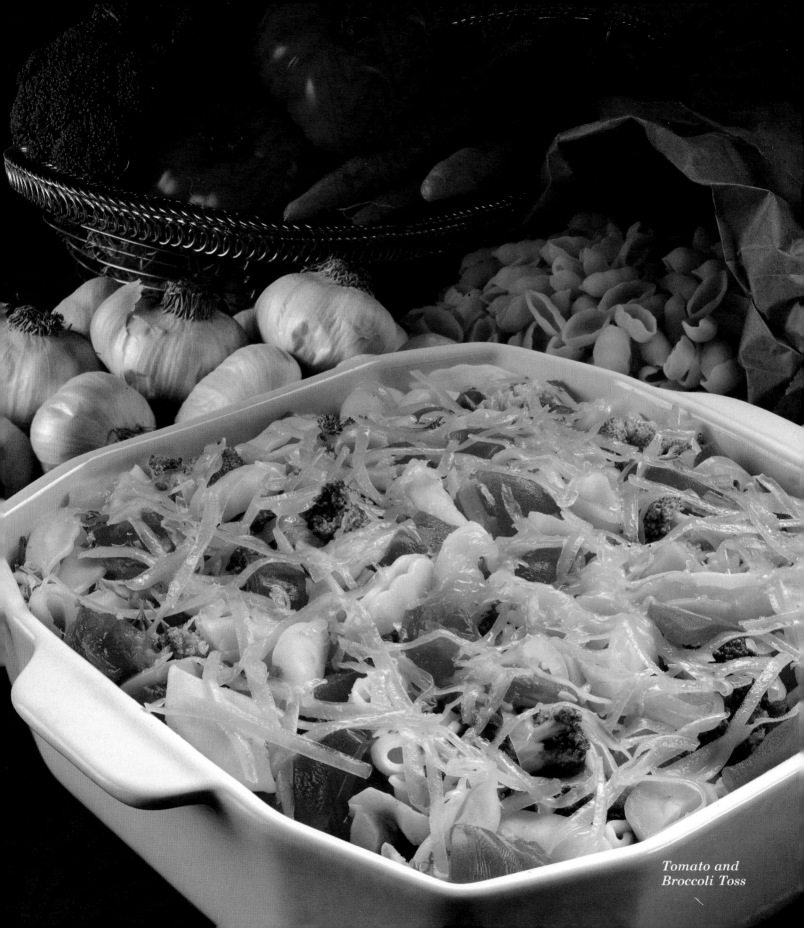

Tomato and Broccoli Toss

TOMATO AND BROCCOLI TOSS

Combine pasta with vegetables for a two-in-one side dish.

2 ounces cavatelli *or* macaroni (about 1 cup)
2 medium tomatoes
1 small onion
  Nonstick spray coating
1 teaspoon dried parsley flakes
1 teaspoon instant chicken bouillon granules
¼ teaspoon dried Italian seasoning, crushed
¼ teaspoon bottled minced garlic *or* dash garlic powder
1 cup frozen cut broccoli
½ cup finely shredded cheddar cheese (2 ounces)

■ Cook pasta according to package directions, *except* use a large saucepan and 4 cups *hot* water. Drain.

■ While pasta is cooking, seed and chop tomatoes. Thinly slice onion. Spray a *cold* large skillet with nonstick coating. Preheat skillet over medium heat. Add onion, then cook till tender but not brown. Add the chopped tomatoes, parsley, bouillon granules, Italian seasoning, and garlic.

■ Heat the mixture till hot, then add broccoli. Cover and cook over medium heat for 4 minutes, stirring occasionally. Stir in pasta. Cover and cook for 2 to 3 minutes more or till broccoli is crisp-tender. To serve, transfer to a serving dish. Sprinkle with cheese. Makes 4 servings.

PER SERVING

Calories	129
Protein	7 g
Carbohydrate	15 g
Fat	5 g
Cholesterol	15 mg
Sodium	461 mg
Potassium	204 mg

TIMETABLE

Total preparation time: 25 minutes

20 minutes or less

DILLED CORN AND PEA PODS

Fresh pea pods are a tasty option to frozen ones—just allow a little extra time to remove the tips and strings. (Pictured on page 122.)

1 cup frozen whole kernel corn
½ cup water
1 small sweet red pepper
1 6-ounce package frozen pea pods
2 teaspoons margarine *or* butter
¼ teaspoon dried dillweed
⅛ teaspoon salt
⅛ teaspoon pepper

■ In a medium saucepan combine frozen corn and water. Bring to boiling, then reduce heat. Cover and simmer for 4 minutes. Meanwhile, cut the red pepper into bite-size strips.

■ Add red pepper and pea pods to saucepan. Cover and cook about 2 minutes or till red pepper and pea pods are crisp-tender. Drain.

■ Add the margarine or butter, dillweed, salt, and pepper to vegetable mixture. Toss till margarine or butter melts and vegetables are coated. Serves 5.

PER SERVING

Calories	60
Protein	2 g
Carbohydrate	10 g
Fat	2 g
Cholesterol	0 mg
Sodium	76 mg
Potassium	152 mg

TIMETABLE

Total preparation time: 15 minutes

POPPY-SEED FRUIT SALAD

Use pineapple yogurt as the base for a creamy, tasty dressing.

1 10½-ounce can mandarin
   orange sections
   (water pack)
1 8-ounce can pineapple
   tidbits (juice pack)
1½ cups small strawberries
   or seedless red grapes
1 medium apple
½ cup pineapple low-fat
   yogurt
½ teaspoon poppy seed
   Lettuce leaves

■ Drain mandarin oranges. Then drain pineapple, reserving *1 tablespoon* of the pineapple juice. If using strawberries, cut them in half. Core apple, then cut into bite-size pieces.

■ For the fruit mixture, in a medium mixing bowl combine orange sections, pineapple, strawberries or grapes, and apple. Toss lightly to mix.

■ For dressing, in a small mixing bowl stir together yogurt, poppy seed, and the reserved pineapple juice.

■ To serve, line salad plates with the lettuce leaves. Arrange fruit mixture on lettuce. Drizzle dressing over fruit. Makes 5 or 6 servings.

PER SERVING

Calories	101
Protein	2 g
Carbohydrate	24 g
Fat	1 g
Cholesterol	1 mg
Sodium	18 mg
Potassium	285 mg

TIMETABLE

Total preparation time:
25 minutes

20 minutes or less

APPLE 'N' CABBAGE SLAW

Whipped dessert topping and creamy cucumber salad dressing make for a rich-tasting coleslaw.

1 large apple
2 cups shredded cabbage
¼ cup raisins
¼ cup frozen whipped dessert
   topping, thawed (see tip,
   page 167)
3 tablespoons reduced-calorie
   creamy cucumber salad
   dressing

■ Core, then chop apple. In a medium mixing bowl combine apple, cabbage, and raisins.

■ For dressing, in a small mixing bowl gently stir together thawed dessert topping and salad dressing. Fold dressing mixture into cabbage mixture. If desired, chill slaw in the freezer for 5 minutes before serving. Makes 6 servings.

PER SERVING

Calories	66
Protein	1 g
Carbohydrate	11 g
Fat	3 g
Cholesterol	0 mg
Sodium	73 mg
Potassium	134 mg

TIMETABLE

Total preparation time:
10 minutes

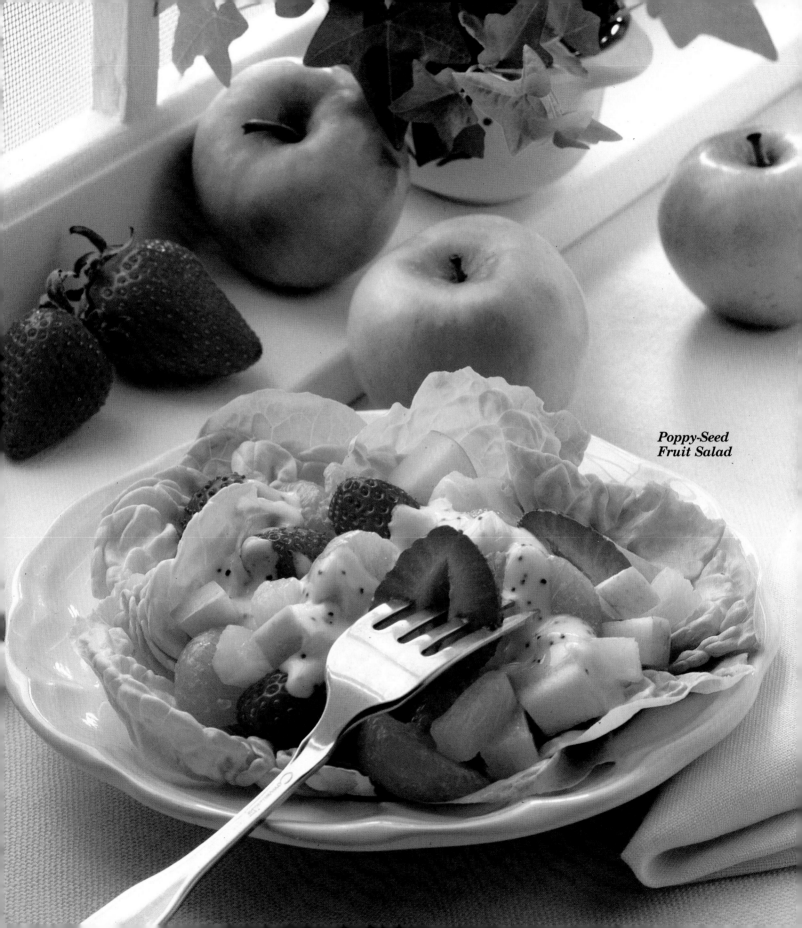

*Poppy-Seed
Fruit Salad*

20 minutes or less

ROMAINE-VEGETABLE SALAD

½ of a small head romaine
2 stalks celery
1 tablespoon white wine
vinegar
1 tablespoon cooking oil
2 teaspoons soy sauce
¼ teaspoon five-spice powder
1 16-ounce package loose-
pack frozen broccoli, red
peppers, bamboo shoots,
and straw mushrooms
2 tablespoons water

■ Clean and tear romaine into bite-size pieces (you should have about 3 cups). Thinly slice celery. Set romaine and celery aside.

■ For dressing, in a custard cup or small mixing bowl stir together vinegar, oil, soy sauce, and five-spice powder. Set dressing aside.

■ In a 12-inch skillet combine frozen vegetables and water. Cook over medium-high heat for 3 to 4 minutes or till thawed and just heated through, stirring occasionally. *Do not drain.* Reduce heat to medium. Stir in dressing, then add romaine and celery. Carefully toss about 30 seconds or till romaine begins to wilt. To serve, immediately spoon romaine mixture onto salad plates. Makes 6 servings.

PER SERVING

Calories	49
Protein	3 g
Carbohydrate	5 g
Fat	2 g
Cholesterol	0 mg
Sodium	149 mg
Potassium	294 mg

TIMETABLE

Total preparation time:
15 minutes

20 minutes or less

GREEK-STYLE SALADS

Mix bottled dressing with a hint of mint and a dash of lemon juice and presto! You've got a new flavor combination.

1 medium tomato
½ of a small red onion
¼ of a small cucumber
4 cups torn mixed salad
greens (see tip, opposite)
¼ cup sliced pitted ripe olives
2 tablespoons reduced-calorie
Italian salad dressing
2 tablespoons lemon juice
1 tablespoon water
½ teaspoon dried mint,
crushed
¼ cup crumbled feta cheese
or 2 tablespoons crumbled
blue cheese

■ Cut the tomato into 8 wedges, then cut the wedges in half crosswise. Slice onion, then separate into rings. Slice cucumber.

■ For salad, in a large bowl combine salad greens, tomato, onion rings, cucumber, and olives. For dressing, in a screw-top jar combine salad dressing, lemon juice, water, and mint. Cover and shake well. Pour over greens mixture. Toss lightly till coated.

■ To serve, spoon greens onto salad plates. Sprinkle salads with feta or blue cheese. Makes 4 servings.

PER SERVING

Calories	59
Protein	2 g
Carbohydrate	5 g
Fat	4 g
Cholesterol	8 mg
Sodium	172 mg
Potassium	241 mg

TIMETABLE

Total preparation time:
15 minutes

20 minutes or less

VEGETABLE TOSS

Tomatoes + cucumber + celery + mushrooms = a cool refreshing addition to your meal. (Pictured on pages 122 and 123.)

3 **medium tomatoes**
½ **of a small cucumber**
½ **of a small stalk celery**
½ **cup sliced fresh mushrooms**
2 **tablespoons frozen sliced green onion (see tip, page 39)**
¼ **cup reduced-calorie Italian salad dressing**
  Dash bottled hot pepper sauce
4 **Bibb *or* Boston lettuce leaves**
  Coarsely ground pepper
½ **cup croutons**

■ Cut each tomato into 8 wedges, then cut the wedges in half crosswise. Slice cucumber and celery.

■ In a medium mixing bowl combine the tomatoes, cucumber, celery, mushrooms, and onion. Pour salad dressing over vegetable mixture. Add hot pepper sauce. Toss lightly till coated.

■ To serve, place lettuce leaves on salad plates. Spoon the vegetable mixture onto the lettuce leaves. Sprinkle with pepper. Top with croutons. Serves 4.

PER SERVING

Calories	61
Protein	2 g
Carbohydrate	9 g
Fat	2 g
Cholesterol	1 mg
Sodium	88 mg
Potassium	264 mg

TIMETABLE

Total preparation time: 15 minutes

THE SALAD BAR HELPER

Let the take-out salad bar at the supermarket lend you a helping hand. Save time, yet enjoy freshness, by choosing sliced and chopped vegetables from the salad bar assortment. Look for torn mixed salad greens, shredded cheese, cut broccoli and cauliflower, and sliced cucumber, celery, carrots, mushrooms, and olives.

It's fun making your own selection, but for maximum freshness, buy only what you need for a day or two. You can always go back for more.

20 minutes or less

LEMONY MUSHROOMS

This refreshing salad is perfect for a summer luncheon.

½ of an 8-ounce carton plain low-fat yogurt
1 tablespoon reduced-calorie mayonnaise *or* salad dressing
1 teaspoon honey
⅛ teaspoon finely shredded lemon peel
½ teaspoon lemon juice
⅛ teaspoon dry mustard
⅛ teaspoon pepper
3 cups sliced fresh mushrooms (8 ounces)
2 tablespoons frozen chopped onion (see tip, page 39)
1 medium tomato
Lettuce leaves
Coarsely ground pepper (optional)

■ In a large mixing bowl stir together yogurt, mayonnaise or salad dressing, honey, lemon peel, lemon juice, mustard, and ⅛ teaspoon pepper. Add mushrooms and frozen onion. Toss lightly till coated.

■ To serve, cut tomato into 8 wedges. Line salad plates with lettuce leaves. Spoon mushroom mixture on top of lettuce. Garnish with the tomato wedges. If desired, sprinkle with coarsely ground pepper. Makes 4 servings.

PER SERVING

Calories	56
Protein	3 g
Carbohydrate	8 g
Fat	2 g
Cholesterol	2 mg
Sodium	46 mg
Potassium	350 mg

TIMETABLE

Total preparation time: 20 minutes

---

20 minutes or less

DILLED PEA SALAD

A surefire complement to grilled chicken or burgers.

1 10-ounce package frozen peas
½ of an 8-ounce can (½ cup) sliced water chestnuts
¼ cup plain low-fat yogurt
1 tablespoon reduced-calorie mayonnaise *or* salad dressing
¾ teaspoon dried dillweed
⅛ teaspoon onion salt
⅛ teaspoon pepper
2 tablespoons chopped pimiento

■ Place frozen peas in a colander. Run *hot water* over peas just till thawed. Drain well. Meanwhile, drain water chestnuts.

■ In a medium mixing bowl stir together yogurt, mayonnaise or salad dressing, dillweed, onion salt, and pepper. Add thawed peas, water chestnuts, and pimiento. Toss lightly till coated. Makes 4 servings.

PER SERVING

Calories	86
Protein	5 g
Carbohydrate	14 g
Fat	2 g
Cholesterol	1 mg
Sodium	165 mg
Potassium	182 mg

TIMETABLE

Total preparation time: 10 minutes

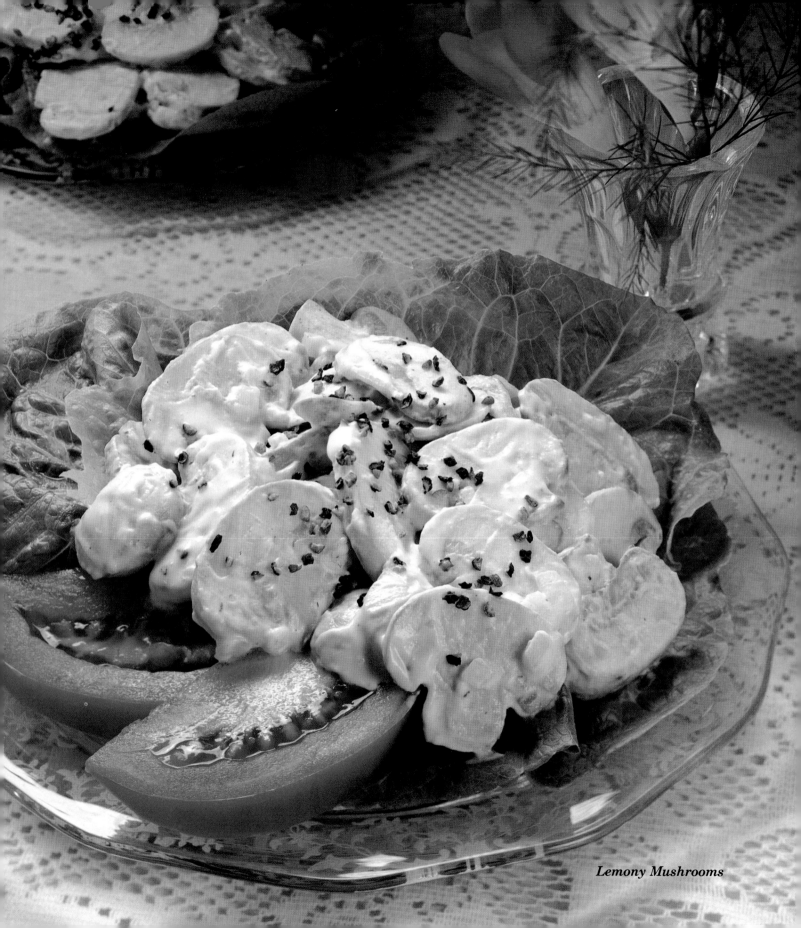

Lemony Mushrooms

BARLEY WITH VEGETABLES

Serve this vegetable-dotted side dish with broiled chicken or fish.

1½ cups water
1 teaspoon instant chicken bouillon granules
⅛ teaspoon pepper
⅛ teaspoon garlic powder
1 small carrot
⅔ cup quick-cooking barley
½ cup frozen sliced green onion (see tip, page 39)
1 tablespoon frozen snipped parsley (see tip, page 39)

■ In a medium saucepan combine water, chicken bouillon granules, pepper, and garlic powder. Bring to boiling. Meanwhile, shred carrot (you should have about ½ cup).

■ Stir carrot, barley, and frozen onion into boiling mixture in saucepan. Return to boiling, then reduce heat. Cover and simmer for 12 to 15 minutes or till barley is tender. Just before serving, stir in parsley. Makes 4 servings.

PER SERVING

Calories	90
Protein	3 g
Carbohydrate	19 g
Fat	0 g
Cholesterol	0 mg
Sodium	100 mg
Potassium	135 mg

TIMETABLE

Total preparation time: 25 minutes

20 minutes or less

VEGETABLE-SAUCED FETTUCCINE

4 ounces fettuccine
1 cup sliced fresh mushrooms
¼ cup frozen chopped onion (see tip, page 39)
2 tablespoons dry red wine *or* water
½ of a medium zucchini
1 15½-ounce jar chunk-style meatless spaghetti sauce
2 tablespoons frozen snipped parsley (see tip, page 39)
½ teaspoon bottled minced garlic *or* ⅛ teaspoon garlic powder

■ Cook pasta according to package directions, *except* use a large saucepan and 5 cups *hot* water. Drain.

■ While pasta is cooking, in a medium saucepan combine mushrooms, onion, and wine or water. Cook, uncovered, over medium-high heat about 3 minutes or till tender. Meanwhile, slice zucchini.

■ Add zucchini, spaghetti sauce, parsley, and garlic to mushroom mixture in saucepan. Bring to boiling, then reduce the heat. Simmer, uncovered, about 5 minutes or till zucchini is tender.

■ To serve, transfer hot pasta to a large serving bowl. Pour sauce over pasta, then toss lightly till coated. Make 6 servings.

PER SERVING

Calories	144
Protein	5 g
Carbohydrate	26 g
Fat	2 g
Cholesterol	0 mg
Sodium	680 mg
Potassium	132 mg

TIMETABLE

Total preparation time: 20 minutes

20 minutes or less

PARSLEY-PESTO-STYLE TOSS

Some for now and some for later: Make a double batch of the pesto, then freeze half to have on hand for another time. (Pictured on pages 122 and 123.)

5 ounces spaghetti
1 cup lightly packed
    fresh parsley sprigs with
    stems (1 ounce)
¼ cup reduced-calorie creamy
    Italian salad dressing
2 teaspoons dried basil,
    crushed
2 tablespoons grated
    Parmesan cheese

■ Cook pasta according to package directions, *except* use a large saucepan and 5 cups *hot* water. Drain.

■ While pasta is cooking, prepare pesto. In a blender container or food processor bowl combine parsley, salad dressing, and basil. Cover and blend or process till smooth. (When necessary, stop and scrape the sides of the container.)

■ Transfer hot pasta to a large serving bowl. Add parsley-pesto mixture to pasta. Toss till pasta is coated. To serve, transfer to a serving dish, then sprinkle pasta with Parmesan cheese. Makes 5 servings.

PER SERVING

Calories	141
Protein	5 g
Carbohydrate	23 g
Fat	3 g
Cholesterol	2 mg
Sodium	366 mg
Potassium	108 mg

TIMETABLE

Total preparation time:
20 minutes

20 minutes or less

HERB BISCUITS

Make to your liking. You pick the flavor of cheese and herb for these tiny biscuits. (Pictured on page 123.)

1 tablespoon grated
    Romano *or* Parmesan
    cheese
½ teaspoon dried basil
    or oregano, crushed
    Dash garlic powder
    Nonstick spray coating
1 4½-ounce package (6)
    refrigerated biscuits
1 tablespoon skim milk

■ Preheat the oven to 450°. Meanwhile, for herb mixture, in a small bowl combine Romano or Parmesan cheese, basil or oregano, and garlic powder.

■ Spray a 7½x3½x2-inch loaf pan with nonstick coating. Using kitchen shears, cut each biscuit into 4 pieces. Place biscuit pieces in the prepared pan. Brush with milk, then sprinkle with herb mixture.

■ Bake in the 450° oven for 8 to 10 minutes or till golden. Makes 6 servings.

PER SERVING

Calories	55
Protein	2 g
Carbohydrate	10 g
Fat	1 g
Cholesterol	1 mg
Sodium	246 mg
Potassium	24 mg

TIMETABLE

Preparation time:
10 minutes

Cooking time:
8 to 10 minutes

SQUASH-APPLE BAKE

Perfect for fall meals when acorn squash and apples are in their prime.

1 ¾-pound acorn squash
2 medium cooking apples
　Lemon juice
2 tablespoons raisins
　Dash ground cinnamon
2 tablespoons reduced-calorie
　　pancake and waffle syrup

■ Preheat the oven to 350°. Meanwhile, cut squash into ½-inch-thick round slices. Core apples. Cut apples into ½-inch-thick round slices. Brush apple slices with lemon juice to prevent browning.

■ In a 1-quart casserole layer squash and apples. Sprinkle with raisins and cinnamon. Bake, covered, in the 350° oven for 50 to 60 minutes or till squash is tender. Before serving, drizzle squash and apples with syrup. Makes 4 servings.

PER SERVING

Calories	106
Protein	1 g
Carbohydrate	27 g
Fat	0 g
Cholesterol	0 mg
Sodium	22 mg
Potassium	413 mg

TIMETABLE

Preparation time:
15 minutes

Cooking time:
50 to 60 minutes

EATING OUT TIPS

It's a challenge to eat right when you dine away from home. There are so many luscious foods ready to tempt the dieter. So, here are some simple suggestions for eating out healthfully and enjoyably without destroying a diet.
● Park your car a few blocks away from the restaurant and walk the rest of the way. Exercise (yes, even a stroll) speeds your metabolism.
● Munch on an apple or orange before a lunch or dinner outing. You'll cut the edge off your appetite and order less food.
● Arrive for a dinner reservation right on time, or even a little late. That way, you'll bypass a before-dinner cocktail. Alcohol stimulates the appetite rather than depressing it.
● Drink two full glasses of water before ordering. Water tricks your stomach into feeling full.
● Make a deal with yourself that you're going to eat only three-fourths of the food on your plate. Then stop and leave the rest.

DRESSED-UP POTATOES

Nonstick spray coating
3 medium baking potatoes
(about 1 pound total)
¼ cup reduced-calorie Italian
salad dressing
1 tablespoon frozen snipped
chives (see tip, page 39)
Pepper

■ Preheat the oven to 350°. Spray an 8x1½-inch-round baking dish with nonstick coating.

■ Scrub potatoes. Cut unpeeled potatoes into ½-inch-thick slices. Toss potatoes and salad dressing in the prepared dish till potatoes are coated. Sprinkle with chives and pepper. Cover with foil.

■ Bake in the 350° oven about 55 minutes or till potatoes are tender. Makes 4 servings.

PER SERVING

Calories	106
Protein	2 g
Carbohydrate	21 g
Fat	2 g
Cholesterol	1 mg
Sodium	11 mg
Potassium	619 mg

TIMETABLE

Preparation time:
10 minutes

Cooking time:
about 55 minutes

POTATO-ONION BAKE

Next time you grill meat, grill vegetables, too. Wrap and seal this potato mixture in an 18x12-inch piece of heavy foil. Cook over medium coals about 25 minutes.

2 medium potatoes
(about 10 ounces total)
1 medium onion
1 tablespoon margarine
or butter
¼ teaspoon ground
coriander *or*
½ teaspoon dried basil,
crushed
¼ teaspoon salt
Dash pepper

■ Preheat the oven to 375°. Meanwhile, scrub potatoes and thinly slice. Peel onion, then cut into wedges. Place potatoes and onion in a 1½-quart casserole.

■ Dot margarine or butter atop vegetables. Sprinkle with coriander or basil, salt, and pepper. Toss gently. Bake, covered, in the 375° oven about 45 minutes. Makes 4 servings.

PER SERVING

Calories	89
Protein	2 g
Carbohydrate	14 g
Fat	3 g
Cholesterol	0 mg
Sodium	172 mg
Potassium	420 mg

TIMETABLE

Preparation time:
10 minutes

Cooking time:
about 45 minutes

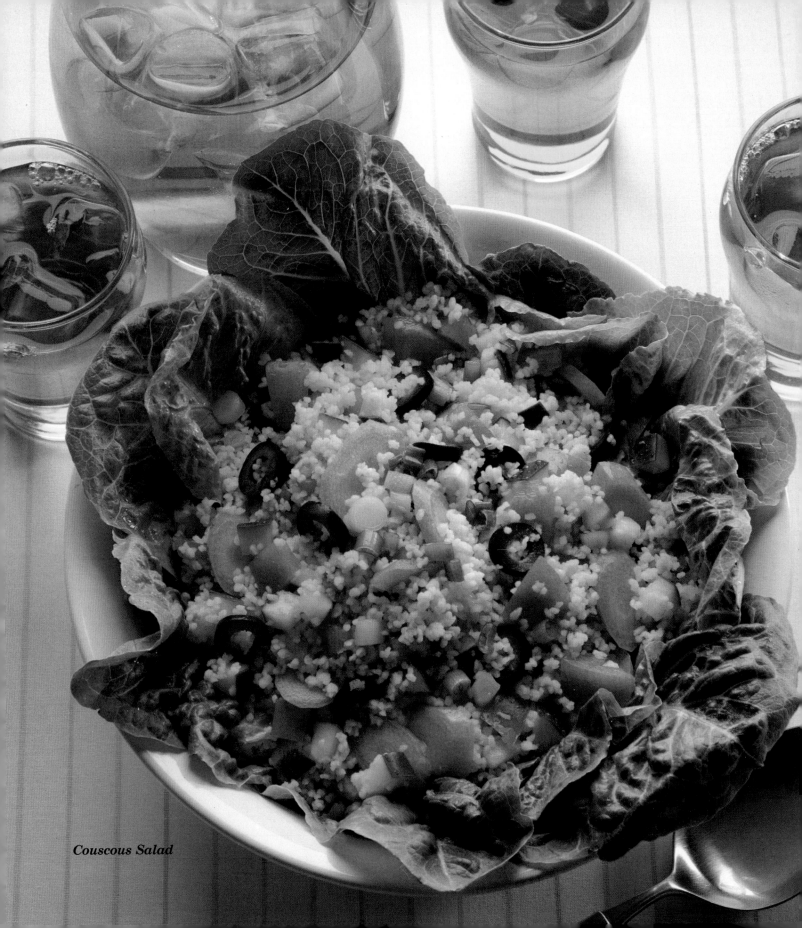

Couscous Salad

COUSCOUS SALAD

An ideal picnic dish, it's o-o-oh so refreshing. Pack the salad in your cooler with plenty of ice to keep it nice and chilly.

1 **small cucumber**
1 **medium tomato**
1 **medium carrot**
½ **cup quick-cooking couscous**
2 **tablespoons frozen sliced green onion (see tip, page 39)**
2 **tablespoons sliced pitted ripe olives**
⅓ **cup reduced-calorie Italian salad dressing**
   Romaine *or* lettuce leaves

■ Chop cucumber and tomato. Slice carrot. In a medium mixing bowl combine cucumber, tomato, carrot, *uncooked* couscous, frozen onion, and olives. Pour salad dressing over vegetable mixture. Cover and chill in the refrigerator for 1 to 1½ hours.

■ To serve, spoon couscous mixture into a bowl lined with romaine or lettuce. Makes 6 servings.

PER SERVING

Calories	69
Protein	2 g
Carbohydrate	12 g
Fat	2 g
Cholesterol	1 mg
Sodium	34 mg
Potassium	142 mg

TIMETABLE

Advance preparation time:
15 minutes

Chilling time:
1 to 1½ hours

APPLE COLESLAW

Don't bother shredding cabbage and carrot if the produce section of your supermarket carries bags of shredded coleslaw mixture.

1 **medium apple**
½ **of a small carrot**
½ **of a small stalk celery**
½ **cup plain low-fat yogurt**
2 **teaspoons sugar**
1 **teaspoon prepared mustard**
⅛ **teaspoon salt**
   Dash pepper
1½ **cups shredded cabbage**
1 **tablespoon frozen sliced green onion (see tip, page 39)**

■ Core and chop apple. Shred carrot. Thinly slice celery. In a medium bowl stir together yogurt, sugar, mustard, salt, and pepper. Add apple, then stir to coat thoroughly. Add carrot, celery, cabbage, and frozen green onion. Toss lightly till vegetables are coated. Cover and chill in the refrigerator for 1 to 1½ hours. Makes 4 servings.

PER SERVING

Calories	61
Protein	2 g
Carbohydrate	12 g
Fat	1 g
Cholesterol	2 mg
Sodium	119 mg
Potassium	233 mg

TIMETABLE

Advance preparation time:
15 minutes

Chilling time:
1 to 1½ hours

EASY TOSSED SALAD

When time is really short, use a purchased reduced- or low-calorie salad dressing instead of the dressing recipes below.

¼ of a small head romaine *or* escarole *or* 3 ounces fresh spinach
¼ of a small head leaf lettuce
½ of a medium cucumber *or* 1 medium carrot
½ cup medium radishes *or* small fresh mushrooms
½ of a small red onion
Desired salad dressing

■ Clean and tear romaine, escarole, or spinach into bite-size pieces (you should have about 2 cups). Tear leaf lettuce into bite-size pieces (you should have about 2 cups). Slice cucumber or carrot and radishes or mushrooms. Slice onion, then separate into rings.

■ In a large salad bowl combine salad greens, cucumber or carrot, radishes or mushrooms, and onion rings. Toss lightly to mix. Cover and chill till serving time. Prepare dressing; cover and chill.

■ To serve, stir or shake dressing, then pour over salad mixture. Toss lightly to coat. Makes 4 servings.

Mexican Dressing: In a small screw-top jar combine 3 tablespoons *salsa*, 1 tablespoon *lemon juice*, ½ teaspoon *sugar*, and ¼ teaspoon *dry mustard*. Cover and shake well. Chill. Makes 4 (1-tablespoon) servings.

Creamy Yogurt Dressing: In a small mixing bowl stir together ¼ cup plain low-fat *yogurt*, 2 tablespoons reduced-calorie *mayonnaise or salad dressing*, ½ teaspoon *sugar*, ½ teaspoon prepared *horseradish*, and dash *pepper*. If necessary, stir in 1 or 2 teaspoons *skim milk* for desired consistency. Cover and chill. Makes 4 (1½-tablespoon) servings.

PER SERVING

Calories	19
Protein	1 g
Carbohydrate	4 g
Fat	0 g
Cholesterol	0 mg
Sodium	7 mg
Potassium	206 mg

TIMETABLE

Advance preparation time: 20 minutes

Chilling time: up to 4 hours

Calories	7

Advance preparation time: 5 minutes

Calories	34

Advance preparation time: 5 minutes

MAKE YOUR OWN HERB VINEGARS

Do yourself a flavor favor—make an herb-flavored vinegar. Heat 2 cups *vinegar* in a stainless steel or enamel saucepan till hot, *but not boiling.* Put 2 cups tightly packed fresh *herb leaves or sprigs* (tarragon, thyme, dill, mint, or basil) into a hot, clean 1-quart jar. Pour hot vinegar over herb. Cover loosely with a glass, plastic, or cork lid till mixture cools. Then cover tightly with the nonmetallic lid and let stand in a cool, dark place for one week before using.

To store, remove herbs from jar. Label jar. Cover tightly with the nonmetallic lid. Place in a cool, dark place for up to three months.

CUCUMBER AND ORANGE SALAD

A fruit and vegetable combination delicately flavored with tarragon.

1 medium cucumber
1 small orange
2 tablespoons orange juice
2 tablespoons tarragon
    vinegar
1 tablespoon salad oil
    Lettuce leaves
2 tablespoons frozen snipped
    parsley (see tip, page 39)

■ Slice cucumber; place in one side of a 9-inch pie plate. Peel the orange. Cut orange in half lengthwise; slice orange halves crosswise into ¼-inch-thick slices. Place next to cucumber slices in pie plate.

■ In a small mixing bowl combine orange juice, vinegar, and salad oil; pour mixture over cucumber and oranges. Cover and chill for 1 to 1½ hours.

■ To serve, line salad plates with lettuce leaves. Arrange orange and cucumber slices on lettuce, alternately overlapping cucumber and orange half-slices. Sprinkle salads with parsley. Makes 4 servings.

PER SERVING

Calories	56
Protein	1 g
Carbohydrate	6 g
Fat	4 g
Cholesterol	0 mg
Sodium	3 mg
Potassium	177 mg

TIMETABLE

Advance preparation time:
10 minutes

Chilling time:
1 to 1½ hours

CURRIED RICE AND CARROT SALAD

¾ cup quick-cooking rice
½ teaspoon curry powder
½ cup canned diced carrots
¼ cup plain low-fat yogurt
2 tablespoons reduced-calorie
    creamy Italian salad
    dressing
1 teaspoon frozen snipped
    chives (see tip, page 39)
4 lettuce leaves

■ In a small saucepan cook rice according to package directions, *except* omit the margarine or butter and add the curry powder. Remove from heat. Stir carrots into cooked rice.

■ In a mixing bowl combine yogurt, salad dressing, and chives. Add the rice-carrot mixture and toss till combined. Press mixture lightly into four 6-ounce custard cups. Cover and chill in the refrigerator for 1 to 2 hours. To serve, line salad plates with lettuce leaves. Unmold rice onto lettuce. Makes 4 servings.

PER SERVING

Calories	97
Protein	2 g
Carbohydrate	18 g
Fat	2 g
Cholesterol	1 mg
Sodium	260 mg
Potassium	102 mg

TIMETABLE

Advance preparation time:
15 minutes

Chilling time:
1 to 2 hours

DILLY LAYERED SALAD

Sprinkle crunchy croutons and fresh tomatoes on the salad just before serving. The rest of the work can be done the day before.

1 cup loose-pack frozen broccoli, cauliflower, and carrots
6 cherry tomatoes
¼ cup plain low-fat yogurt
3 tablespoons reduced-calorie mayonnaise *or* salad dressing
1 tablespoon skim milk
¾ teaspoon dried dillweed
3 cups torn mixed salad greens (see tip, page 137)
1 cup sliced fresh mushrooms
2 tablespoons frozen sliced green onion (see tip, page 39)
¼ cup cheese-flavored croutons

■ Place frozen vegetables in a colander. Run *hot water* over them just till thawed. Drain well. Meanwhile, cut tomatoes into quarters. Place tomatoes in a covered container, then chill.

■ For the dressing, in a small mixing bowl stir together yogurt, mayonnaise or salad dressing, skim milk, and dillweed. Set dressing aside.

■ To assemble salad, in a 6- to 6½-cup clear glass salad bowl layer torn mixed greens, thawed vegetables, mushrooms, and onion. Spread dressing over top of salad. Cover and chill for up to 24 hours. Before serving, top with tomatoes and croutons. Serves 4.

PER SERVING

Calories	79
Protein	3 g
Carbohydrate	8 g
Fat	4 g
Cholesterol	1 mg
Sodium	121 mg
Potassium	306 mg

TIMETABLE

Advance preparation time: 15 minutes

Chilling time: up to 24 hours

BERRY-ORANGE SALAD MOLDS

Short on time? Then cut the chilling time for the individual salads from 2 hours to 20 or 30 minutes by quick-chilling the salads in the freezer before unmolding.

1½ teaspoons unflavored gelatin
½ cup cold water
½ of a 10½-ounce can mandarin orange sections (water pack)
3 tablespoons frozen orange juice concentrate
2 tablespoons honey
½ cup frozen unsweetened whole strawberries
Curly endive

■ In a small saucepan soften gelatin in cold water. Heat and stir till gelatin dissolves. Remove from heat. Meanwhile, drain oranges; set oranges aside.

■ Pour gelatin into a blender container. Add frozen juice concentrate and honey. Cover and blend just till mixed. Add frozen berries, one at a time, blending till pureed. Divide mandarin oranges among 4 individual molds *or* place oranges in a 2- to 3-cup mold, reserving 4 sections for garnish, if desired. Add the blended mixture to each mold, stirring gently to mix in the oranges. Chill salads in the refrigerator about 2 hours or till firm.

■ To serve, line individual salad plates with curly endive. Unmold individual salads onto the plates. *Or,* unmold larger mold onto endive on a serving plate. If desired, garnish with reserved oranges. Serves 4.

PER SERVING

Calories	82
Protein	2 g
Carbohydrate	19 g
Fat	0 g
Cholesterol	0 mg
Sodium	7 mg
Potassium	209 mg

TIMETABLE

Advance preparation time: 15 minutes

Chilling time: 2 to 24 hours

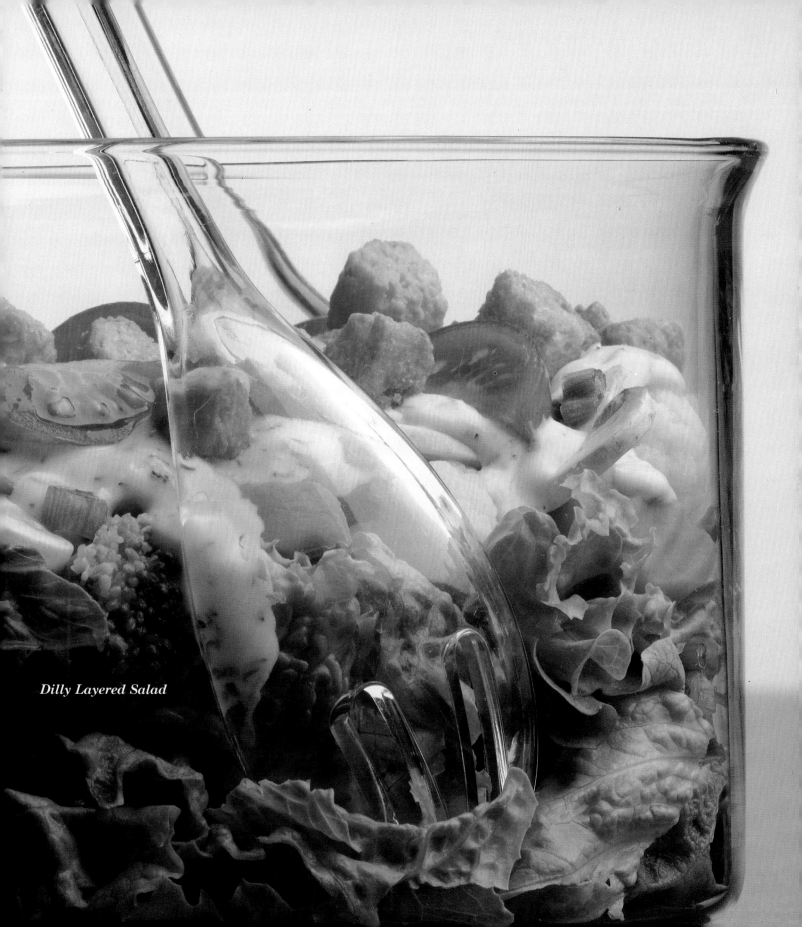

Dilly Layered Salad

CONFETTI CORN SALAD

A side dish with just that sparkle of color and flavor a calorie-trimmed meal deserves.

1   10-ounce package frozen whole kernel corn
2   teaspoons cornstarch
1   teaspoon sugar
1   teaspoon dry mustard
2   tablespoons vinegar
1   tablespoon prepared horseradish
½   of a medium carrot
½   cup frozen chopped sweet red pepper (see tip, page 39) *or* one 4-ounce jar pimiento pieces
½   cup frozen chopped green pepper (see tip, page 39)
2   tablespoons frozen sliced green onion (see tip, page 39)
6   lettuce cups

■ Cook corn according to package directions, then drain. Meanwhile, for dressing, in a small saucepan combine cornstarch, sugar, mustard, and ¼ teaspoon *salt*. Gradually stir in ⅓ cup *cold water*. Cook and stir over medium-high heat till thickened and bubbly. Then cook and stir for 2 minutes more. Remove from heat. Stir in vinegar and horseradish.

■ Coarsely shred carrot. If using pimiento, drain. In a medium mixing bowl combine corn, carrot, frozen red pepper or pimiento, frozen green pepper, and green onion. Pour dressing over corn mixture. Stir till coated. Cover and chill in the refrigerator for 6 to 24 hours, stirring occasionally. Stir mixture before serving. Serve in lettuce cups. Makes 6 servings.

PER SERVING

Calories	61
Protein	2 g
Carbohydrate	14 g
Fat	1 g
Cholesterol	0 mg
Sodium	97 mg
Potassium	202 mg

TIMETABLE

Advance preparation time: 20 minutes

Chilling time: 6 to 24 hours

DIJON SLAW

1   small carrot
1   cup cherry tomatoes
2   cups shredded cabbage
¼   cup frozen chopped green pepper (see tip, page 39)
2   tablespoons frozen sliced green onion (see tip, page 39)
2   tablespoons white wine vinegar
2   tablespoons Dijon-style mustard
2   tablespoons water
1   tablespoon salad oil
¼   teaspoon salt
¼   teaspoon dried basil, crushed
¼   teaspoon pepper

■ Thinly slice carrot and cut cherry tomatoes in half. In a medium bowl combine carrot, tomatoes, cabbage, frozen green pepper, and green onion.

■ For dressing, in a screw-top jar combine vinegar, mustard, water, salad oil, salt, basil, and pepper. Cover and shake well. Pour dressing over cabbage mixture. Toss lightly to coat. Cover. Chill in the refrigerator for 6 to 24 hours. Toss mixture lightly before serving. Makes 6 servings.

PER SERVING

Calories	44
Protein	1 g
Carbohydrate	4 g
Fat	3 g
Cholesterol	0 mg
Sodium	246 mg
Potassium	164 mg

TIMETABLE

Advance preparation time: 15 minutes

Chilling time: 6 to 24 hours

CURRIED CABBAGE SALAD

Raisins or currants add a pleasant bit of sweetness to this coleslaw mixture.

2 tablespoons reduced-calorie mayonnaise *or* salad dressing
2 tablespoons plain low-fat yogurt
½ teaspoon curry powder
½ of a small carrot
1½ cups shredded cabbage
2 tablespoons raisins *or* currants

■ For dressing, in a medium mixing bowl stir together mayonnaise or salad dressing, yogurt, and curry powder. Coarsely shred carrot.

■ Add carrot, cabbage, and raisins or currants to dressing in bowl. Toss to coat. Cover. Chill in the refrigerator for 6 to 24 hours. Toss mixture before serving. Makes 4 servings.

PER SERVING

Calories	50
Protein	1 g
Carbohydrate	7 g
Fat	2 g
Cholesterol	0 mg
Sodium	55 mg
Potassium	141 mg

TIMETABLE

Advance preparation time: 10 minutes

Chilling time: 6 to 24 hours

PACK A SALAD FOR LUNCH

Create your own take-along salads. Use plastic bags for wrapping the salad ingredients, packing the juicy ones, like tomato wedges, separately. Tear leafy greens into bite-size pieces and include a variety of other vegetables, such as green pepper strips, broccoli or cauliflower flowerets, and sliced onion, radish, zucchini, cucumber, or carrots.

For a hearty main-dish salad, pack a small can of water-pack tuna, or a small package of very thinly sliced chicken, ham, or turkey into your lunch box.

Pour your favorite reduced- or low-calorie dressing into a tiny airtight container. Then, pack everything into an insulated lunch box containing a frozen ice pack.

Be sure to take along a paper bowl or plate and a plastic fork. At lunchtime, toss the ingredients together for a fresh-tasting salad.

20 minutes or less

HERBED VEGETABLE SOUP

½ **of a small carrot**
¾ **cup loose-pack frozen broccoli, French-style green beans, onions, and red pepper**
1 **14½-ounce can beef broth *or* chicken broth**
½ **teaspoon dried minced onion**
½ **teaspoon dried basil, crushed**
¼ **teaspoon bottled minced garlic *or* dash garlic powder**

■ Shred carrot (you should have about ¼ cup). In a 1-quart microwave-safe casserole combine carrot, frozen vegetables, *¼ cup* of the beef or chicken broth, onion, basil, and garlic. Micro-cook, covered, on 100% power (high) for 3 to 5 minutes or just till vegetables are tender.

■ Stir in the remaining beef or chicken broth. Cook, covered, on high for 2 to 4 minutes more or till boiling. Makes 2 servings.

PER SERVING

Calories	36
Protein	3 g
Carbohydrate	5 g
Fat	1 g
Cholesterol	0 mg
Sodium	682 mg
Potassium	254 mg

TIMETABLE

Preparation time:
5 minutes

Cooking time:
5 to 9 minutes

---

20 minutes or less

NO-FUSS ONION SOUP

Keep all of the ingredients on hand for this quick, side-dish soup.

1½ **cups frozen chopped onion (see tip, page 39)**
1 **10½-ounce can condensed beef broth**
¾ **cup water**
½ **teaspoon Worcestershire sauce**
⅛ **teaspoon garlic powder**
⅓ **cup cheese-flavored croutons**

■ In a 1½-quart microwave-safe casserole combine frozen onion, beef broth, water, Worcestershire sauce, and garlic powder. Micro-cook, covered, on 100% power (high) for 8 to 10 minutes or till onions are tender and mixture is bubbling over entire surface; stir twice. Pass croutons. Makes 3 servings.

PER SERVING

Calories	74
Protein	6 g
Carbohydrate	11 g
Fat	1 g
Cholesterol	0 mg
Sodium	589 mg
Potassium	257 mg

TIMETABLE

Preparation time:
5 minutes

Cooking time:
8 to 10 minutes

20 minutes or less

ORANGE-SAUCED VEGETABLES

2 cups loose-pack frozen
   broccoli, baby carrots,
   and water chestnuts *or*
   other frozen mixed
   vegetable combination
½ teaspoon finely shredded
   orange peel
¼ cup orange juice
1 tablespoon Dijon-style
   mustard
1 teaspoon soy sauce

■ In a 1-quart microwave-safe casserole cook vegetables according to package microwave directions.

■ While vegetables are cooking, in a small mixing bowl combine orange peel, orange juice, mustard, and soy sauce. Stir with a fork or wire whisk till combined. Drain vegetables. Toss with orange juice mixture. Serve immediately. Makes 4 servings.

PER SERVING

Calories	45
Protein	2 g
Carbohydrate	9 g
Fat	0 g
Cholesterol	0 mg
Sodium	221 mg
Potassium	240 mg

TIMETABLE

Total preparation time:
about 15 minutes

20 minutes or less

PARMESAN TOMATO SLICES

A little extra cooking time is needed to heat the tomatoes if they come right from the refrigerator. Allow 4 to 6 minutes on high, turning the dish after 2 minutes.

3 medium tomatoes (about 1
   pound)
¼ cup plain low-fat yogurt
2 tablespoons reduced-calorie
   mayonnaise *or* salad
   dressing
¼ teaspoon dried basil,
   crushed
⅛ teaspoon lemon-pepper
   seasoning
¼ cup grated Parmesan cheese

■ Cut tomatoes into ½-inch-thick slices. Place tomato slices in an 8x8x2-inch microwave-safe baking dish, overlapping slightly, if necessary. In a small mixing bowl stir together yogurt, mayonnaise or salad dressing, basil, and lemon-pepper seasoning.

■ Dollop yogurt mixture on top of tomato slices. Sprinkle with parmesan cheese. Micro-cook, uncovered, on 100% power (high) for 3 to 4 minutes or till heated through, giving dish a half-turn after 2 minutes. Makes 4 servings.

PER SERVING

Calories	82
Protein	4 g
Carbohydrate	7 g
Fat	5 g
Cholesterol	6 mg
Sodium	178 mg
Potassium	282 mg

TIMETABLE

Preparation time:
10 minutes

Cooking time:
3 to 4 minutes

SIMPLE SQUASH

What looks like golden strands of pasta, but tastes like delicious cooked squash? Spaghetti squash, of course.

1	2¼- to 2¾-pound spaghetti squash
½	cup finely shredded *or* grated Parmesan cheese (2 ounces)
1	tablespoon frozen snipped parsley (see tip, page 39)
¼	teaspoon garlic powder
¼	teaspoon pepper

■ Pierce squash in several places (see photo 1). Place squash in a 10x6x2-inch microwave-safe baking dish. Micro-cook, uncovered, on 100% power (high) for 8 to 12 minutes or till squash is tender, turning squash over after 5 minutes. Let stand for 5 minutes.

■ Halve cooked squash lengthwise, then scoop out and discard seeds. Using a fork, shred and separate squash pulp into strands and place in a medium bowl (see photo 2). Sprinkle squash with *half* of the Parmesan cheese, the parsley, garlic powder, and pepper. Toss lightly to mix. Sprinkle squash with the remaining cheese and toss lightly again. Serves 4.

PER SERVING		TIMETABLE
Calories	**100**	Preparation time: 10 minutes
Protein	7 g	
Carbohydrate	9 g	Cooking time: 8 to 12 minutes
Fat	4 g	
Cholesterol	10 mg	Standing time: 5 minutes
Sodium	233 mg	
Potassium	451 mg	

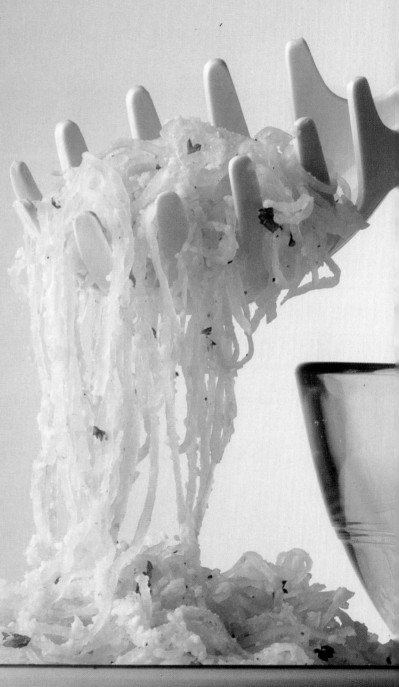

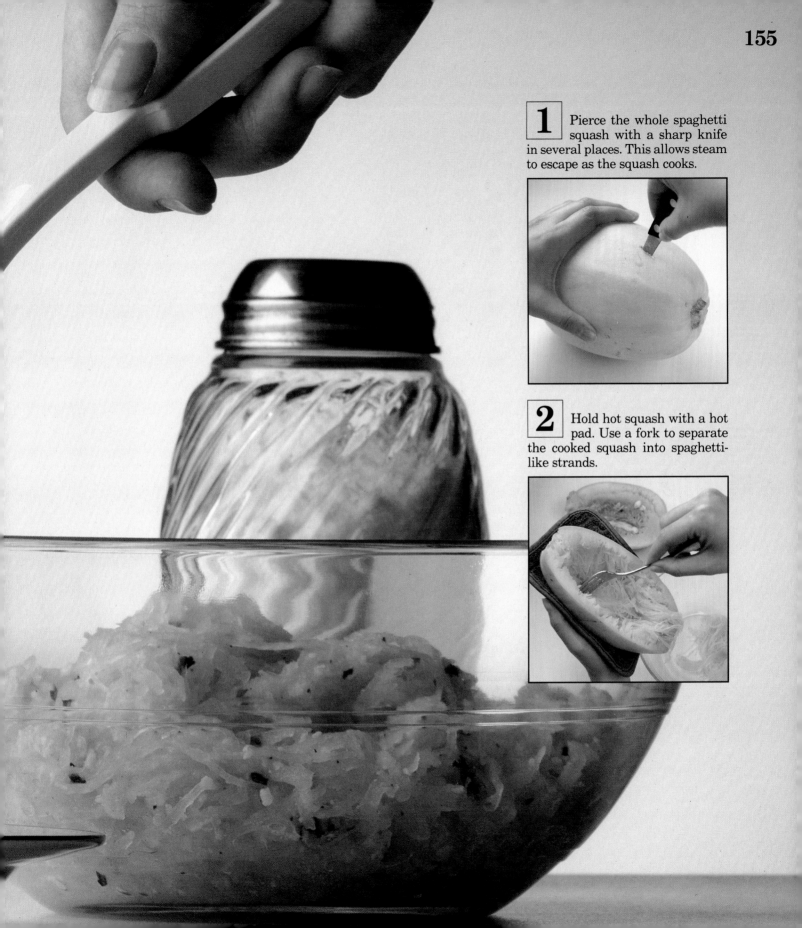

1 Pierce the whole spaghetti squash with a sharp knife in several places. This allows steam to escape as the squash cooks.

2 Hold hot squash with a hot pad. Use a fork to separate the cooked squash into spaghetti-like strands.

20 minutes or less

CREAMY DILLED SPINACH

Fix an old favorite, creamed spinach, in a delicious new way. This yogurt-creamed, microwave version is ready in about 15 minutes.

1 10-ounce package frozen chopped spinach
2 tablespoons frozen sliced green onion (see tip, page 39)
1 teaspoon margarine *or* butter
1 teaspoon cornstarch
⅛ teaspoon dried dillweed
⅓ cup water
½ teaspoon instant chicken bouillon granules
¼ cup plain low-fat yogurt
1 teaspoon all-purpose flour

■ Place frozen spinach in a 1- or 1½-quart microwave-safe casserole. Cook according to package microwave directions. Drain well. Return the drained spinach to casserole.

■ In a 2-cup microwave-safe measure combine onion and margarine or butter. Micro-cook, uncovered, on 100% power (high) for 1 to 2 minutes or till onion is tender. Stir in cornstarch and dillweed. Then stir in water and bouillon granules. Cook, uncovered, on high for 1 to 2 minutes or till thickened and bubbly, stirring every 30 seconds. Stir mixture into drained spinach in the casserole.

■ Stir together yogurt and flour. Stir into spinach mixture. Cook, uncovered, on high for 1 to 2 minutes more or till bubbly. Makes 4 servings.

PER SERVING

Calories	42
Protein	3 g
Carbohydrate	5 g
Fat	1 g
Cholesterol	1 mg
Sodium	118 mg
Potassium	380 mg

TIMETABLE

Total preparation time: about 15 minutes

20 minutes or less

HERBED VEGETABLES

A trio of herbs, plus a little garlic and Parmesan, turn vegetables into a lip-smacking side dish—all for a mere 53 calories.

1 medium tomato
1 small zucchini
½ cup frozen chopped onion (see tip, page 39)
1 teaspoon margarine *or* butter
½ teaspoon bottled minced garlic
1 9-ounce package frozen Italian-style green beans
¼ teaspoon salt
¼ teaspoon dried marjoram, crushed
¼ teaspoon dried basil, crushed
¼ teaspoon dried thyme, crushed
⅛ teaspoon pepper
1 tablespoon grated Parmesan cheese

■ Coarsely chop tomato; thinly slice zucchini. Set vegetables aside.

■ In a 1½-quart microwave-safe casserole combine onion, margarine or butter, and garlic. Micro-cook, covered, on 100% power (high) for 2 minutes.

■ Add green beans, salt, marjoram, basil, thyme, and pepper to onion mixture. Cook, covered, on high for 7 to 9 minutes or till beans are nearly crisp-tender, stirring twice.

■ Stir tomato and zucchini into green bean mixture. Micro-cook, covered, on high for 2 to 4 minutes or till heated through, stirring once. Sprinkle with Parmesan cheese. Makes 4 servings.

PER SERVING

Calories	53
Protein	3 g
Carbohydrate	8 g
Fat	2 g
Cholesterol	1 mg
Sodium	179 mg
Potassium	269 mg

TIMETABLE

Total preparation time: 20 minutes

20 minutes or less

ASPARAGUS WITH HONEY-MUSTARD SAUCE

¾ pound fresh asparagus *or*
    one 10-ounce package
    frozen asparagus spears
2 tablespoons water
¼ cup plain low-fat yogurt
1 teaspoon honey
1 teaspoon Dijon-style
    mustard
    Dash pepper

■ If using fresh asparagus, wash and break off woody bases. In an 8x8x2-inch microwave-safe baking dish combine fresh asparagus and the 2 tablespoons water. Cover with vented microwave-safe plastic wrap. Micro-cook on 100% power (high) for 4 to 6 minutes or till crisp-tender, turning the dish once. (If using frozen asparagus, cook according to package microwave directions.) Cover asparagus and let stand while preparing sauce.

■ In a 1-cup microwave-safe measure stir together yogurt, honey, mustard, and pepper. Cook on high about 45 seconds or till heated through, stirring every 15 seconds. *Do not boil.*

■ Drain asparagus. To serve, transfer asparagus to a serving platter. Pour sauce over asparagus. Serves 3.

PER SERVING

Calories	47
Protein	5 g
Carbohydrate	8 g
Fat	1 g
Cholesterol	1 mg
Sodium	66 mg
Potassium	394 mg

TIMETABLE

Total preparation time:
10 minutes

KOHLRABI AND COUSCOUS

1 medium kohlrabi
    (about 9 ounces)
2 medium carrots
2 tablespoons water
½ cup chicken broth
⅓ cup quick-cooking couscous
2 tablespoons grated
    Parmesan cheese

■ Remove and discard the leaves, stems, and woody tops from kohlrabi. Peel and cut kohlrabi into ½-inch cubes. Thinly slice carrots. Place kohlrabi, carrots, and water in a 1½-quart microwave-safe casserole. Micro-cook, covered, on 100% power (high) for 6 to 8 minutes or till vegetables are tender, rotating dish after 3 minutes. Drain and set aside.

■ In the same casserole combine chicken broth and couscous. Cook, covered, on high for 2 to 3 minutes or till broth is absorbed. Add kohlrabi mixture and Parmesan cheese to couscous mixture in casserole. Toss lightly till mixed. Cook, covered, on high about 1 minute or till heated through. Makes 6 servings.

PER SERVING

Calories	53
Protein	3 g
Carbohydrate	9 g
Fat	1 g
Cholesterol	2 mg
Sodium	114 mg
Potassium	165 mg

TIMETABLE

Total preparation time:
25 minutes

20 minutes or less

HORSERADISH-SAUCED VEGETABLES

1 **16-ounce package loose-pack frozen French-style green beans, broccoli, mushrooms, and red pepper**
2 **tablespoons frozen sliced green onion (see tip, page 39)**
1 **tablespoon water**
⅓ **cup reduced-calorie mayonnaise *or* salad dressing**
2 **to 3 tablespoons skim milk**
2 **teaspoons prepared horseradish**
⅛ **teaspoon salt**
⅛ **teaspoon pepper**
1 **4-ounce can mushroom stems and pieces**

■ In a 1½-quart microwave-safe casserole combine frozen vegetables, onion, and water. Micro-cook, covered, on 100% power (high) for 8 to 10 minutes or till vegetables are crisp-tender, stirring once. Drain and set aside.

■ While vegetables are cooking, in a small mixing bowl stir together mayonnaise or salad dressing, milk, horseradish, salt, and pepper. Drain mushrooms. Add mayonnaise mixture and mushrooms to vegetables in casserole. Stir to combine. Cook, uncovered, on high for 2 to 4 minutes or till heated through. Makes 5 servings.

PER SERVING

Calories	93
Protein	2 g
Carbohydrate	9 g
Fat	6 g
Cholesterol	0 mg
Sodium	568 mg
Potassium	196 mg

TIMETABLE

Preparation time:
5 minutes

Cooking time:
10 to 14 minutes

20 minutes or less

CHEESE-TOPPED POTATOES

Making 6 servings is easy. Double the ingredients and use a 2-quart casserole. Then, micro-cook the potato mixture for 14 to 17 minutes.

1 **large potato (about 8 ounces)**
1½ **cups shredded cabbage**
2 **tablespoons water**
1 **tablespoon frozen snipped chives (see tip, page 39)**
1 **teaspoon margarine *or* butter**
¼ **cup finely shredded cheddar cheese (1 ounce)**

■ Peel potato; cut into ½-inch cubes (you should have about 1½ cups). In a 1-quart microwave-safe casserole combine potato, cabbage, and water. Micro-cook, covered, on 100% power (high) for 8 to 10 minutes or till potato is tender, stirring once. Drain.

■ Stir in chives and margarine or butter. Add salt and pepper to taste. Sprinkle with cheese. Serves 3.

PER SERVING

Calories	118
Protein	4 g
Carbohydrate	16 g
Fat	5 g
Cholesterol	10 mg
Sodium	84 mg
Potassium	510 mg

TIMETABLE

Preparation time:
5 minutes

Cooking time:
8 to 10 minutes

WILTED ROMAINE SALAD

Cooking just till the greens begin to wilt is important. The outcome? A luscious wilted (not cooked) salad.

½ of a small head romaine *or* 3 ounces fresh spinach
1 medium orange
1 tablespoon soy sauce
¼ teaspoon dry mustard
⅛ teaspoon garlic powder
Dash ground ginger
½ cup sliced water chestnuts
2 tablespoons frozen sliced green onion (see tip, page 39)
½ cup sliced fresh mushrooms
1 teaspoon cooked bacon pieces

■ Clean and tear romaine or spinach into bite-size pieces (you should have about 3½ cups). Cut half of the orange into thin slices, then halve the slices crosswise; set aside. Squeeze juice from other half of orange (you should have about 3 tablespoons juice).

■ In a 1½-quart microwave-safe casserole combine orange juice, soy sauce, mustard, garlic powder, and ginger. Stir in romaine or spinach, water chestnuts, and green onion. Toss lightly to coat. Micro-cook, covered, on 100% power (high) for 1 to 1½ minutes or till romaine just begins to wilt, stirring once. Add mushrooms and toss. Spoon mixture onto salad plates. Sprinkle with bacon pieces. Garnish with reserved orange half-slices. Makes 4 servings.

PER SERVING

Calories	44
Protein	2 g
Carbohydrate	8 g
Fat	1 g
Cholesterol	1 mg
Sodium	279 mg
Potassium	209 mg

TIMETABLE

Total preparation time: 15 minutes

GET KIDS INVOLVED IN GOOD NUTRITION

It's important to establish good eating habits early in a child's life. And, here are a few ways to involve kids in good nutrition:
• Discuss what makes a healthful meal. Then set up guidelines for family meals to include a vegetable, fruit, whole grain, milk, and protein food. Let them help with menu planning.
• Allow your children to help prepare the food. Depending on their ages, let them stir together a yogurt fruit salad, toss a vegetable salad, or mash the potatoes.
• Put their green thumbs to work in a small garden. Carrots, green beans, lettuce, and spinach the kids grow themselves will have new appeal.

De-light-ful Desserts

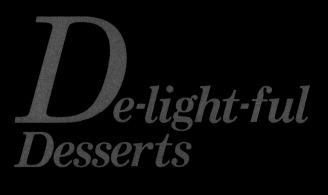

Being on a diet doesn't have to mean giving up desserts! Our recipes prove that you can stick to a diet and eat dessert, too. Each is light in calories—150 calories or less per serving—yet takes little effort to prepare.

Go ahead. Satisfy your sweet tooth with a delicious dessert. You'll find plenty to choose from.

Cheese-Topped Pears
(see recipe, page 185)

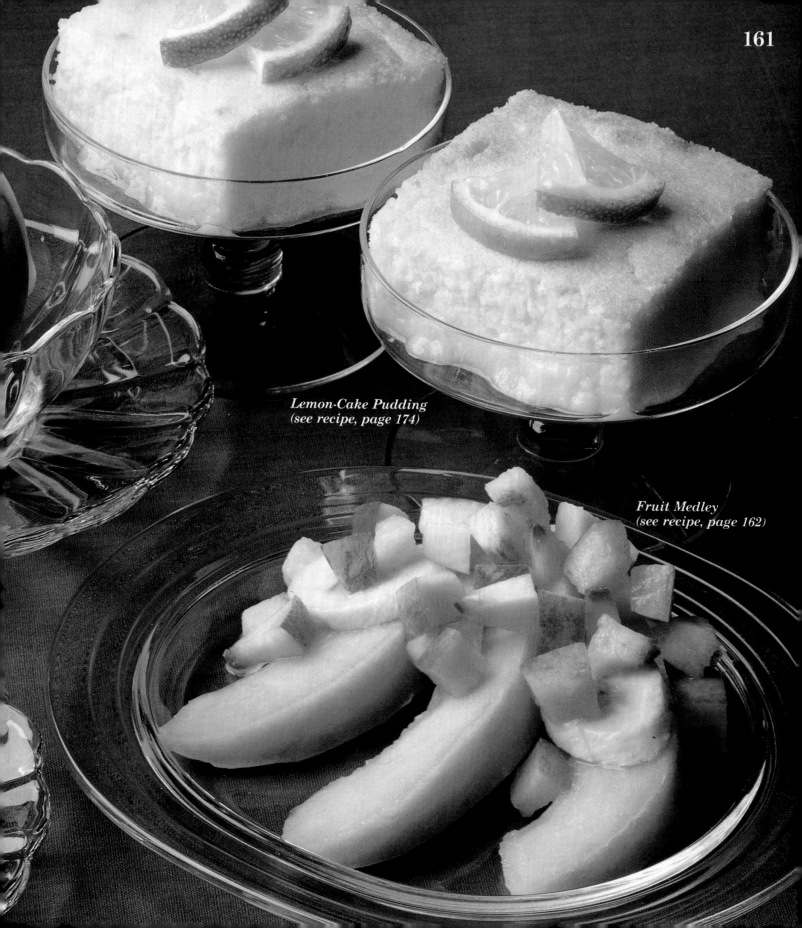

Lemon-Cake Pudding
(see recipe, page 174)

Fruit Medley
(see recipe, page 162)

FRUIT MEDLEY

Toast pine nuts in a small, preheated skillet for 1 minute over medium heat. They add only 34 calories to each serving. (Pictured on page 161.)

3 tablespoons orange juice
1 tablespoon lime *or* lemon
   juice
1 tablespoon honey
1 large nectarine *or* peach
1 large banana
1 cantaloupe *or* ½ of a
   honeydew melon
2 tablespoons pine nuts,
   toasted (optional)
   Lime peel (optional)

■ In a small bowl combine orange juice, lime or lemon juice, and honey.

■ Pit and coarsely chop nectarine. (*Or,* peel peach, if desired, and coarsely chop.) Add nectarine or peach to fruit juice mixture. Bias-slice banana into ¼-inch pieces; add to fruit juice mixture.

■ Remove seeds from cantaloupe or honeydew melon, then cut into 12 thin slices. Cut off peel. On 4 individual dessert plates fan the melon slices. Top each serving with ¼ of the fruit mixture. If desired, sprinkle with pine nuts and garnish with a lime peel curl. Makes 4 servings.

PER SERVING

Calories	113
Protein	2 g
Carbohydrate	28 g
Fat	1 g
Cholesterol	0 mg
Sodium	13 mg
Potassium	631 mg

TIMETABLE

Total preparation time:
25 minutes

ORANGE-PEACH GELATIN

This delicate dessert has a scrumptious peach color and flavor.

¾ cup water
1 4-serving-size package
   low-calorie orange-
   flavored gelatin
½ cup ice cubes
2 cups frozen unsweetened
   peach slices (8 ounces)
½ of a 4-ounce container
   frozen whipped dessert
   topping, thawed (see tip,
   page 167)

■ Bring water to boiling. Place gelatin and boiling water in a blender container. Cover and blend at low speed till gelatin is dissolved. Add the ice cubes to the blender container. Cover and blend till ice is chopped and melted.

■ Add frozen peaches to mixture in blender. Cover and blend until smooth. Pour mixture into a mixing bowl and fold in the dessert topping. Spoon gelatin mixture into 6 dessert dishes. Chill for 5 minutes in the freezer, then chill for 15 minutes in the refrigerator. Makes 6 servings.

PER SERVING

Calories	51
Protein	1 g
Carbohydrate	6 g
Fat	2 g
Cholesterol	0 mg
Sodium	5 mg
Potassium	104 mg

TIMETABLE

Total preparation time:
30 minutes

20 minutes or less

BLUEBERRIES 'N' CREAM

Don't stop with blueberries! Try the creamy cheese sauce over fresh nectarines, peaches, strawberries, or any combination that sounds good.

½ of an 8-ounce container reduced-calorie soft-style cream cheese
½ of an 8-ounce carton plain low-fat yogurt
2 tablespoons reduced-calorie orange marmalade
2 cups fresh blueberries

■ In a small mixer bowl beat cream cheese till softened. Add yogurt and marmalade. Beat till smooth.

■ Rinse blueberries and drain thoroughly. Place ½ *cup* of the blueberries in each of 4 dessert dishes.

■ Spoon the cream cheese mixture over the blueberries in the serving dishes. Serve immediately. Makes 4 servings.

PER SERVING

Calories	132
Protein	5 g
Carbohydrate	17 g
Fat	5 g
Cholesterol	18 mg
Sodium	197 mg
Potassium	198 mg

TIMETABLE

Total preparation time: 10 minutes

20 minutes or less

SPICY PEACHES

Save even more time—prepare this recipe in your microwave oven and serve it from the same dish!

2 tablespoons brown sugar
1 tablespoon rum
1 teaspoon margarine *or* butter
1 teaspoon lime *or* lemon juice
¼ teaspoon ground allspice *or* ground cinnamon
2 cups frozen unsweetened peach slices (8 ounces)
¼ cup plain low-fat yogurt

■ In a medium saucepan combine brown sugar, rum, margarine or butter, lime or lemon juice, and allspice or cinnamon.

■ Cook and stir over medium heat till mixture is bubbly. Add frozen peach slices. Cook, uncovered, till peaches are thawed, stirring occasionally.

■ To serve, spoon the warm fruit into 4 dessert dishes. Dollop with yogurt. Makes 4 servings.

Microwave oven: In a 1-quart microwave-safe casserole combine brown sugar, rum, margarine or butter, lime or lemon juice, and allspice or cinnamon. Micro-cook, uncovered, on 100% power (high) for 30 to 45 seconds or till margarine is melted; stir to mix well. Add frozen peach slices. Toss to coat. Cook, uncovered, on high for 3 to 3½ minutes or till peaches are thawed, stirring twice. Serve as above.

PER SERVING

Calories	78
Protein	1 g
Carbohydrate	14 g
Fat	1 g
Cholesterol	1 mg
Sodium	24 mg
Potassium	174 mg

TIMETABLE

Total preparation time: 10 minutes

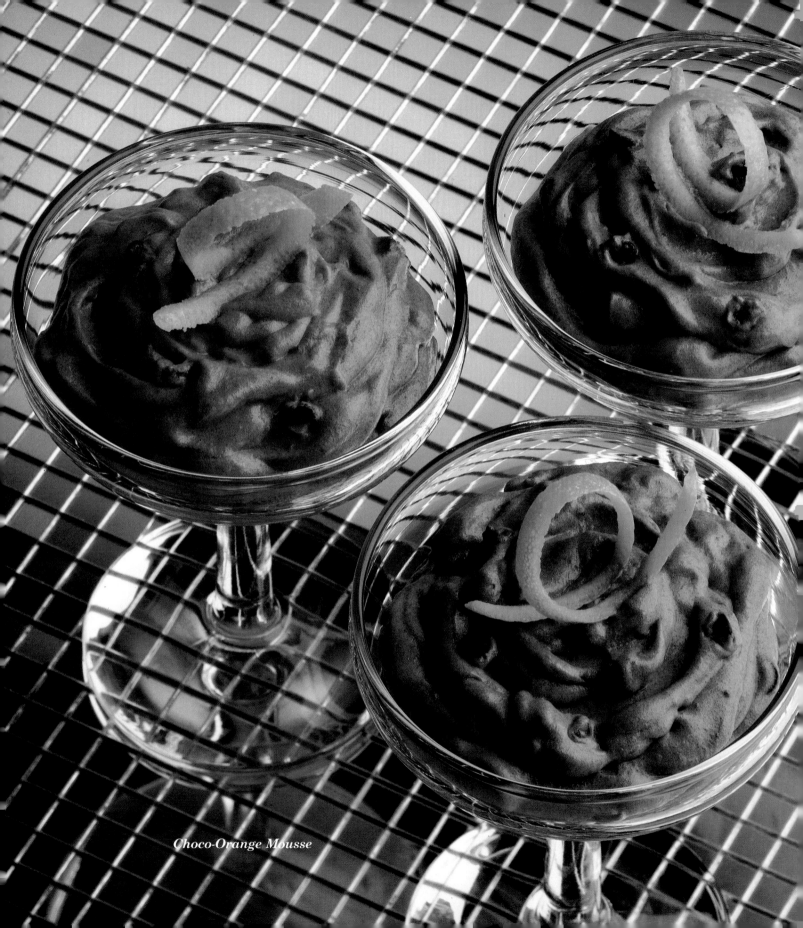

Choco-Orange Mousse

CHOCO-ORANGE MOUSSE

Take a bite and savor the velvety richness—guilt free.

1 1.4-ounce envelope whipped
    dessert topping mix
1½ cups cold skim milk
½ cup orange juice
1 4-serving-size package
    reduced-calorie *instant*
    chocolate pudding mix
3 tablespoons miniature
    semisweet chocolate
    pieces
    Orange peel curls (optional)

■ In a small mixer bowl combine topping mix and ½ *cup* of the milk. Beat with an electric mixer on high speed about 2 minutes or till mixture forms stiff peaks (tips stand straight).

■ Add the remaining milk, orange juice, and pudding mix. Beat with an electric mixer on low speed just till mixed. Then beat on medium speed about 2 minutes more or till well mixed. Fold in the miniature chocolate pieces.

■ Spoon the mixture into 6 dessert dishes. Quick-chill in the freezer about 20 minutes before serving. Garnish with orange peel curls, if desired. Serves 6.

Vanilla-Orange Mousse: Prepare Choco-Orange Mousse as above, *except* substitute one 4-serving-size package *reduced-calorie instant vanilla pudding mix* for the chocolate pudding mix.

PER SERVING

Calories	116
Protein	3 g
Carbohydrate	16 g
Fat	5 g
Cholesterol	1 mg
Sodium	280 mg
Potassium	169 mg

TIMETABLE

Preparation time:
10 minutes

Chilling time:
about 20 minutes

Calories	116

20 minutes or less

PEACH-A-BERRY FROST

Indulge your sweet tooth the next time you feel an ice cream craving coming on.

1 cup frozen unsweetened
    peach slices (4 ounces)
½ cup skim milk
¼ cup loose-pack frozen red
    raspberries
1 tablespoon honey
¼ teaspoon vanilla

■ In a blender container or food processor bowl combine frozen peaches, milk, frozen raspberries, honey, and vanilla. Cover and blend or process till fruit mixture is smooth. Pour fruit mixture into 2 dessert dishes; serve immediately. Makes 2 servings.

PER SERVING

Calories	85
Protein	3 g
Carbohydrate	20 g
Fat	0 g
Cholesterol	1 mg
Sodium	32 mg
Potassium	242 mg

TIMETABLE

Total preparation time:
10 minutes

20 minutes or less

DOUBLE-BERRY DELIGHTS

This red, white, and blueberry dessert is a star-spangled hit.

3 tablespoons sugar
2 teaspoons cornstarch
1 cup fresh *or* frozen
    blueberries
⅓ cup orange juice
2 ounces Neufchâtel cheese
1 tablespoon powdered sugar
2 teaspoons skim milk
2 cups fresh *or* loose-pack
    frozen red raspberries
Orange peel (optional)

■ In a small saucepan combine sugar and cornstarch. Stir in ½ *cup* of the fresh or frozen blueberries and the orange juice. Cook and stir till mixture is thickened and bubbly, then cook and stir for 2 minutes more.

■ Remove from heat and stir in remaining blueberries. Cover and chill in the refrigerator while preparing the cheese mixture.

■ For cheese mixture, in a small mixer bowl beat Neufchâtel cheese till softened. Beat in powdered sugar and milk.

■ To serve, in 6 dessert dishes alternately layer raspberries and blueberry mixture. Drizzle cheese mixture atop each serving. Garnish with orange peel, if desired. Makes 6 servings.

PER SERVING

Calories	96
Protein	2 g
Carbohydrate	18 g
Fat	3 g
Cholesterol	7 mg
Sodium	40 mg
Potassium	124 mg

TIMETABLE

Total preparation time:
20 minutes

20 minutes or less

STRAWBERRY CREAM

¾ cup low-fat cottage cheese
1 cup frozen unsweetened
    whole strawberries
1 cup vanilla ice milk
1 teaspoon frozen, finely
    shredded orange peel
    (see tip, page 66)
Assorted fresh fruit
    (optional)

■ Place cottage cheese in a blender container. Cover and blend till smooth. Add frozen strawberries, ice milk, and orange peel. Cover and blend till smooth, stopping to scrape down sides as necessary.

■ Pour strawberry mixture into 4 stemmed glasses and serve at once. Garnish with a small piece of fresh fruit, if desired. Makes 4 servings.

PER SERVING

Calories	97
Protein	7 g
Carbohydrate	12 g
Fat	2 g
Cholesterol	8 mg
Sodium	198 mg
Potassium	163 mg

TIMETABLE

Total preparation time:
10 minutes

CHEESY LEMON PUDDING

This luscious lemon treat is light eating at its best. Enjoy every bite without cheating on your diet.

1 cup low-fat ricotta cheese
2 tablespoons frozen lemonade concentrate
1 4-serving-size package reduced-calorie *instant* vanilla pudding mix
Ground nutmeg (optional)

■ In a small bowl combine ricotta cheese and lemonade concentrate. Set aside. Prepare pudding according to package directions, using *skim milk*.

■ Divide *half* of the pudding among 5 dessert dishes. Top each with some of the ricotta mixture. Pour remaining pudding atop ricotta mixture in the dishes. Sprinkle lightly with ground nutmeg, if desired. Makes 5 servings.

PER SERVING

Calories	134
Protein	9 g
Carbohydrate	15 g
Fat	4 g
Cholesterol	17 mg
Sodium	325 mg
Potassium	229 mg

TIMETABLE

Total preparation time: 10 minutes

APRICOTS WITH RASPBERRY TOPPER

½ of an 8-ounce carton lemon, pineapple, *or* vanilla low-fat yogurt
½ cup fresh *or* loose-pack frozen raspberries
1 tablespoon coconut *or* sliced almonds
1 16-ounce can unpeeled apricot halves in light syrup

■ In a small bowl combine the lemon, pineapple, or vanilla yogurt and the fresh or frozen raspberries. In a small skillet toast coconut over high heat about 2 minutes or till lightly browned; stir constantly to brown evenly. Set aside.

■ Drain apricot halves. Then cut each apricot half in half again. Divide apricots among 4 dessert dishes. Spoon ¼ of the yogurt mixture over apricots in each dessert dish. Sprinkle with toasted coconut or almonds. Makes 4 servings.

PER SERVING

Calories	68
Protein	2 g
Carbohydrate	14 g
Fat	1 g
Cholesterol	1 mg
Sodium	32 mg
Potassium	258 mg

TIMETABLE

Total preparation time: 10 minutes

THAWING AHEAD

Get in the habit of placing frozen whipped dessert topping in your refrigerator as soon as you buy it. Or, put the topping in your refrigerator the night before you plan to use it. Then the topping will be thawed and ready to use. If you don't need it, refreeze the topping.

20 minutes or less

LEMON-YOGURT BLUEBERRIES

For a change of taste, serve the lemon-yogurt sauce atop melon balls, strawberries, or kiwi fruit slices.

2 teaspoons frozen lemonade concentrate
½ cup vanilla low-fat yogurt
⅓ cup frozen whipped dessert topping, thawed (see tip, page 167)
2 cups blueberries
Lemon slices (optional)

■ In a small bowl stir frozen lemonade concentrate into yogurt. Fold in thawed dessert topping.

■ Divide blueberries among 4 dessert dishes. Spoon ¼ of the yogurt mixture atop berries in each dish. Garnish with lemon slices, if desired. Serves 4.

PER SERVING

Calories	92
Protein	2 g
Carbohydrate	17 g
Fat	2 g
Cholesterol	2 mg
Sodium	26 mg
Potassium	135 mg

TIMETABLE

Total preparation time: 10 minutes

20 minutes or less

GLAZED PAPAYA

Be sure the papaya is ripe before using it. You'll know it's ready when it yields to gentle pressure.

1 papaya
3 tablespoons reduced-calorie apple jelly
2 teaspoons lime juice
⅛ teaspoon ground ginger
Lime slices

■ Preheat the oven to 375°. Meanwhile, peel, seed, and cut papaya lengthwise into eighths. Place papaya slices in a shallow baking pan.

■ For glaze, in a small saucepan melt jelly over low heat. Stir in lime juice and ginger. Brush *half* of the glaze over the papaya slices. Bake in the 375° oven for 8 to 10 minutes. Remove from oven and brush papaya slices with the remaining glaze. Divide papaya slices between 2 or 3 dessert plates. Pass lime slices to serve with papaya. Makes 2 or 3 servings.

PER SERVING

Calories	97
Protein	1 g
Carbohydrate	25 g
Fat	0 g
Cholesterol	0 mg
Sodium	40 mg
Potassium	451 mg

TIMETABLE

Preparation time: 10 minutes

Cooking time: 8 to 10 minutes

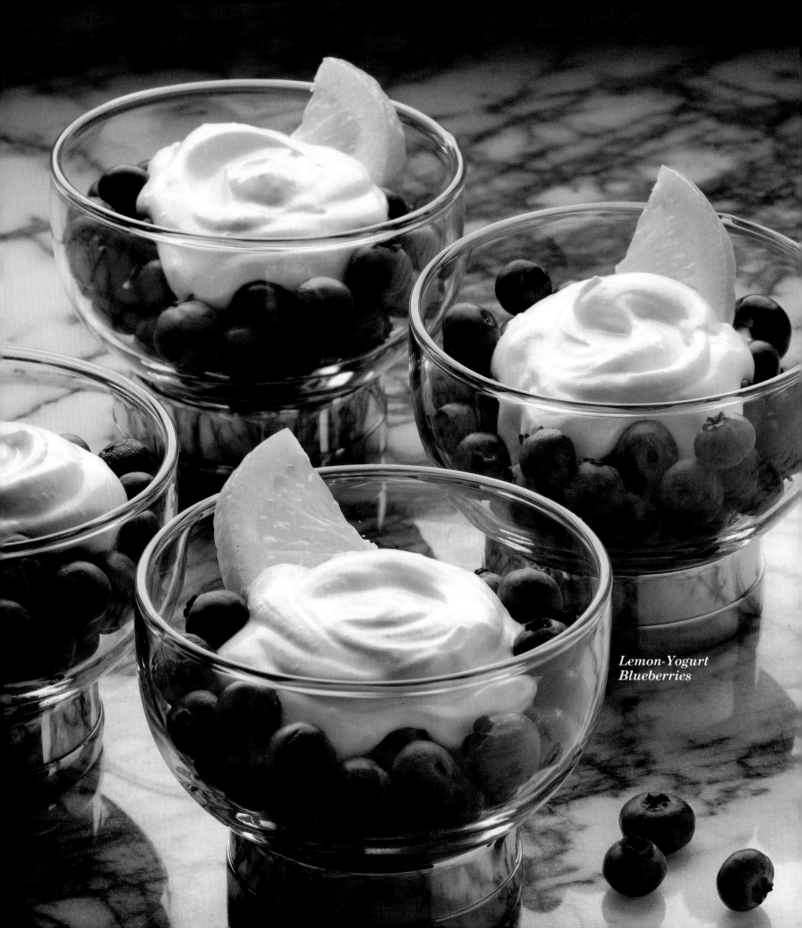

Lemon-Yogurt Blueberries

20 minutes or less

CHOCOLATE TOPPING

Spoon this smooth, milk chocolaty sauce over small scoops of ice milk or fresh fruit for a calorie-trimmed treat.

1 tablespoon sugar
1 tablespoon cornstarch
1 cup skim milk
3 tablespoons semisweet
    chocolate pieces
1 teaspoon vanilla

■ In a small saucepan combine sugar and cornstarch. Stir in milk. Cook and stir over medium heat till mixture thickens and bubbles. Then cook and stir for 2 minutes more.

■ Remove mixture from the heat and stir in the semisweet chocolate pieces and vanilla. (If necessary, beat smooth with a rotary beater.) Serve warm. (*Or*, if served chilled, stir till smooth before serving.) Makes 8 (2-tablespoon) servings.

PER SERVING

Calories	41
Protein	1 g
Carbohydrate	6 g
Fat	1 g
Cholesterol	1 mg
Sodium	16 mg
Potassium	63 mg

TIMETABLE

Total preparation time:
10 minutes

20 minutes or less

POACHED APPLES AND ORANGES

¾ cup water
¼ cup sugar
 2 medium oranges
 2 medium apples
 2 tablespoons orange liqueur
    Fresh mint sprigs (optional)

■ In a medium saucepan combine water and sugar. Bring mixture to boiling. Meanwhile, peel oranges and cut each into 6 slices; set aside. Core apples and cut each into 8 wedges; cut each wedge in half. Add apples to mixture in saucepan.

■ Return mixture to boiling, then reduce the heat. Cover and simmer for 5 to 6 minutes or just till apples are tender, gently turning occasionally. Add oranges during the last minute of cooking to heat through.

■ Remove fruit from the saucepan with a slotted spoon, reserving liquid in saucepan. Divide fruit among 4 dessert dishes. Stir orange liqueur into reserved liquid in saucepan; spoon over fruit in dessert dishes. Garnish with fresh mint springs, if desired. Serve warm. Makes 4 servings.

PER SERVING

Calories	143
Protein	1 g
Carbohydrate	37 g
Fat	0 g
Cholesterol	0 mg
Sodium	0 mg
Potassium	198 mg

TIMETABLE

Total preparation time:
20 minutes

STUFFED APPLES

Here's a top-of-the-stove "baked" apple that's tops in taste!

1 **6-ounce can unsweetened pineapple juice**
⅛ **teaspoon ground cinnamon**
4 **small cooking apples**
4 **pitted dates**

■ In a medium saucepan combine the pineapple juice and cinnamon.

■ Remove core and a strip of peel from the top of each apple. Place apples in the pineapple juice mixture in the saucepan. Stuff center of each apple with *1* pitted date. Bring mixture to boiling, then reduce the heat. Cover and simmer for 10 minutes or till apples are tender when tested with a fork.

■ To serve, spoon apples and juice into dessert dishes. Makes 4 servings.

PER SERVING

Calories	105
Protein	0 g
Carbohydrate	27 g
Fat	0 g
Cholesterol	0 mg
Sodium	1 mg
Potassium	225 mg

TIMETABLE

Total preparation time:
20 minutes

FLAVORED BEVERAGES FOR DESSERT

Instead of something sweet for dessert, try a steaming cup of coffee or tea to end the meal.

For a special treat, brew one of the flavored dessert coffee blends. Check the selection of dessert coffees available in specialty coffee shops. You'll find they range from flavored regular coffees to decaffeinated blends. Some coffees are flavored with spices or vanilla, others are flavored with nuts or chocolate. Dress up the coffee with a dollop of thawed, frozen whipped dessert topping and a sprinkling of ground cinnamon or nutmeg. (A tablespoon of the whipped dessert topping adds about 15 calories.)

Flavored teas are another possible meal ending. Look for spice- and fruit-flavored varieties at the supermarket.

LEMON PUFF

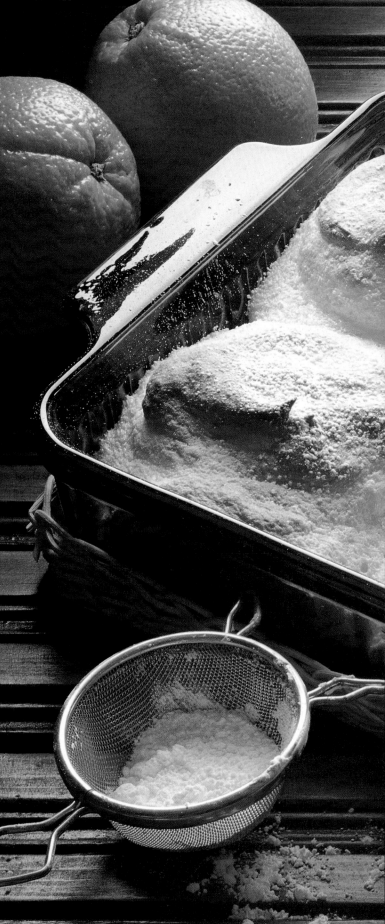

As easily as a chameleon changes color, this fluffy dessert can change flavor. Go from lemon to orange by substituting orange juice and peel for the lemon.

Nonstick spray coating
4 eggs
2 teaspoons all-purpose flour
½ teaspoon frozen, finely shredded lemon peel
    (see tip, page 66)
2 tablespoons lemon juice
1 teaspoon vanilla
3 tablespoons sugar
1 tablespoon powdered sugar

■ Preheat the oven to 375°. Meanwhile, generously spray an 8x8x2-inch baking dish with nonstick coating. Set aside. Separate eggs, reserving 2 of the egg yolks for another use. Beat the remaining yolks with an electric mixer on high speed about 2 minutes or till well combined. Fold in flour; set aside.

■ Wash and dry beaters thoroughly. In a large mixer bowl beat egg whites, lemon peel, lemon juice, and vanilla with an electric mixer on medium speed till soft peaks form (tips curl). Gradually add the 3 tablespoons sugar while beating at high speed till stiff peaks form (tips stand straight).

■ Fold some of the egg white mixture into yolk mixture (see photo 1). Then, gently fold yolk mixture into remaining stiffly beaten egg whites. Spoon mixture into prepared baking dish, forming 4 even mounds.

■ Bake in the 375° oven for 8 to 10 minutes or till golden and a knife inserted near the center comes out clean (see photo 2). Sift powdered sugar atop. Serve immediately. Makes 4 servings.

PER SERVING		TIMETABLE
Calories	**96**	Preparation time: 25 minutes
Protein	5 g	
Carbohydrate	13 g	Cooking time:
Fat	3 g	8 to 10 minutes
Cholesterol	136 mg	
Sodium	55 mg	
Potassium	64 mg	

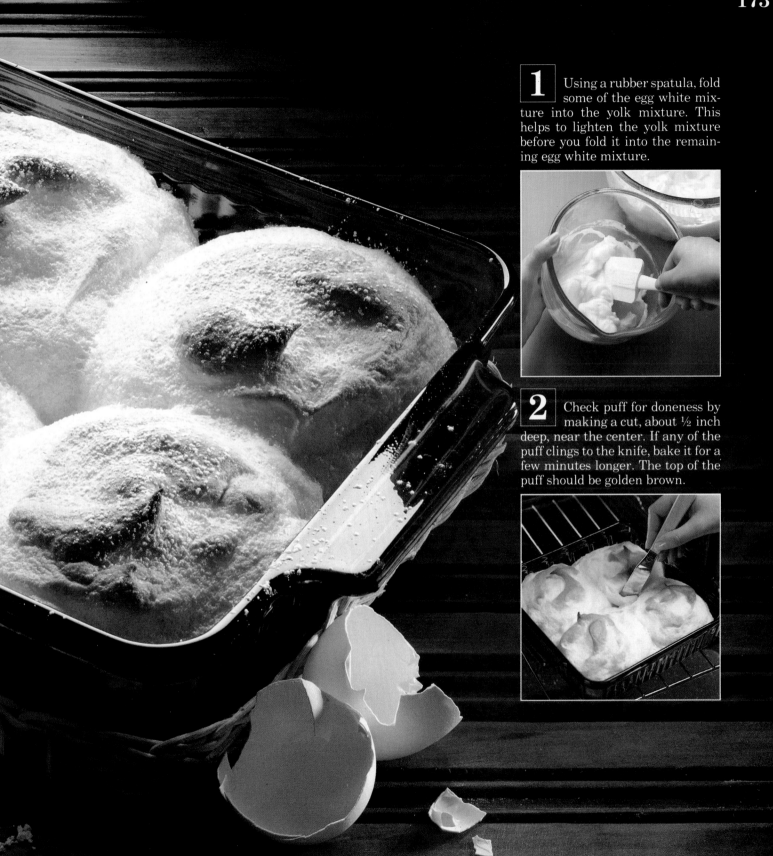

1 Using a rubber spatula, fold some of the egg white mixture into the yolk mixture. This helps to lighten the yolk mixture before you fold it into the remaining egg white mixture.

2 Check puff for doneness by making a cut, about ½ inch deep, near the center. If any of the puff clings to the knife, bake it for a few minutes longer. The top of the puff should be golden brown.

MOCHA SOUFFLÉ

6 egg whites
⅓ cup sugar
3 tablespoons unsweetened cocoa powder
2 tablespoons cornstarch
1 teaspoon instant coffee crystals
1 cup evaporated skim milk
2 teaspoons vanilla
Nonstick spray coating
1 tablespoon sugar
½ teaspoon cream of tartar

■ Preheat the oven to 375°. Place egg whites in a large mixer bowl; let stand at room temperature. Meanwhile, in a saucepan combine the ⅓ cup sugar, cocoa powder, cornstarch, and coffee crystals. Stir in milk. Cook and stir mocha mixture over medium heat till mixture is thickened and bubbly. Remove from heat. Stir in vanilla. Cover surface of mixture with clear plastic wrap. Set aside.

■ Spray a 2-quart soufflé dish with nonstick coating. Coat sides and bottom of dish with the 1 tablespoon sugar. Set aside. Beat egg whites and cream of tartar till stiff peaks form (tips stand straight). Fold some of the egg whites into the mocha mixture to lighten (see photo 1, page 173). Then, gently fold mocha mixture into remaining stiffly beaten egg whites. Pour into prepared soufflé dish.

■ Bake in the 375° oven for 20 to 25 minutes or till a knife inserted near the center comes out clean. Serve immediately. Makes 6 servings.

PER SERVING

Calories	116
Protein	7 g
Carbohydrate	22 g
Fat	1 g
Cholesterol	2 mg
Sodium	118 mg
Potassium	209 mg

TIMETABLE

Preparation time:
20 minutes

Cooking time:
20 to 25 minutes

LEMON-CAKE PUDDING

A sensational sponge cake with an extra-special pudding sauce takes a bit of time and trouble, but good things come to those who wait. (Pictured on page 161.)

⅔ cup sugar
¼ cup all-purpose flour
Dash salt
1 teaspoon frozen, finely shredded lemon peel (see tip, page 66)
2 tablespoons lemon juice
1 tablespoon liquid margarine
3 egg yolks
1 8-ounce carton plain low-fat yogurt
½ cup skim milk
3 egg whites
Lime slices (optional)

■ Preheat the oven to 350°. Meanwhile, in a mixing bowl combine sugar, flour, and salt. Stir in lemon peel, lemon juice, and liquid margarine.

■ In another mixing bowl beat egg yolks thoroughly with a rotary beater; beat in yogurt and skim milk. Add to lemon mixture.

■ Beat egg whites till stiff peaks form (tips stand straight); fold into lemon mixture. Pour batter into an *ungreased* 8x8x2-inch baking pan. Place baking pan in a larger pan; place on an oven rack and pour *hot water* into larger pan to a depth of 1 inch.

■ Bake in the 350° oven about 40 minutes or till set. Garnish with small lime slices, if desired. Serve warm. Makes 9 servings.

PER SERVING

Calories	128
Protein	4 g
Carbohydrate	20 g
Fat	4 g
Cholesterol	93 mg
Sodium	71 mg
Potassium	111 mg

TIMETABLE

Preparation time:
25 minutes

Cooking time:
about 40 minutes

APPLE CRUNCH

3 medium cooking apples
  (1 pound total)
¼ cup apple *or* orange juice
1 tablespoon brown sugar
1 teaspoon cornstarch
⅓ cup granola

■ Preheat the oven to 350°. Meanwhile peel, core, and thinly slice the apples. Combine apple or orange juice, brown sugar, and cornstarch. Toss with apples. Place apple mixture in a 1-quart casserole. Cover and bake in the 350° oven for 40 to 45 minutes or till apples are very tender. Sprinkle the granola over the apple mixture just before serving. Makes 4 servings.

PER SERVING

Calories	126
Protein	1 g
Carbohydrate	26 g
Fat	3 g
Cholesterol	0 mg
Sodium	2 mg
Potassium	192 mg

TIMETABLE

Preparation time: 10 minutes
Cooking time: 40 to 45 minutes

PEACH-A-BERRY CUSTARD

Strawberries, raspberries, blueberries, blackberries—try 'em all atop this peach of a baked custard.

¾ cup frozen unsweetened
  peach slices (about 4
  ounces)
2 eggs
1 cup skim milk
2 tablespoons sugar
1 teaspoon vanilla
  Fresh berries

■ Preheat the oven to 325°. Meanwhile, chop the peach slices and place on paper towels to thaw and drain thoroughly.

■ While peaches are draining, in a medium mixing bowl beat eggs. Beat in milk, sugar, and vanilla till well combined. Divide peaches among four 6-ounce custard cups. Then place custard cups into a 9x9x2 inch baking pan. Pour egg-milk mixture atop peaches in custard cups.

■ Pour *hot water* into the pan around custard cups to a depth of 1 inch. Bake in the 325° oven about 40 minutes or till a knife inserted near the center comes out clean. Transfer custard cups from pan of water to a wire rack. Let stand for 15 minutes. Garnish with fresh berries. Makes 4 servings.

PER SERVING

Calories	108
Protein	6 g
Carbohydrate	15 g
Fat	3 g
Cholesterol	139 mg
Sodium	66 mg
Potassium	247 mg

TIMETABLE

Preparation time: 15 minutes
Cooking time: about 40 minutes
Standing time: 15 minutes

SPICY FRUIT CUP

Change the fruits in this dessert for another taste treat. Substitute an apple for the pear and sliced kiwi fruit for the strawberries.

1   8-ounce can pineapple
    chunks (juice pack)
½   cup orange juice
2   tablespoons dry white wine
⅛   teaspoon ground cinnamon
    Dash ground nutmeg
1   medium pear
1   cup fresh strawberries
1   11-ounce can mandarin
    orange sections
1   8-ounce can grapefruit
    sections (juice pack)

■ In a medium mixing bowl stir together *undrained* pineapple, orange juice, wine, cinnamon, and nutmeg. Core and slice the pear. Halve the strawberries. Drain mandarin orange sections and grapefruit.

■ Add the pear, strawberries, orange sections, and grapefruit to the pineapple mixture. Cover and chill fruit mixture for up to 6 hours. Divide the fruit mixture among 6 dessert dishes. Makes 6 servings.

PER SERVING

Calories	85
Protein	1 g
Carbohydrate	21 g
Fat	0 g
Cholesterol	0 mg
Sodium	5 mg
Potassium	269 mg

TIMETABLE

Advance preparation time:
10 minutes

Chilling time:
3 to 6 hours

COCONUT PUDDING

2   tablespoons coconut
2   tablespoons sugar
1   tablespoon cornstarch
1   cup skim milk
1   tablespoon margarine
    or butter
1   teaspoon vanilla
1   11-ounce can mandarin
    orange sections

■ In a small saucepan toast the coconut over high heat for 2 to 3 minutes or till lightly browned; stir constantly to brown evenly. Remove coconut from the pan and set aside.

■ In the same saucepan stir together the sugar and cornstarch. Stir in the milk. Cook and stir till mixture is thickened and bubbly. Then cook and stir for 2 minutes more. Remove from heat. Stir in the margarine or butter and vanilla.

■ Drain the mandarin oranges and divide among 4 dessert dishes. Spoon ¼ of the pudding mixture over mandarin oranges in each dish. Cover and chill pudding for 4 to 6 hours. Before serving, sprinkle each serving with some of the toasted coconut. Serves 4.

PER SERVING

Calories	108
Protein	3 g
Carbohydrate	17 g
Fat	4 g
Cholesterol	1 mg
Sodium	72 mg
Potassium	182 mg

TIMETABLE

Advance preparation time:
15 minutes

Chilling time:
4 to 6 hours

BERRY-FULL COMPOTE

A honey-ginger fruit compote that has options! How about canned pears or peaches packed in light syrup instead of the apricots.

¼ teaspoon finely shredded
   lime peel
2 tablespoons lime juice
2 tablespoons honey
⅛ teaspoon ground ginger
1 16-ounce can unpeeled
   apricot halves in light
   syrup
½ cup fresh or frozen
   blueberries

■ In a medium bowl stir together lime peel, lime juice, honey, and ginger. Drain apricots. Add apricots and blueberries to honey mixture in bowl and toss gently to coat. Cover and chill for up to 4 hours.

■ To serve, spoon fruit and juice into 4 small dessert dishes. Makes 4 servings.

PER SERVING

Calories	116
Protein	1 g
Carbohydrate	31 g
Fat	0 g
Cholesterol	0 mg
Sodium	6 mg
Potassium	187 mg

TIMETABLE

Advance preparation time:
10 minutes

Chilling time:
1 to 4 hours

COFFEE PUDDING

Avoiding caffeine? Use decaffeinated instant coffee crystals.

1 tablespoon instant coffee
   crystals
1¾ cups skim milk
1 4-serving-size package
   reduced-calorie *instant*
   vanilla pudding mix
½ cup frozen whipped dessert
   topping, thawed (see tip,
   page 167)
2 tablespoons slivered
   almonds (toasted, if
   desired)

■ In a small mixer bowl dissolve coffee crystals in milk. Add pudding mix and prepare according to pudding package directions.

■ Pour pudding into 4 small dessert dishes. Cover surface of pudding with clear plastic wrap. Chill for several hours or overnight.

■ Before serving, dollop pudding with dessert topping and sprinkle with almonds. Makes 4 servings.

PER SERVING

Calories	112
Protein	4 g
Carbohydrate	14 g
Fat	4 g
Cholesterol	2 mg
Sodium	323 mg
Potassium	232 mg

TIMETABLE

Advance preparation time:
10 minutes

Chilling time:
3 to 24 hours

PAPAYA ICE

Make the ice with 1½ cups fresh or frozen unsweetened strawberries if a papaya is unavailable.

½ cup sugar
1 teaspoon unflavored gelatin
½ cup water
1 papaya (about 1 pound)
4 teaspoons lemon juice
   Lemon *or* lime slices
      (optional)
   Fresh mint sprigs (optional)

■ In a small saucepan stir together sugar and gelatin. Add water. Cook and stir over low heat till sugar and gelatin are dissolved; set aside.

■ Meanwhile, peel, seed, and cut up papaya to make about 1¾ cups papaya cubes. In a blender container or food processor bowl combine sugar mixture, papaya, and lemon juice. Cover and blend or process till smooth. Pour fruit mixture into a small mixer bowl.

■ Cover and freeze fruit mixture for 2 to 3 hours or till almost firm. Beat with an electric mixer on medium speed about 2 minutes or till mixture is fluffy. Transfer mixture to a 7½x3½x2-inch or 8x4x2-inch loaf pan. Cover; freeze for at least 4 hours or till firm.

■ To serve, let stand for 10 minutes at room temperature. Scrape or scoop into dessert dishes. If desired, garnish with thin lemon or lime slices or a fresh mint sprig. Makes 4 servings.

PER SERVING

Calories	128
Protein	2 g
Carbohydrate	31 g
Fat	0 g
Cholesterol	0 mg
Sodium	4 mg
Potassium	164 mg

TIMETABLE

Advance preparation time:
20 minutes

Freezing times:
2 to 3 hours
4 to 24 hours

Final preparation time:
15 minutes

CRANBERRY-APPLE FLUFF

Scoop the cranberry juice concentrate out of the can while it's still frozen to help chill the gelatin mixture.

1½ cups water
2 teaspoons lemon juice
1 envelope unflavored gelatin
¼ teaspoon ground cinnamon
½ cup dried apples
½ of a 6-ounce can (⅓ cup)
      frozen cranberry juice
      cocktail concentrate
   Red food coloring
2 egg whites
½ cup frozen whipped dessert
      topping, thawed (see tip,
      page 167)
   Fresh mint sprigs

■ In a small saucepan combine *1 cup* of the water, lemon juice, gelatin, and cinnamon; let stand for 5 minutes. Meanwhile, finely chop apples. Stir apples into saucepan. Cook and stir mixture over low heat till gelatin is dissolved.

■ Remove mixture from heat. Stir in remaining ½ cup water, cranberry juice cocktail concentrate, and a few drops food coloring. Quick-chill in a bowl of ice water about 10 minutes or till partially set (consistency of unbeaten egg whites), stirring frequently.

■ When mixture is partially set, beat egg whites till soft peaks form (tips curl). Gradually add gelatin mixture, beating till fluffy. By hand, fold in whipped dessert topping. Spoon mixture into serving dishes. Chill for at least 2 hours or overnight. If desired, garnish with a fresh mint sprig. Makes 6 servings.

PER SERVING

Calories	65
Protein	2 g
Carbohydrate	11 g
Fat	2 g
Cholesterol	0 mg
Sodium	29 mg
Potassium	71 mg

TIMETABLE

Advance preparation time:
25 minutes

Chilling time:
2 to 24 hours

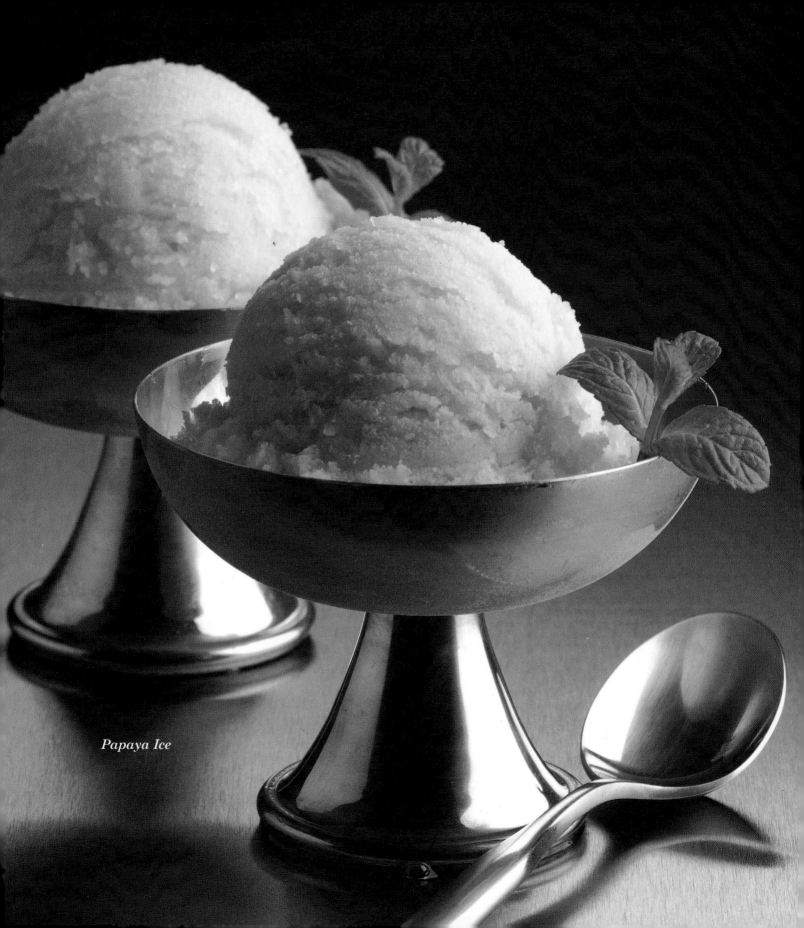

Papaya Ice

CHILLY JAVA SOUFFLÉ

Creamy and rich-tasting—all the characteristics of an undietlike dessert!

¼ cup cold water
1 envelope unflavored gelatin
½ of an 8-ounce container reduced-calorie soft-style cream cheese
1 cup skim milk
3 tablespoons sugar
2 teaspoons instant coffee crystals
1 teaspoon vanilla
2 egg whites
½ of a 4-ounce container frozen whipped dessert topping, thawed (see tip, page 167)
Ground nutmeg

■ In a small saucepan stir together the water and gelatin; let stand for 1 minute. Cook and stir over low heat until the gelatin is dissolved.

■ Place cream cheese in a blender container or food processor bowl. Pour gelatin mixture over cheese. Cover and blend or process until smooth. Add milk, sugar, coffee crystals, and vanilla; cover and blend or process until smooth. Pour into a bowl and quick-chill gelatin mixture in the freezer for 5 minutes or till partially set (consistency of unbeaten egg whites), stirring frequently.

■ While mixture is chilling, in a small mixer bowl beat egg whites till soft peaks form (tips curl). Fold beaten egg whites into gelatin mixture along with the thawed topping. Pour mixture into a 5-cup soufflé dish or a 5-cup mold. Cover and chill for at least 4 hours or till firm. Sprinkle with nutmeg. Serves 6.

PER SERVING

Calories	119
Protein	6 g
Carbohydrate	12 g
Fat	6 g
Cholesterol	12 mg
Sodium	148 mg
Potassium	119 mg

TIMETABLE

Advance preparation time: 30 minutes

Chilling time: 4 to 24 hours

PINEAPPLE-YOGURT PUDDING

2 tablespoons coconut
Nonstick spray coating
2 tablespoons graham cracker crumbs
1 15¼-ounce can crushed pineapple (juice pack)
1 teaspoon unflavored gelatin
⅛ teaspoon ground nutmeg
1 8-ounce carton vanilla low-fat yogurt

■ In a medium skillet toast coconut over high heat for 2 to 3 minutes or till lightly browned; stir constantly to brown evenly. Remove coconut from skillet; set aside. Spray a 1- or 1½-quart soufflé dish with nonstick coating. Coat bottom and sides of dish with the graham cracker crumbs; set aside.

■ Drain pineapple; reserve ¾ *cup* juice. (Add water if necessary to equal ¾ cup.) In a small saucepan combine reserved juice, gelatin, and nutmeg; let stand for 1 minute. Stir over medium heat till gelatin dissolves. Pour gelatin mixture into a small mixer bowl. Quick-chill mixture in a bowl of ice water about 10 minutes or till partially set (consistency of unbeaten egg whites); stir frequently. Beat gelatin mixture with an electric mixer on high speed for 3 minutes or till fluffy. Fold in yogurt and pineapple. Spoon mixture into the prepared dish. Sprinkle with coconut. Chill in the refrigerator for at least 4 hours or till firm. Makes 6 servings.

PER SERVING

Calories	94
Protein	3 g
Carbohydrate	19 g
Fat	1 g
Cholesterol	2 mg
Sodium	42 mg
Potassium	184 mg

TIMETABLE

Advance preparation time: about 30 minutes

Chilling time: 4 to 24 hours

APRICOT FLUFF

2 tablespoons sugar
1½ teaspoons unflavored
    gelatin
¼ cup cold water
¼ cup orange juice
1 5½-ounce can (⅔ cup)
    apricot nectar
¼ cup nonfat dry milk powder
¼ cup cold water
4 canned unpeeled apricot
    halves in light syrup,
    drained and cut up
    (optional)

■ In a small saucepan stir together the sugar and gelatin. Stir in ¼ cup water and orange juice. Cook and stir over low heat till gelatin and sugar are dissolved. Remove from heat and stir in apricot nectar.

■ Pour the gelatin mixture into a bowl and quick-chill in a bowl of ice water about 10 minutes or till partially set (consistency of unbeaten egg whites), stirring frequently.

■ In a small *cold* mixer bowl combine milk powder and the ¼ cup *cold* water. Beat with an electric mixer on high speed until stiff peaks form (tips stand straight). Fold the gelatin mixture into the whipped milk. If desired, place fruit in bottom of 4 dessert dishes. Spoon gelatin mixture into dishes. Cover and chill for at least 1 hour or till set. Makes 4 servings.

PER SERVING

Calories	86
Protein	4 g
Carbohydrate	18 g
Fat	0 g
Cholesterol	1 mg
Sodium	39 mg
Potassium	192 mg

TIMETABLE

Advance preparation time:
20 minutes

Chilling time:
at least 1 hour

CHOCOLATE ICE MILK

WE want you to have a bowl of creamy chocolate ice milk as much as YOU do!

1 tablespoon sugar
1½ teaspoons unflavored
    gelatin
½ cup cold water
¾ cup evaporated skim milk
¼ cup chocolate-flavored
    syrup
1 teaspoon vanilla
½ of a 4-ounce container
    frozen whipped dessert
    topping, thawed (see tip,
    page 167)

■ In a small saucepan combine the sugar and gelatin. Stir in cold water. Cook and stir over low heat till gelatin and sugar are dissolved.

■ Pour the gelatin mixture into a bowl and stir in the evaporated milk, chocolate-flavored syrup, and vanilla. Quick-chill in a bowl of ice water for 5 to 10 minutes till well chilled.

■ Beat the gelatin mixture with a rotary beater about 1 minute or till fluffy. Fold in the thawed whipped dessert topping. Beat smooth with a rotary beater, if necessary.

■ Pour mixture into an 8x4x2-inch loaf pan and freeze for 6 to 24 hours or till firm. Scoop into dessert dishes. Makes 6 servings.

PER SERVING

Calories	98
Protein	4 g
Carbohydrate	16 g
Fat	3 g
Cholesterol	1 mg
Sodium	46 mg
Potassium	142 mg

TIMETABLE

Advance preparation time:
20 minutes

Freezing time:
6 to 24 hours

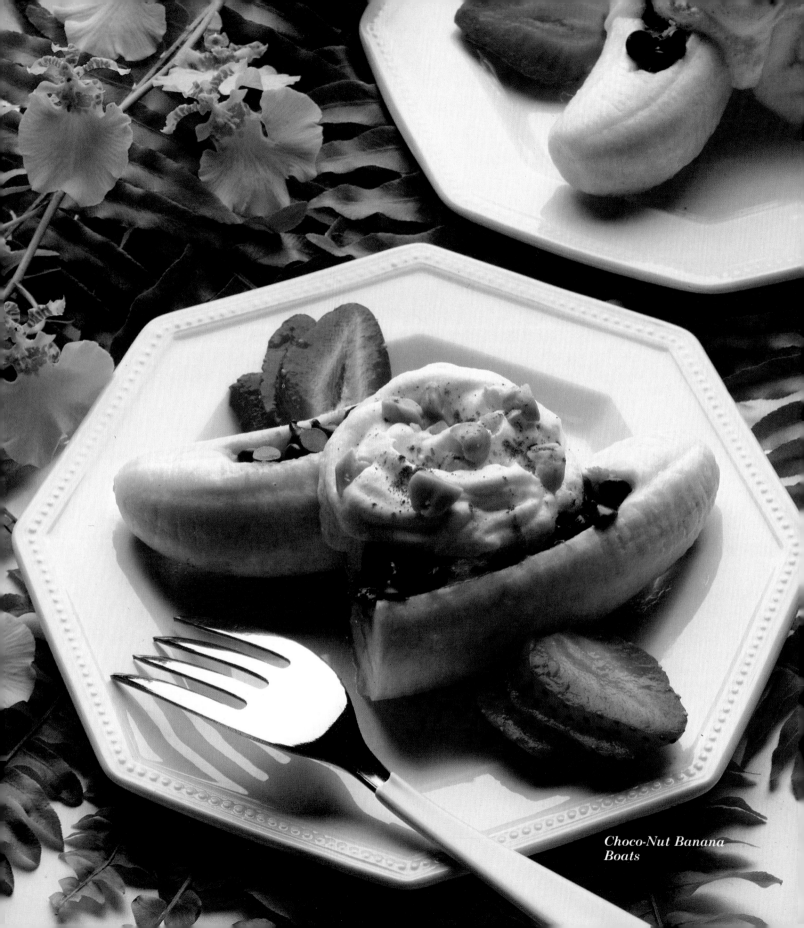

Choco-Nut Banana Boats

20 minutes or less

CHOCO-NUT BANANA BOATS

The chocolate pieces won't look melted at the end of micro-cooking, but they really will be.

2 tablespoons miniature semi-sweet chocolate pieces
⅛ to ¼ teaspoon frozen, finely shredded orange peel (see tip, page 66)
4 small firm bananas
Orange juice
¼ cup frozen whipped dessert topping, thawed (see tip, page 167)
1 tablespoon chopped peanuts
Ground cinnamon
Fresh strawberries (optional)

■ In a small bowl toss together chocolate pieces and orange peel; set aside. Peel bananas; brush with a little orange juice. Arrange bananas in an 8x8x2-inch microwave-safe baking dish. With the tip of a spoon, hollow out a very shallow lengthwise groove in each banana. Divide the chocolate mixture among the bananas, spooning mixture into the grooves.

■ Cover with vented microwave-safe plastic wrap. Micro-cook on 100% power (high) about 2 minutes or till bananas are warm and chocolate is soft.

■ To serve, halve bananas crosswise and place *2* halves on each dessert plate. Top each serving with some of the dessert topping and nuts. Sprinkle lightly with cinnamon. Garnish with fresh strawberries, if desired. Serve immediately. Makes 4 servings.

PER SERVING

Calories	126
Protein	2 g
Carbohydrate	23 g
Fat	5 g
Cholesterol	0 mg
Sodium	12 mg
Potassium	338 mg

TIMETABLE

Preparation time:
10 minutes

Cooking time:
about 2 minutes

---

20 minutes or less

QUICK FRUIT MÉLANGE

⅓ cup seedless red or green grapes
1 8-ounce can pear slices (juice pack)
1 teaspoon margarine *or* butter
1 teaspoon honey
⅛ teaspoon ground cinnamon
Dash ground nutmeg
1 medium orange
1 medium banana

■ Halve grapes. Place in a 1-quart microwave-safe casserole. Add *undrained* pear slices, margarine or butter, honey, cinnamon, and nutmeg. Micro-cook, uncovered, on 100% power (high) for 2½ to 4½ minutes or till boiling, stirring once.

■ While pear mixture is cooking, peel and slice orange; quarter the slices. Slice banana into ½-inch-thick slices. Add orange and banana to hot fruit; cover and let stand about 3 minutes to heat through. Makes 4 servings.

PER SERVING

Calories	94
Protein	1 g
Carbohydrate	22 g
Fat	1 g
Cholesterol	0 mg
Sodium	14 mg
Potassium	259 mg

TIMETABLE

Preparation time:
5 minutes

Cooking time:
2½ to 4½ minutes

Standing time:
about 3 minutes

20 minutes or less

YOGURT-TOPPED APPLES

To save about 19 calories a serving, skip the yogurt and marmalade topping.

2 **tablespoons raisins**
⅛ **teaspoon ground nutmeg**
2 **large cooking apples (7 to 8 ounces each)**
1 **teaspoon margarine *or* butter**
¼ **cup vanilla low-fat yogurt**
1 **tablespoon reduced-calorie orange marmalade**

■ For filling, in a small bowl combine raisins and nutmeg; set aside. Peel apples if desired. Remove core from apples and cut each apple in half crosswise. Place apples cut side up in an 8x8x2-inch microwave-safe baking dish. Spoon filling into centers of apple halves; dot with margarine or butter.

■ Cover the dish with waxed paper. Micro-cook the apples on 100% power (high) for 4 to 5 minutes or till tender, giving dish a half-turn and spooning the cooking liquid over apples after 2 minutes.

■ While apples are cooking, prepare yogurt sauce. For sauce, in a small mixing bowl stir together yogurt and orange marmalade.

■ To serve, place apples in 4 dessert dishes; spoon cooking liquid atop. Drizzle yogurt sauce over apples. Serve warm. Makes 4 servings.

PER SERVING

Calories	100
Protein	1 g
Carbohydrate	22 g
Fat	2 g
Cholesterol	1 mg
Sodium	28 mg
Potassium	191 mg

TIMETABLE

Preparation time: 5 minutes
Cooking time: 4 to 5 minutes

ATTENTION, MICROWAVE OWNERS

Microwave recipes were tested in countertop microwave ovens that provide 600 to 700 watts of cooking power. The cooking times are approximate because microwave ovens vary by manufacturer.

20 minutes or less

CHEESE-TOPPED PEARS

Chilly pears from the refrigerator need a little more cooking time than pears at room temperature. (Pictured on pages 160 and 161.)

4　small pears (1 to 1¼ pounds total)
¼　of an 8-ounce container reduced-calorie soft-style cream cheese
2　tablespoons plain low-fat yogurt
1　tablespoon sugar
1　drop mint extract (optional)
　　Ground nutmeg *or* ground cinnamon (optional)

■ Core pears from bottom, leaving stems in place. Lay pears in a 2-quart microwave-safe casserole. Micro-cook the pears, covered, on 100% power (high) for 4 to 6 minutes or till tender, rearranging pears once.

■ While pears are cooking, in a small mixing bowl beat together cream cheese, yogurt, sugar, and mint extract, if desired, till smooth.

■ To serve, remove pears from casserole and place in 4 dessert dishes. Spoon some of the cheese mixture over each pear. Sprinkle with nutmeg or cinnamon, if desired. Serve warm. Makes 4 servings.

PER SERVING

Calories	117
Protein	2 g
Carbohydrate	22 g
Fat	3 g
Cholesterol	9 mg
Sodium	85 mg
Potassium	185 mg

TIMETABLE

Preparation time:
10 minutes

Cooking time:
4 to 6 minutes

GLACÉED NECTARINES

1　tablespoon sugar
1　teaspoon cornstarch
1　5½-ounce can (⅔ cup) apricot nectar
⅛　teaspoon frozen, finely shredded lemon peel (see tip, page 66)
¼　teaspoon vanilla
1½　cups fresh strawberries
1　medium nectarine

■ For glaze, in a 2-cup microwave-safe measure stir together sugar and cornstarch. Stir in apricot nectar and lemon peel; mix well.

■ Micro-cook, uncovered, on 100% power (high) for 1½ to 2½ minutes or till mixture is thickened and bubbly, stirring every 30 seconds. Cook for 30 seconds more; stir in vanilla. Pour into a bowl and quick-chill the glaze in a bowl of ice water for 15 to 20 minutes, stirring frequently.

■ While glaze is cooling, slice strawberries and thinly slice nectarine. Arrange fruit in 4 dessert dishes. Spoon glaze over fruit. Makes 4 servings.

PER SERVING

Calories	73
Protein	1 g
Carbohydrate	18 g
Fat	0 g
Cholesterol	0 mg
Sodium	2 mg
Potassium	216 mg

TIMETABLE

Total preparation time:
30 minutes

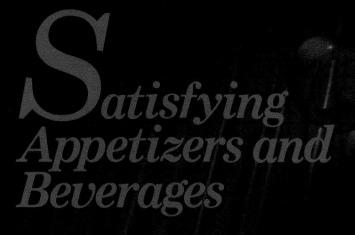

Satisfying Appetizers and Beverages

You're not alone. The temptation to snack between meals seems to strike everyone who's dieting.

The recipes on the next few pages give you some quick, make-ahead, and microwave snack and drink ideas.

Don't forget to add the calories from these treats to your daily tally.

Citrus-Crab Cocktail (see recipe, page 188)

Cheese-Tomato Popcorn
(see recipe, page 189)

Apple-Tomato Sipper
(see recipe, page 201)

Wonton Chips
(see recipe, page 188)

20 minutes or less

CITRUS-CRAB COCKTAIL

Place the canned fruit in the refrigerator the night before, or quick-chill it in the freezer for 15 minutes before using. (Pictured on page 186.)

¼ cup plain low-fat yogurt
2 tablespoons cocktail sauce
6 ounces crab-flavored fish pieces *or* one 6-ounce can crabmeat
1 10½-ounce can mandarin orange sections (water pack), chilled
Leaf lettuce

■ For dressing, in a small mixing bowl stir together yogurt and cocktail sauce. For crab-flavored fish pieces, cut into bite-size pieces, if necessary. If using canned crabmeat, drain, remove cartilage, and cut into bite-size pieces. Drain orange sections.

■ To serve, line cocktail cups or glasses with lettuce. Then arrange crabmeat and orange sections in cups. Drizzle dressing over crabmeat and orange sections. Makes 4 servings.

PER SERVING

Calories	95
Protein	11 g
Carbohydrate	9 g
Fat	2 g
Cholesterol	39 mg
Sodium	195 mg
Potassium	289 mg

TIMETABLE

Total preparation time: 15 minutes

---

20 minutes or less

WONTON CHIPS

Sweet or savory—whatever your craving, these crispy chips come to the rescue. (Pictured on page 187.)

12 wonton skins
2 teaspoons liquid margarine, *or* margarine *or* butter, melted
Nonstick spray coating
¼ teaspoon seasoned salt *or* ½ teaspoon cinnamon sugar

■ Preheat the oven to 400°. Meanwhile, lightly brush 1 side of wonton skins with liquid margarine or melted margarine or butter. Cut *each* wonton skin in half diagonally, forming 24 triangles.

■ Spray a 15x10x1-inch baking pan with nonstick coating. Arrange triangles, margarine side up, in a single layer in the pan. Lightly sprinkle with seasoned salt or cinnamon sugar. Bake in the 400° oven for 5 to 7 minutes or till golden brown and crisp. Makes 4 servings.

PER SERVING

Calories	79
Protein	2 g
Carbohydrate	12 g
Fat	2 g
Cholesterol	0 mg
Sodium	188 mg
Potassium	21 mg

TIMETABLE

Preparation time: 5 minutes

Cooking time: 5 to 7 minutes

20 minutes or less

LIGHT-AS-A-FEATHER SNACK MIX

3 tablespoons margarine *or* butter
¼ teaspoon garlic powder
¼ teaspoon lemon-pepper seasoning *or* dried basil, crushed
6 plain rice cakes
2 cups bite-size shredded wheat biscuits
1 cup bite-size fish-shape crackers

■ If desired, preheat the oven to 300°. Meanwhile, in a small saucepan combine margarine or butter, garlic powder, and lemon-pepper seasoning or basil. Cook over low heat till margarine or butter is melted.

■ While margarine is melting, break rice cakes into bite-size pieces and place in an extra-large mixing bowl. Add shredded wheat biscuits and crackers.

■ Drizzle melted margarine mixture over the cereal mixture. Toss till coated. Serve immediately. *Or,* if desired, spread cereal mixture in a 15x10x1-inch baking pan and bake in the 300° oven about 30 minutes, stirring once. Makes 16 (½-cup) servings.

PER SERVING

Calories	66
Protein	1 g
Carbohydrate	9 g
Fat	3 g
Cholesterol	1 mg
Sodium	68 mg
Potassium	33 mg

TIMETABLE

Total preparation time: 10 minutes

20 minutes or less

CHEESE-TOMATO POPCORN

So full of flavor, yet so few calories. (Pictured on page 187.)

2 tablespoons unpopped popcorn
1 tablespoon margarine *or* butter
½ of a single-serving-size envelope (4 teaspoons) *instant* tomato soup mix
1 teaspoon grated American cheese food *or* Parmesan cheese

■ To pop popcorn, place popcorn in a large skillet. Cover and cook over medium-high heat, shaking skillet constantly till all the popcorn is popped. *Or,* pop the popcorn in a hot-air popper according to manufacturer's directions.

■ Transfer popcorn to a serving bowl. Then place margarine or butter in the hot skillet to melt. Drizzle melted margarine or butter over popcorn. Sprinkle with tomato soup mix and American cheese food or Parmesan cheese. Toss till well coated. Makes 3 (1⅓-cup) servings.

Pesto Popcorn: Prepare Cheese-Tomato Popcorn as directed above, *except* omit soup mix and cheese food. Stir 1 tablespoon grated *Parmesan cheese;* 2 teaspoons dried *parsley flakes;* ¼ teaspoon dried *basil,* crushed; and ⅛ teaspoon *garlic powder* into the melted margarine. Drizzle over popcorn. Toss till well coated. Makes 3 (1⅓-cup) servings.

PER SERVING

Calories	90
Protein	2 g
Carbohydrate	10 g
Fat	5 g
Cholesterol	1 mg
Sodium	270 mg
Potassium	92 mg

TIMETABLE

Total preparation time: 15 minutes

Calories	75

Total preparation time: 15 minutes

20 minutes or less

PEPPERCORN DIP

Pep up cream cheese with green, pickled peppercorns.

1 tablespoon dried whole green peppercorns
1 8-ounce container reduced-calorie soft-style cream cheese
3 tablespoons skim milk
1 tablespoon lemon juice
¼ teaspoon garlic powder

■ Using a mortar and pestle, crush peppercorns.

■ For dip, in a small mixer bowl combine crushed peppercorns, cream cheese, milk, lemon juice, and garlic powder. Beat mixture with an electric mixer on medium speed till smooth.

■ To serve, transfer dip to a small serving bowl. Serve with assorted raw vegetable dippers (see tip, below). Makes 10 (2-tablespoon) servings of dip.

PER SERVING

Calories	53
Protein	3 g
Carbohydrate	2 g
Fat	4 g
Cholesterol	13 mg
Sodium	131 mg
Potassium	59 mg

TIMETABLE

Total preparation time: 15 minutes

20 minutes or less

DIETER'S GUACAMOLE

It's fiesta time! Use bright red tomatoes as festive bowls for the creamy dip.

2 medium tomatoes
1 ripe medium avocado
1 cup low-fat cottage cheese
1 tablespoon lemon juice
¼ teaspoon bottled minced garlic *or* dash garlic powder
⅛ teaspoon salt
Few dashes bottled hot pepper sauce

■ Cut a thin slice off stem ends of tomatoes. Using a spoon, hollow out tomatoes, leaving ¼- to ½-inch-thick shells. Discard seeds; chop tomato pulp and tops. Set tomato shells and pulp aside. Halve, seed, and peel avocado, then cut avocado into chunks. In a blender container or food processor bowl combine the avocado chunks, cottage cheese, lemon juice, garlic, salt, and hot pepper sauce. Cover and blend or process till mixture is smooth. Stir in chopped tomato.

■ To serve, spoon avocado mixture into tomato shells; refill as needed. Serve with homemade tortilla chips (see recipe, page 30) or vegetable dippers (see tip, below). Makes 16 (2-tablespoon) servings of dip.

PER SERVING

Calories	35
Protein	2 g
Carbohydrate	2 g
Fat	2 g
Cholesterol	1 mg
Sodium	76 mg
Potassium	113 mg

TIMETABLE

Total preparation time: 10 minutes

VEGETABLE DIPPERS

Put away those high-calorie chips, and pull out the vegetables. We suggest accompanying the dips in this chapter with an assortment of raw vegetables. Carrots, celery, broccoli, cauliflower, and mushrooms are all good choices.

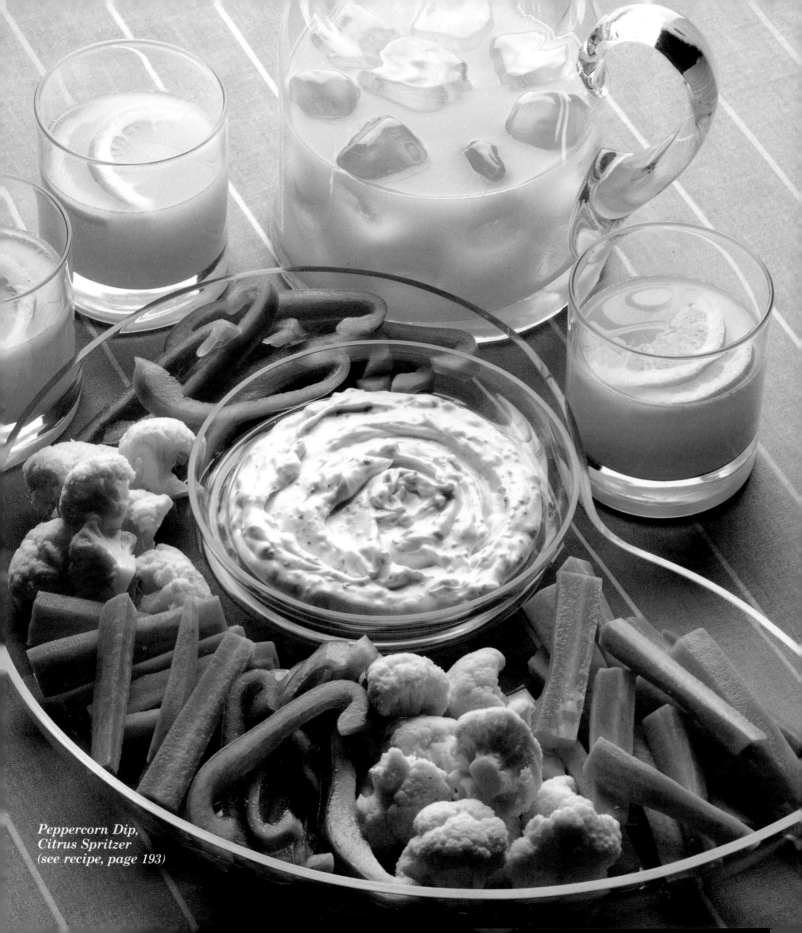

Peppercorn Dip,
Citrus Spritzer
(see recipe, page 193)

20 minutes or less

SALSA DIP

Add a few dashes of pepper sauce for mild salsa, or several dashes for hot salsa.

1 **16-ounce can Mexican-style stewed tomatoes**
2 **tablespoons tomato paste**
¼ **cup frozen chopped onion (see tip, page 39)**
¼ **cup frozen chopped green pepper (see tip, page 39)**
1 **tablespoon red wine vinegar**
¼ **teaspoon salt**
¼ **teaspoon bottled minced garlic *or* dash garlic powder**
Few to several dashes bottled hot pepper sauce

■ Cut up tomatoes, if necessary. In a bowl stir together *undrained* tomatoes, tomato paste, onion, green pepper, vinegar, salt, garlic, and pepper sauce. Let stand at room temperature about 15 minutes, stirring occasionally. *Or*, cover and chill overnight. Serve with homemade tortilla chips (see recipe, page 30) as dippers. Makes 16 (2-tablespoon) servings of dip.

PER SERVING

Calories	11
Protein	0 g
Carbohydrate	3 g
Fat	0 g
Cholesterol	0 mg
Sodium	122 mg
Potassium	96 mg

TIMETABLE

Total preparation time: 20 minutes

20 minutes or less

APPLE-ORANGE CIDER

When it's cold outside, warm up with a hot, fruity drink.

2 **cups orange juice**
½ **of a 6-ounce can (⅓ cup) frozen apple juice concentrate**
⅔ **cup water**
2 **tablespoons apple brandy**

■ In a medium saucepan combine orange juice, apple juice concentrate, and water. Cook over medium heat for 8 to 10 minutes or till hot, stirring occasionally. Stir in brandy and serve. Makes 5 (5-ounce) servings.

Microwave oven: In a 4-cup microwave-safe measure combine orange juice, apple juice concentrate, and water. Micro-cook, uncovered, on 100% power (high) for 6 to 7 minutes or till hot, stirring every 2 minutes. Stir in brandy and serve.

PER SERVING

Calories	88
Protein	1 g
Carbohydrate	18 g
Fat	0 g
Cholesterol	0 mg
Sodium	5 mg
Potassium	266 mg

TIMETABLE

Preparation time: 5 minutes

Cooking time: 8 to 10 minutes

NUTTY COFFEE

Peanut butter in coffee? It's delicious!

½ **cup cold water**
2 **teaspoons instant coffee crystals**
1¼ **cups skim milk**
1 **tablespoon peanut butter**
1 **tablespoon honey**
   Ice cubes (optional)

■ In a blender container combine water and coffee crystals. Cover and blend till coffee crystals are dissolved. Add milk, peanut butter, and honey. Cover and blend till smooth.

■ To serve, for an iced drink, pour mixture over ice in glasses. *Or,* for a hot drink, pour mixture into a small saucepan; heat through. Makes 3 (5-ounce) servings.

PER SERVING

Calories	90
Protein	5 g
Carbohydrate	12 g
Fat	3 g
Cholesterol	2 mg
Sodium	78 mg
Potassium	233 mg

TIMETABLE

Total preparation time:
10 minutes

CITRUS SPRITZER

It's like a wine spritzer, but with orange juice added. (Pictured on page 191.)

2 **cups orange juice**
½ **cup dry white wine**
   Ice cubes
1 **cup carbonated water**
   Orange and lemon slices, halved (optional)

■ In a pitcher or serving bowl stir together orange juice and wine. Then add ice cubes. Slowly add carbonated water. If desired, garnish with orange and lemon half-slices. Makes 7 (4-ounce) servings.

PER SERVING

Calories	45
Protein	1 g
Carbohydrate	8 g
Fat	0 g
Cholesterol	0 mg
Sodium	1 mg
Potassium	130 mg

TIMETABLE

Total preparation time:
5 minutes

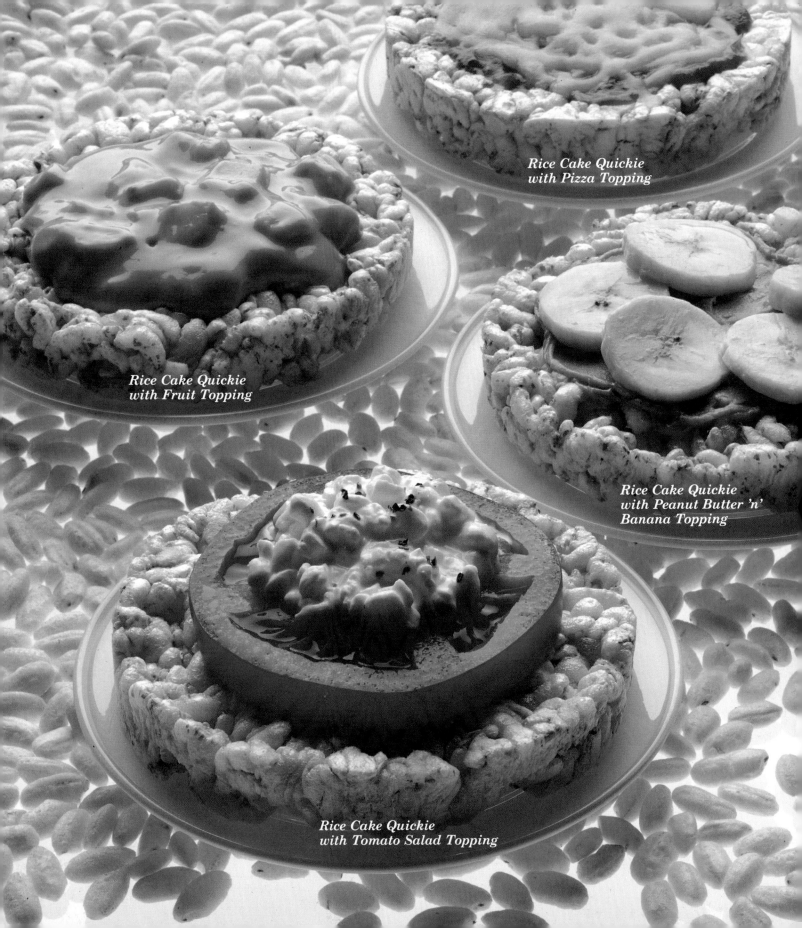

*Rice Cake Quickie
with Pizza Topping*

*Rice Cake Quickie
with Fruit Topping*

*Rice Cake Quickie
with Peanut Butter 'n'
Banana Topping*

*Rice Cake Quickie
with Tomato Salad Topping*

20 minutes or less

RICE CAKE QUICKIES

Plain rice cakes are a great diet food—only 35 calories each. For a fast pick-me-up, eat one plain or add one of these low-calorie toppings.

1 **plain rice cake**
 Desired topping (see recipes, below)

■ If necessary, preheat the broiler. Meanwhile, prepare rice cake with desired topping. Then heat rice cake as directed. Makes 1 serving.

PER SERVING (plain)	
Calories	35
Protein	1 g
Carbohydrate	7 g
Fat	0 g
Cholesterol	0 mg
Sodium	35 mg
Potassium	20 mg

Pizza Topping: Spread rice cake with 1 tablespoon canned *pizza sauce.* Sprinkle with 2 tablespoons shredded *mozzarella cheese.* Broil 3 to 4 inches from the heat for 1 to 2 minutes or till the cheese is melted. *Or,* micro-cook on 100% power (high) for 15 to 30 seconds or till cheese is melted.

Calories	48

Total preparation time: about 5 minutes

Cheesy Cinnamon Topping: Spread rice cake with 1 tablespoon reduced-calorie soft-style *cream cheese.* Combine ½ teaspoon *sugar* and dash ground *cinnamon.* Sprinkle mixture over cream cheese. Serve immediately. *Or,* broil 3 to 4 inches from the heat for 1 to 2 minutes or till cheese is warm. *Or,* micro-cook on 100% power (high) for 10 to 20 seconds or till warm.

Calories	41

Total preparation time: about 5 minutes

Garlic-Cheese Topping: Spread rice cake with 1 teaspoon *margarine or butter.* Sprinkle lightly with *garlic powder,* then sprinkle with 1 tablespoon grated *Parmesan cheese.* Broil 3 to 4 inches from the heat about 1 minute or till cheese is light brown.

Calories	63

Total preparation time: about 5 minutes

Tomato Salad Topping: Top rice cake with 1 *tomato slice.* Combine 1 tablespoon low-fat *cottage cheese* and 1 teaspoon *reduced-calorie creamy buttermilk salad dressing.* Spoon cottage cheese mixture on top of tomato. Sprinkle with *pepper.*

Calories	27

Total preparation time: 5 minutes

Fruit Topping: Stir together 2 tablespoons *strawberry or raspberry low-fat yogurt;* 1 tablespoon chopped fresh *peach, nectarine, strawberries, or raspberries;* 1 teaspoon *Grape Nuts cereal;* and several drops of *vanilla.* Spread on rice cake, then serve immediately.

Calories	44

Total preparation time: 5 minutes

Peanut Butter 'n' Banana Topping: Spread rice cake with 1½ teaspoons *peanut butter.* Place 4 or 5 slices of *banana* on top of peanut butter.

Calories	75

Total preparation time: 5 minutes

CARROT-CHEESE LOG

Spread the colorful cheese on cucumber slices, a refreshing, low-calorie alternative to crackers.

2 medium carrots
½ of an 8-ounce container reduced-calorie soft-style cream cheese
3 tablespoons grated Parmesan cheese
¼ teaspoon fines herbes, crushed
1 small cucumber
¼ cup Grape Nuts cereal

■ Finely shred the carrots. In a small mixing bowl stir together carrots, cream cheese, Parmesan cheese, and fines herbes. Cover and chill cheese mixture for at least 1 hour or overnight.

■ Just before serving, slice cucumber. Slightly crush cereal. Shape cheese mixture into a 7-inch-long log, then roll cheese log in the crushed cereal to coat. Serve with cucumber slices. Makes 5 servings.

PER SERVING

Calories	103
Protein	5 g
Carbohydrate	10 g
Fat	5 g
Cholesterol	16 mg
Sodium	245 mg
Potassium	210 mg

TIMETABLE

Advance preparation time:
20 minutes

Chilling time:
at least 1 hour

Final preparation time:
5 minutes

PRONTO PÂTÉ

With the help of your food processor, you can whip up this easy spread in a jiffy.

1 small carrot
1 8-ounce package turkey pastrami
¼ cup frozen chopped onion (see tip, page 39)
2 tablespoons reduced-calorie creamy Italian salad dressing
½ teaspoon dry mustard
½ teaspoon prepared horseradish
½ teaspoon Worcestershire sauce
Parsley sprigs

■ Place the steel blade in a food processor. Peel and cut carrot into 1-inch pieces. Place carrot in the food processor bowl. Cover and process till finely chopped. Cut up pastrami. Then add pastrami and onion to food processor bowl. Cover and process till finely chopped. Add Italian salad dressing, mustard, horseradish, and Worcestershire sauce. Cover and process till smooth.

■ Line a small bowl or a 2-cup mold with clear plastic wrap. Spoon mixture into bowl or mold. Cover and chill for at least 6 hours or overnight.

■ To serve, invert pâté onto a serving platter. Remove plastic wrap. Garnish with parsley. Serve with melba toast rounds or sliced rye party bread. Makes 12 (2-tablespoon) servings of spread.

PER SERVING

Calories	37
Protein	5 g
Carbohydrate	1 g
Fat	2 g
Cholesterol	10 mg
Sodium	198 mg
Potassium	74 mg

TIMETABLE

Advance preparation time:
15 minutes

Chilling time:
at least 6 hours

Final preparation time:
5 minutes

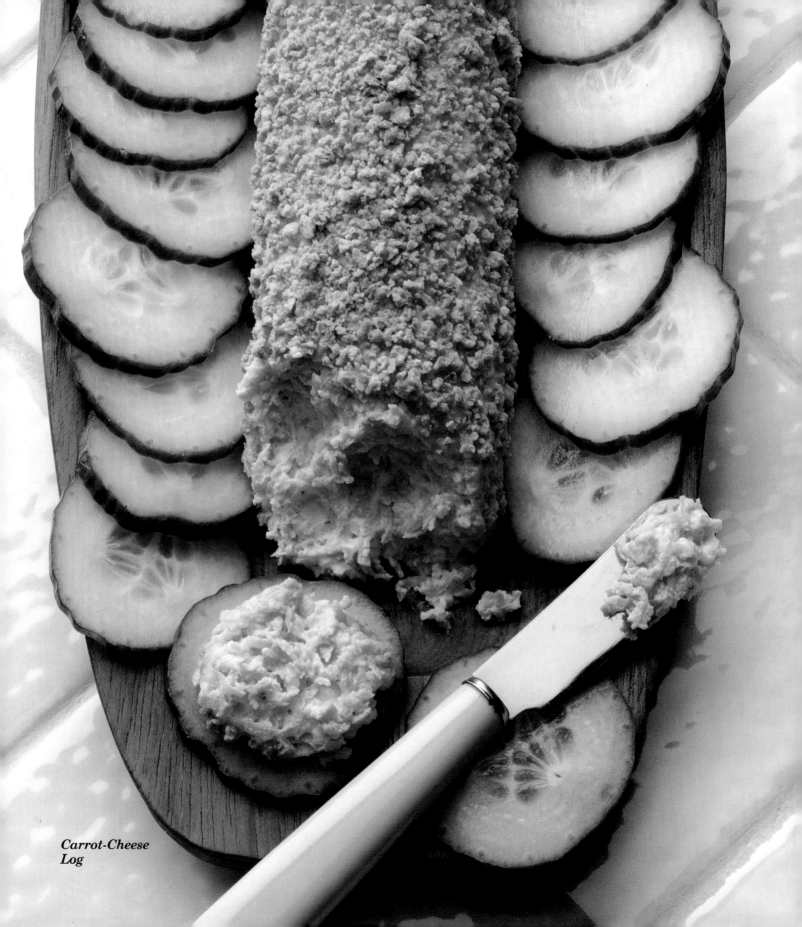

*Carrot-Cheese
Log*

HERBED YOGURT CHEESE

Check the carton: You'll need low-fat yogurt that doesn't contain gelatin to make a thick, creamy cheese.

1 8-ounce carton plain low-fat yogurt (made without gelatin)
⅛ teaspoon dried basil, oregano, Italian seasoning, thyme, *or* marjoram, crushed, *or* ½ teaspoon snipped fresh basil, oregano, thyme, *or* marjoram
1 tablespoon grated Parmesan cheese
   Cheesecloth for cooking

■ In a small mixing bowl stir together yogurt and herb. Then stir in Parmesan cheese.

■ Set a small colander or funnel over a small bowl. Place a double layer of clean cheesecloth for cooking in the colander or funnel. Then spoon the yogurt mixture into cheesecloth-lined colander or funnel. Cover and place in the refrigerator for at least 8 hours or overnight to allow yogurt to drain.

■ To serve, carefully invert yogurt cheese onto a serving plate. Remove cheesecloth and discard whey (liquid). Use cheese as a spread for assorted raw vegetables (see tip, page 190), crackers, or bagels. Store, covered, in the refrigerator for up to 1 week. Makes 8 (1-tablespoon) servings.

PER SERVING

Calories	22
Protein	2 g
Carbohydrate	2 g
Fat	1 g
Cholesterol	2 mg
Sodium	34 mg
Potassium	68 mg

TIMETABLE

Advance preparation time: 5 minutes

Chilling time: at least 8 hours

ARTICHOKE-PARMESAN DIP

½ of a 14-ounce can (3 or 4) artichoke hearts
1 cup low-fat cottage cheese
2 tablespoons frozen snipped chives (see tip, page 39)
2 tablespoons skim milk
¼ teaspoon seasoned salt
¼ teaspoon dried basil, crushed
¼ teaspoon bottled minced garlic *or* dash garlic powder
   Dash bottled hot pepper sauce
2 tablespoons grated Parmesan cheese

■ Drain and finely chop artichoke hearts; set artichokes aside. In a blender container or food processor bowl combine cottage cheese, chives, milk, seasoned salt, basil, garlic, and hot pepper sauce. Cover and blend or process till smooth. Stir in the artichokes and Parmesan cheese.

■ Transfer dip to a small serving bowl. Cover and chill for at least 4 hours (mixture will thicken as it chills). Serve with assorted raw vegetable dippers (see tip, page 190). Makes 14 (2-tablespoon) servings.

PER SERVING

Calories	22
Protein	3 g
Carbohydrate	2 g
Fat	1 g
Cholesterol	2 mg
Sodium	117 mg
Potassium	22 mg

TIMETABLE

Advance preparation time: 15 minutes

Chilling time: at least 4 hours

MARINATED MUSHROOMS

Two for one: Served alone, the herbed mushrooms and tomatoes make a tasty appetizer; tossed with greens, they make a simple, elegant salad.

- 8 ounces small whole fresh mushrooms (4 cups)
- 3 tablespoons white wine vinegar
- 2 tablespoons water
- 1 tablespoon salad oil
- 1 teaspoon sugar
- ½ teaspoon salt
- ½ teaspoon dried oregano, crushed
- ½ teaspoon dried basil, crushed
- ⅛ teaspoon garlic powder
- 12 cherry tomatoes

■ Gently wash mushrooms, then trim ends from stems. In a medium nonmetallic mixing bowl combine vinegar, water, oil, sugar, salt, oregano, basil, and garlic powder. Stir in mushrooms. Cover and chill for at least 8 hours, stirring occasionally. (Mushrooms can be stored in the refrigerator for up to 4 days.)

■ Just before serving, cut tomatoes in half, then add tomatoes to mushrooms. Toss lightly till coated. Using a slotted spoon, transfer the mushrooms and tomatoes to a serving bowl. Makes 6 servings.

PER SERVING

Calories	36
Protein	1 g
Carbohydrate	3 g
Fat	2 g
Cholesterol	0 mg
Sodium	182 mg
Potassium	191 mg

TIMETABLE

Advance preparation time: 10 minutes

Chilling time: at least 8 hours

Final preparation time: 5 minutes

BANANA-FRUIT POPS

Kids will love these fruity treats, too! Keep them on hand for the whole family.

- 2 tablespoons sugar
- 1 teaspoon unflavored gelatin
- ½ cup low-calorie cranberry juice cocktail
- 2 ripe medium bananas
- 1 8-ounce can crushed pineapple (juice pack)
- ½ teaspoon frozen, finely shredded orange peel, (see tip, page 66)
- Few drops red food coloring (optional)
- 9 3-ounce paper drinking cups
- 9 wooden sticks

■ In a medium saucepan combine sugar and unflavored gelatin. Stir in cranberry juice cocktail. Heat and stir till sugar and gelatin are dissolved. Set gelatin mixture aside to cool slightly. Meanwhile, peel and mash bananas. Stir banana, *undrained* pineapple, orange peel, and food coloring, if desired, into partially cooled gelatin mixture.

■ Spoon mixture into the paper drinking cups. Cover cups with small pieces of foil. Insert a wooden stick through center of foil into each pop. Freeze for at least 8 hours before serving. Makes 9 servings.

PER SERVING

Calories	55
Protein	1 g
Carbohydrate	14 g
Fat	0 g
Cholesterol	0 mg
Sodium	1 mg
Potassium	136 mg

TIMETABLE

Advance preparation time: 20 minutes

Freezing time: 8 hours

20 minutes or less

NACHO SNACK CAKE

Nachos are no longer diet no-nos. Just use a low-calorie rice cake instead of high-calorie chips.

1 tablespoon cheese spread
    with jalapeño peppers
1 plain rice cake
    Sliced green onion
    (optional)
    Chopped tomato (optional)

■ Spread cheese on top of rice cake. Place on a microwave-safe plate or paper towel. Micro-cook, uncovered, on 100% power (high) for 10 to 15 seconds, till cheese is bubbly. If desired, top with onion and tomato. Makes 1 serving.

PER SERVING

Calories	84
Protein	4 g
Carbohydrate	8 g
Fat	4 g
Cholesterol	10 mg
Sodium	213 mg
Potassium	62 mg

TIMETABLE

Preparation time:
5 minutes

Cooking time:
10 to 15 seconds

20 minutes or less

SHRIMP WITH HOT 'N' SPICY CRANBERRY DIP

1 16-ounce package frozen
    peeled and deveined
    shrimp *or* 16 ounces crab-
    flavored fish sticks
1 8-ounce can jellied
    cranberry sauce
1½ teaspoons lemon juice
1½ teaspoons Worcestershire
    sauce
1 teaspoon prepared
    horseradish
⅛ teaspoon ground red pepper
¼ teaspoon bottled minced
    garlic *or* dash garlic
    powder

■ If using shrimp, in a large saucepan on the range top bring 4 cups *hot water* to boiling. Add shrimp and bring to boiling, then reduce heat. Cover and simmer for 1 to 3 minutes or till shrimp turn pink. Drain. Place shrimp in a bowl of *ice water* to chill quickly. *Or,* if using crab-flavored fish sticks, cut them into 1-inch pieces.

■ While shrimp are cooking, in a 2-cup microwave-safe measure combine cranberry sauce, lemon juice, Worcestershire sauce, horseradish, red pepper, and garlic. Micro-cook, uncovered, on 100% power (high) for 2 to 4 minutes or till hot, stirring after every 1½ minutes. Serve warm sauce with shrimp or fish sticks as dippers. Makes 8 servings.

PER SERVING

Calories	95
Protein	10 g
Carbohydrate	12 g
Fat	1 g
Cholesterol	85 mg
Sodium	98 mg
Potassium	135 mg

TIMETABLE

Preparation time:
10 minutes

Cooking time:
2 to 4 minutes

20 minutes or less

MOCHA COCOA

Cinnamon adds a spice of niceness to this cocoa.

2 tablespoons sugar
2 tablespoons unsweetened
   cocoa powder
1 teaspoon instant coffee
   crystals
¼ teaspoon ground cinnamon
2¾ cups skim milk

■ In a 4-cup microwave-safe measure combine sugar, cocoa powder, coffee crystals, and cinnamon. Stir in milk. Micro-cook, uncovered, on 100% power (high) for 5 to 7 minutes or till mixture is hot. Makes 4 (7-ounce) servings.

PER SERVING

Calories	90
Protein	6 g
Carbohydrate	16 g
Fat	1 g
Cholesterol	3 mg
Sodium	106 mg
Potassium	303 mg

TIMETABLE

Preparation time:
5 minutes

Cooking time:
5 to 7 minutes

20 minutes or less

APPLE-TOMATO SIPPER

A simply splendid, but easy, fix-up. (Pictured on pages 186 and 187.)

⅓ cup apple juice *or* apple
   cider
⅓ cup vegetable juice cocktail
   or tomato juice
   Dash ground cinnamon
   Stick cinnamon (optional)

■ In a microwave-safe mug combine apple juice or apple cider, vegetable juice cocktail or tomato juice, and ground cinnamon.

■ Micro-cook, uncovered, on 100% power (high) for 1 to 2 minutes or till hot. If desired, serve with stick cinnamon as a stirrer. Makes 1 serving.

PER SERVING

Calories	54
Protein	1 g
Carbohydrate	13 g
Fat	0 g
Cholesterol	0 mg
Sodium	294 mg
Potassium	251 mg

TIMETABLE

Total preparation time:
5 minutes

14 Days of Planned Menus

Looking for a good way to stick with your diet for 14 days straight? Try this two-week menu plan. Or, select a particular day's menu that fits your tastes and needs. Each of the daily menus is designed to fit the busy cook's schedule.

You'll find that the calories listed with each menu item are for a single recipe serving or the serving amount described.

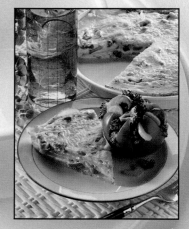

First Day

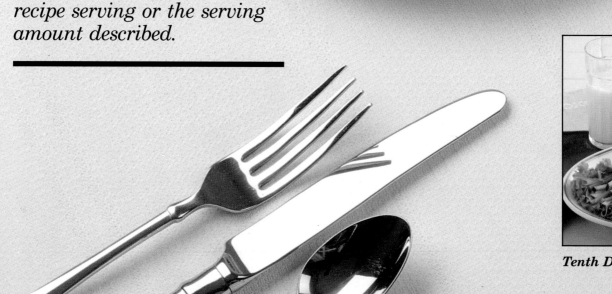

Tenth Day

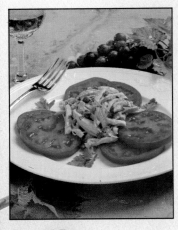

Second Day

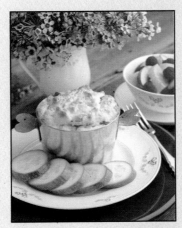

Third Day

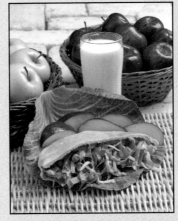

Fourth Day

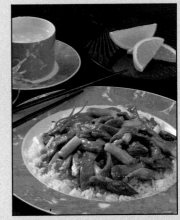

Fifth Day

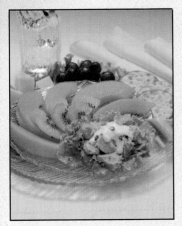

Sixth Day

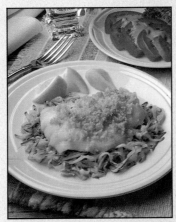

Seventh Day

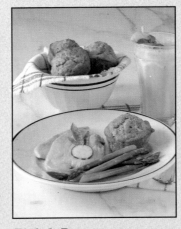

Eighth Day

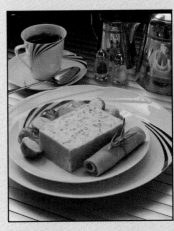

Ninth Day

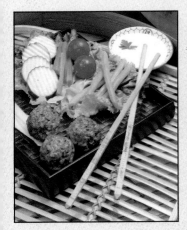

Eleventh Day

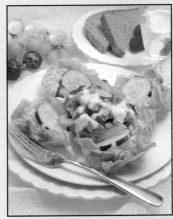

Twelfth Day

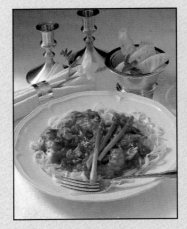

Thirteenth Day

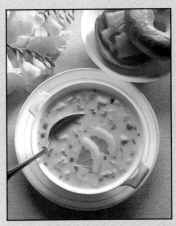

Fourteenth Day

First Day

■ BRUNCH

*Potato-Egg Bake	**199**
*Broccoli-Tomato Cup	**35**
1 slice whole wheat bread	**70**
1 teaspoon margarine *or* butter	**34**
½ cup fresh black raspberries topped with 2 tablespoons whipped dessert topping	**60**
1 cup skim milk	**85**
Iced tea	**0**
Total calories	**483**

■ DINNER

1 broiled loin lamb chop (about 5 ounces uncooked, lean only)	**140**
1 cup cooked brown rice	**230**
1 cup cooked carrots	**70**
1½ cups torn fresh spinach	**15**
1 tablespoon reduced-calorie creamy cucumber salad dressing	**30**
1 whole wheat roll	**85**
2 kiwi fruits, peeled and sliced	**90**
1 cup skim milk	**85**
Total calories	**745**

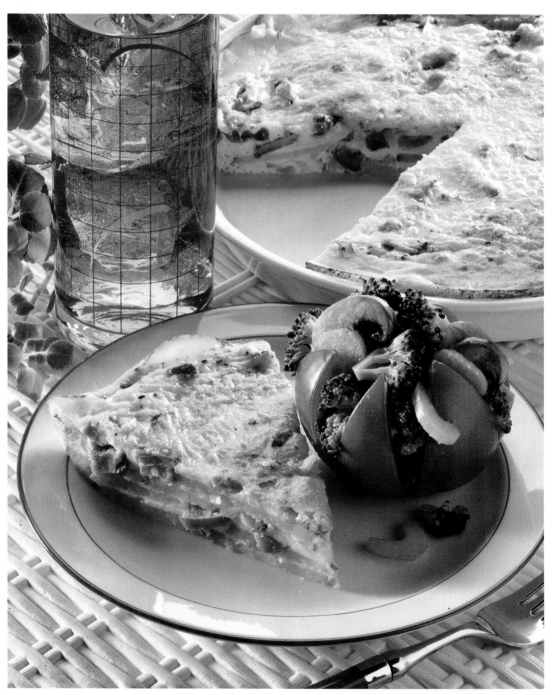

Potato-Egg Bake, Broccoli-Tomato Cup

POTATO-EGG BAKE

Reminiscent of quiche, but without the crust.

1 large potato (about 8 ounces)
¼ cup frozen chopped onion (see tip, page 39)
¼ cup frozen chopped green pepper (see tip, page 39)
4 slices Canadian-style bacon (about 2 ounces total)
8 eggs
⅓ cup skim milk
½ teaspoon dried basil, crushed
¼ teaspoon salt
⅛ teaspoon pepper
   Few dashes bottled hot pepper sauce
½ cup shredded cheddar cheese (2 ounces)
2 tablespoons chopped pimiento
   Nonstick spray coating

■ Preheat the oven to 350°. Meanwhile, scrub potato, then thinly slice (you should have about 1½ cups). In a medium saucepan cook potato, covered, in about 1 cup lightly salted *boiling water* for 6 to 8 minutes or till nearly tender. Add the frozen onion and green pepper to potato in saucepan. Simmer about 2 minutes more or till vegetables are tender. Drain well.

■ While vegetables are cooking, cut Canadian-style bacon into julienne strips; set aside. In a medium mixing bowl use a wire whisk to beat together eggs, milk, basil, salt, pepper, and hot pepper sauce. Stir in *¼ cup* of the cheese and pimiento.

■ Spray a 9-inch glass pie plate or quiche dish with nonstick coating. Arrange vegetables in bottom of the dish. Then sprinkle with Canadian-style bacon. Pour egg mixture over vegetables and bacon in dish. Sprinkle with the remaining cheese. Bake in the 350° oven for 20 to 25 minutes or till a knife inserted near the center comes out clean. Makes 6 servings.

PER SERVING

Calories	199
Protein	14 g
Carbohydrate	10 g
Fat	11 g
Cholesterol	382 mg
Sodium	429 mg
Potassium	393 mg

TIMETABLE

Preparation time:
20 minutes

Cooking time:
20 to 25 minutes

20 minutes or less

BROCCOLI-TOMATO CUPS

Plump red tomatoes attractively encase the salads.

1½ cups broccoli flowerets (see tip, page 137)
¼ cup water
⅛ teaspoon salt
1 stalk celery
1 cup sliced fresh mushrooms
¼ cup reduced-calorie Italian salad dressing
6 small tomatoes

■ In a medium saucepan combine the broccoli, water, and salt. Bring to boiling, then reduce heat. Cover and simmer about 5 minutes or till nearly tender. Then, drain well and transfer broccoli to a large bowl of *ice water* to chill quickly. Let stand about 2 minutes. Drain well. Meanwhile, slice celery.

■ In a bowl combine broccoli, celery, and mushrooms. Pour dressing over vegetable mixture. Toss till coated. Cover and chill till just before serving.

■ While vegetable mixture is chilling, for tomato cups, cut out ½ *inch* of the core from *each* tomato. Then invert tomatoes. For each, cut from top to, *but not quite through,* stem end, making 6 wedges. To serve, for each tomato, spread wedges slightly apart, then fill tomatoes with vegetable mixture. Serves 6.

PER SERVING

Calories	35
Protein	2 g
Carbohydrate	6 g
Fat	1 g
Cholesterol	1 mg
Sodium	69 mg
Potassium	297 mg

TIMETABLE

Total preparation time:
20 minutes

Second Day

■ BREAKFAST

1½ cups wheat flakes	150
¾ cup sliced fresh strawberries	35
1 cup skim milk	85
Total calories	**270**

■ LUNCH

*Tomato 'n' Chicken Salad	178
2 sesame bread-sticks	212
10 seedless red *or* green grapes	35
Ice water	0
Total calories	**425**

■ DINNER

*Citrus Fish	104
½ cup cooked noodles	100
1 cup cooked broccoli	50
2½ cups tossed salad (1 cup romaine, ¼ of a green pepper, ½ of a carrot, ½ of a tomato, ¼ of a cucumber)	52
2 tablespoons reduced-calorie Italian salad dressing	12
1 slice whole wheat bread	70
1 cup skim milk	85
Total calories	**473**

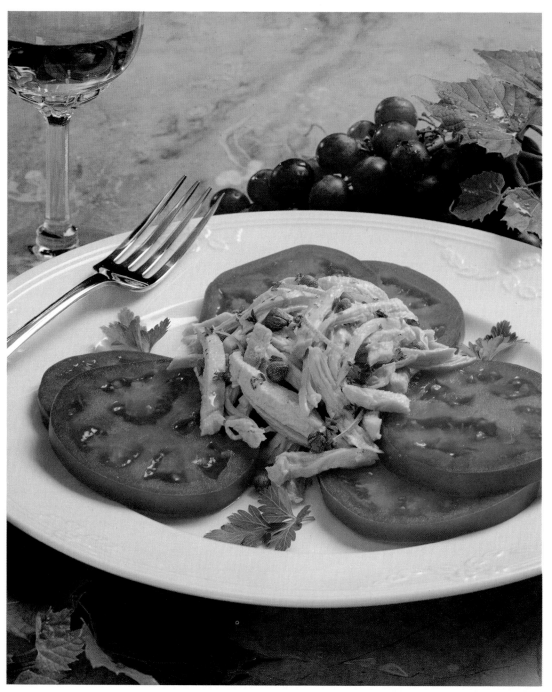

Tomato 'n' Chicken Salad

TOMATO 'N' CHICKEN SALADS

8 ounces boned skinless
    chicken breast halves
    or turkey breast
    tenderloin steaks
⅓ cup dry white wine
1 1-inch square lime peel
    Fresh parsley
2 teaspoons lime juice
1 teaspoon capers, drained
2 medium tomatoes

■ Place poultry in a medium skillet. Pour in wine. Bring to boiling, then reduce heat. Cover and simmer for 9 to 12 minutes or till poultry is tender and no longer pink. Remove poultry, reserving the liquid.

■ Simmer the liquid, uncovered, over medium heat about 2 minutes or till reduced to ¼ *cup.* Meanwhile, cut the lime peel into julienne strips. Snip enough parsley to make *2 tablespoons.*

■ For marinade, in a medium mixing bowl combine the ¼ cup cooking liquid, lime peel, parsley, lime juice, and capers. Cut poultry into julienne strips, then add it to marinade in bowl. Toss lightly till coated. Cover; marinate in the refrigerator for 2 to 8 hours, tossing poultry occasionally with marinade.

■ For salads, slice tomatoes. Arrange tomato slices on plates. Using a slotted spoon, transfer poultry to plates. Then drizzle *each* salad with marinade. If desired, garnish with parsley sprigs. Makes 2 servings.

PER SERVING

Calories	178
Protein	27 g
Carbohydrate	6 g
Fat	2 g
Cholesterol	66 mg
Sodium	83 mg
Potassium	504 mg

TIMETABLE

Advance preparation time:
20 minutes

Chilling time:
2 to 8 hours

Final preparation time:
5 minutes

CITRUS FISH

A hint of orange and marjoram complements the flavor of fish.

1 16-ounce package frozen
    cod *or* haddock fillets
⅔ cup orange juice
2 tablespoons frozen sliced
    green onion (see tip,
    page 39)
2 tablespoons frozen snipped
    parsley (see tip, page 39)
1 tablespoon cooking oil
1 teaspoon frozen, finely
    shredded orange peel
    (see tip, page 66)
½ teaspoon paprika
¼ teaspoon dried marjoram,
    crushed
    Dash salt
    Nonstick spray coating

■ Place the frozen block of fish in a shallow dish. For marinade, in a small mixing bowl combine orange juice, frozen onion, parsley, oil, orange peel, paprika, marjoram, and salt. Pour marinade over fish. Cover and marinate fish in the refrigerator for 5 to 8 hours, spooning marinade over fish once or twice.

■ To cook, preheat the broiler. Meanwhile, spray the *cold* rack of an unheated broiler pan with nonstick coating. Drain fish, reserving the marinade. Cut the thawed block of fish into 4 serving-size pieces. Place fish on the rack. Brush fish with some marinade.

■ Broil fish 4 inches from the heat for 8 to 12 minutes or till the fish flakes easily with a fork, brushing occasionally with marinade. Makes 4 servings.

PER SERVING

Calories	104
Protein	20 g
Carbohydrate	1 g
Fat	2 g
Cholesterol	42 mg
Sodium	86 mg
Potassium	457 mg

TIMETABLE

Advance preparation time:
10 minutes

Chilling time:
5 to 8 hours

Final preparation time:
8 to 12 minutes

Third Day

◼ BREAKFAST

½ of a grapefruit	40
½ cup low-fat cottage cheese	103
8 wheat wafers	70
Coffee *or* tea	0
Total calories	**213**

◼ LUNCH

2 cups canned minestrone soup	160
Cheese sandwich (2 slices whole wheat bread; 1-ounce slice American cheese; dark green lettuce leaves; 1 teaspoon prepared mustard)	255
2 fresh medium plums	70
1 cup skim milk	85
Total calories	**570**

◼ DINNER

*Spinach 'n' Ham Soufflé	196
1 cup sliced zucchini	36
1 whole wheat roll	85
1 teaspoon margarine *or* butter	34
*Rainbow Compote	60
Coffee *or* tea	0
Total calories	**411**

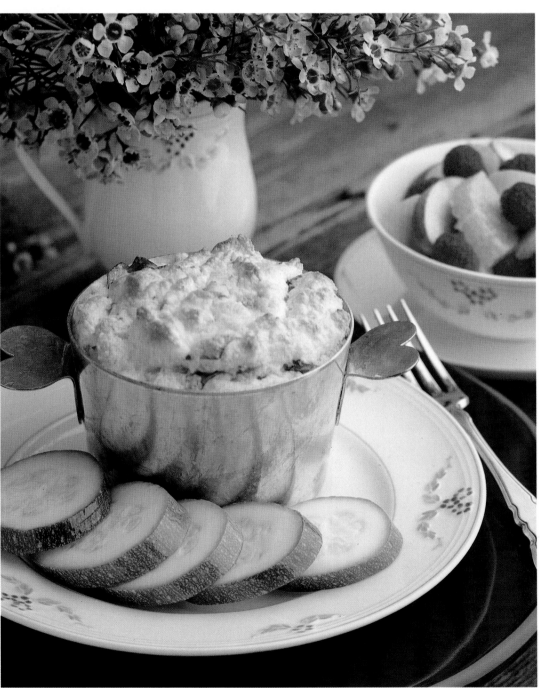

Spinach 'n' Ham Soufflé, Rainbow Compote

SPINACH 'N' HAM SOUFFLÉS

You choose the size: Make four individual soufflés or one large one.

4 eggs
2½ ounces fresh spinach
    (2 cups loosely packed)
½ of a 10¾-ounce can (⅔ cup)
    condensed cream of
    chicken soup
½ cup shredded cheddar
    cheese (2 ounces)
2 ounces ground fully
    cooked ham (about ½ cup)

■ Preheat the oven to 300°. Meanwhile, separate eggs; set aside. Wash and discard stems from spinach, then chop (you should have about ¾ cup). Set aside.

■ In a saucepan combine soup and cheese. Cook and stir just till cheese melts, then remove from heat. In a small mixing bowl, slightly beat yolks. Then *gradually* stir in soup mixture. Stir in spinach and ham.

■ In a large mixer bowl, beat egg whites till stiff peaks form (tips stand straight). Gradually fold in spinach mixture. *For individual soufflés, pour mixture into 4 ungreased 14- or 15-ounce soufflé dishes. Bake in the 300° oven for 25 to 30 minutes or till knife inserted near the center comes out clean. Serves 4.

***For 1 large soufflé:** Use an ungreased 1½-quart soufflé dish. Make a collar for dish by measuring top circumference of dish and adding 6 inches. Cut a 12-inch-wide piece of foil to this length. Fold foil lengthwise into thirds. Lightly butter 1 side of foil. Attach foil, buttered side in, around outside of dish so that foil extends about 2 inches above dish. Fold foil ends until foil fits dish. Pour egg mixture into dish. Bake in the 300° oven for 45 to 50 minutes or till done.

PER SERVING

Calories	196
Protein	14 g
Carbohydrate	4 g
Fat	13 g
Cholesterol	300 mg
Sodium	641 mg
Potassium	245 mg

TIMETABLE

Preparation time:
25 minutes

Cooking time:
25 to 30 minutes

RAINBOW COMPOTE

Use a variety of fruit to get the rainbow of color.

¼ of a medium honeydew
    melon *or* cantaloupe
1 cup fresh raspberries
    or strawberries, *or* 2
    nectarines *or* peaches,
    or a combination
1 medium orange
½ cup unsweetened pineapple
    juice *or* orange juice
⅛ teaspoon ground cinnamon
    Dash ground nutmeg

■ Remove seeds and peel from honeydew melon or cantaloupe, then cut into cubes. If using strawberries, cut them in half; cover and chill berries. If using nectarines or peaches, peel, if desired, then remove pits and cut fruit into slices. Peel orange. Slice orange crosswise into ½-inch slices, then quarter slices.

■ In a medium bowl combine pineapple or orange juice, cinnamon, and nutmeg. Add melon; nectarines or peaches, if using; and orange. Toss lightly till coated. Cover and chill till serving time.

■ To serve, add raspberries or strawberries, if using. Toss lightly. Makes 4 servings.

PER SERVING

Calories	60
Protein	1 g
Carbohydrate	15 g
Fat	0 g
Cholesterol	0 mg
Sodium	4 mg
Potassium	238 mg

TIMETABLE

Preparation time:
15 minutes

Chilling time:
about 25 mintues

Fourth Day

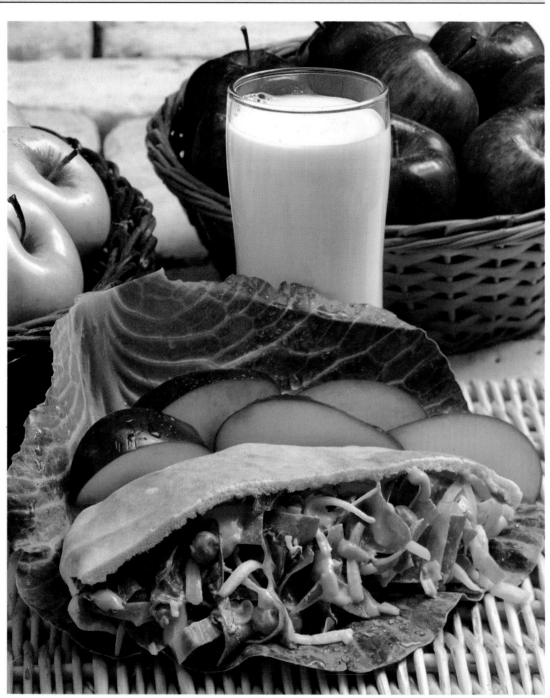

■ **BREAKFAST**

½ of a whole wheat English muffin, toasted	70
1 tablespoon peanut butter	95
1 fresh peach *or* small nectarine	35
1 cup skim milk	85
Total calories	**285**

■ **LUNCH**

*Corned Beef Pocket	368
1 medium apple	80
1 cup skim milk	85
Total calories	**533**

■ **DINNER**

*Lemon-Pepper Chicken	154
*Barley with Vegetables, *recipe, page 140*	90
1 cup cooked cut asparagus	45
½ cup ice milk	93
Coffee *or* tea	0
Total calories	**382**

Save a few extra minutes by buying shredded cabbage for the Corned Beef Pockets.

Corned Beef Pocket

20 minutes or less

CORNED BEEF POCKETS

Corned beef and cabbage in a pita.

¼ cup frozen peas
1 2½-ounce package very
  thinly sliced corned beef
1 cup shredded cabbage
3 tablespoons reduced-calorie
  Thousand Island salad
  dressing
2 tablespoons shredded
  mozzarella cheese
¼ teaspoon caraway seed
1 large pita bread round
2 cabbage *or* lettuce leaves,
  (optional)

■ Place frozen peas in a colander. Run *hot water* over peas just till thawed. Drain well, then transfer to a medium mixing bowl.

■ Chop corned beef, then add it to peas in bowl. Add shredded cabbage, Thousand Island dressing, cheese, and caraway seed. Stir till well combined.

■ To serve, cut pita in half crosswise. Open pockets, then spoon the cabbage mixture into the pockets. If desired, serve the stuffed pitas on top of cabbage or lettuce leaves. Makes 2 servings.

PER SERVING

Calories	**368**
Protein	18 g
Carbohydrate	32 g
Fat	19 g
Cholesterol	41 mg
Sodium	651 mg
Potassium	161 mg

TIMETABLE

Total preparation time:
10 minutes

---

20 minutes or less

LEMON-PEPPER CHICKEN

1 tablespoon margarine
  or butter
1 tablespoon frozen snipped
  parsley (see tip, page 39)
1 tablespoon lemon juice
½ teaspoon lemon-pepper
  seasoning
½ teaspoon bottled minced
  garlic *or* ⅛ teaspoon
  garlic powder
¼ teaspoon salt
4 boned skinless chicken
  breast halves *or* turkey
  breast tenderloin steaks
  (about 1 pound total)
  Paprika

■ Preheat the broiler. Meanwhile, in a small saucepan melt margarine or butter. Stir in parsley, lemon juice, lemon-pepper seasoning, garlic, and salt. Place poultry on the unheated rack of a broiler pan. Brush with *half* of the lemon mixture.

■ Broil poultry 4 inches from the heat for 4 minutes. Turn poultry over and brush with remaining lemon mixture. Broil for 4 to 5 minutes more or till poultry is tender and no longer pink.

■ To serve, transfer poultry to a serving platter. Sprinkle with paprika. Makes 4 servings.

PER SERVING

Calories	**154**
Protein	26 g
Carbohydrate	1 g
Fat	4 g
Cholesterol	66 mg
Sodium	242 mg
Potassium	312 mg

TIMETABLE

Preparation time:
10 minutes

Cooking time:
8 to 9 minutes

Fifth Day

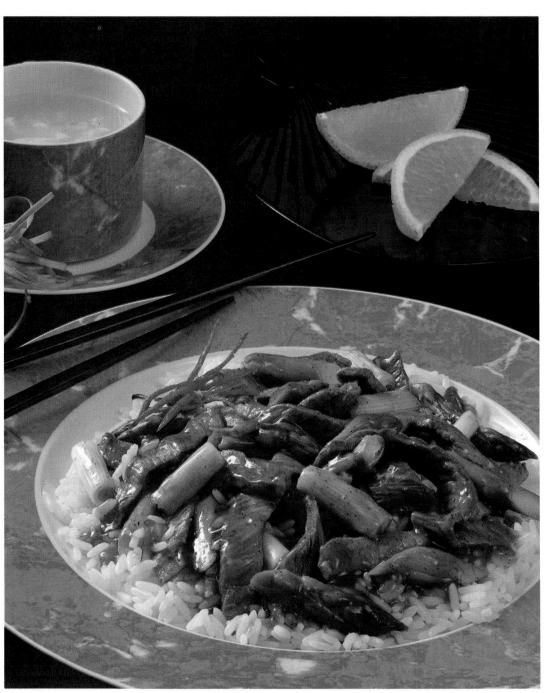

◼ BREAKFAST

¾ cup fresh red raspberries	45
1 poached egg	80
2 slices whole wheat bread, toasted	140
2 teaspoons margarine *or* butter	67
Coffee *or* tea	0
Total calories	**332**

◼ LUNCH

*Bulgur Tacos, *recipe, page 72*	258
2 fresh apricots	34
1 cup skim milk	85
Total calories	**377**

◼ DINNER

*Ginger Soup	63
*Peppery Beef Stir-Fry	306
1 medium orange	60
1 fortune cookie	37
Tea	0
Total calories	**466**

During the 20 minutes the meat is marinating for the Peppery Beef Stir-Fry, prepare the Ginger Soup and slice the orange.

Peppery Beef Stir-Fry, Ginger Soup

PEPPERY BEEF STIR-FRY

Some like it hot and some like it not so hot. If you don't like spicy foods, use only ⅛ teaspoon each of the peppers.

¾ **pound boneless beef top round steak**
2 **tablespoons water**
2 **tablespoons soy sauce**
1 **tablespoon sugar**
1 **teaspoon bottled minced garlic** *or* **¼ teaspoon garlic powder**
⅛ **to ¼ teaspoon ground red pepper**
⅛ **to ¼ teaspoon ground black pepper**
8 **ounces fresh asparagus spears** *or* **1 small sweet red pepper** *and* **1 small green pepper**
6 **green onions**
⅓ **cup cold water**
1½ **teaspoons cornstarch**
1½ **cups quick-cooking rice Nonstick spray coating**
2 **teaspoons cooking oil**

■ Trim fat from meat. Thinly slice meat across the grain into bite-size strips. In a bowl stir together 2 tablespoons water, soy sauce, sugar, garlic, red pepper, and black pepper. Add meat. Toss till coated. Cover and marinate at room temperature for 20 minutes.

■ While beef is marinating, cut asparagus or peppers and onions into 1-inch pieces. In a bowl stir together ⅓ cup water and cornstarch; set aside. Cook rice according to package directions, *except* omit butter.

■ Spray a *cold* wok or large skillet with nonstick coating. Preheat the wok or skillet over high heat. If using asparagus, stir-fry for 3 minutes. Add onions and sweet peppers (if using), and stir-fry about 1½ minutes more or till vegetables are nearly tender. Remove vegetables from wok.

■ Add oil to hot wok, then add beef mixture. Stir-fry for 2 to 3 minutes or till brown. Push meat from center of wok. Stir cornstarch mixture, then add it to center of wok. Cook and stir till thickened and bubbly. Then cook and stir for 1 minute more. Stir in vegetables. Cover and cook for 1 minute more. Stir before serving. Serve over rice. Makes 4 servings.

PER SERVING

Calories	306
Protein	24 g
Carbohydrate	38 g
Fat	6 g
Cholesterol	54 mg
Sodium	828 mg
Potassium	441 mg

TIMETABLE

Preparation time:
25 minutes

Cooking time:
6 to 11 minutes

20 minutes or less

GINGER SOUP

Just add a few ingredients to canned broth for an easy Oriental-style soup.

2 **14½-ounce cans chicken broth**
2 **tablespoons frozen sliced green onion (see tip, page 39)**
1 **teaspoon lime juice**
¼ **teaspoon ground ginger**
1 **ounce fine noodles (½ cup)**

■ In a medium saucepan combine the chicken broth, frozen onion, lime juice, and ginger. Bring to boiling.

■ Break noodles slightly while adding them to broth mixture, then reduce heat. Simmer soup, uncovered, about 5 minutes or till noodles are tender. Serves 4.

PER SERVING

Calories	63
Protein	5 g
Carbohydrate	6 g
Fat	2 g
Cholesterol	7 mg
Sodium	653 mg
Potassium	197 mg

TIMETABLE

Preparation time:
5 minutes

Cooking time:
about 10 minutes

Sixth Day

■ BREAKFAST

*Spicy Oatmeal Mix	201
1 medium banana	105
1 cup skim milk	85
Total calories	**391**

■ LUNCH

*Fruit and Tuna Plate	231
3 crackers	69
1 tomato, sliced	25
Sparkling water	0
Total calories	**325**

■ DINNER

*Spanish Chicken Bake, *recipe, page 79*	234
1 cup cooked broccoli	50
1½ cups torn mixed salad greens	15
1 tablespoon reduced-calorie creamy cucumber salad dressing	30
1 fresh peach *or* small nectarine	35
1 cup skim milk	85
Total calories	**449**

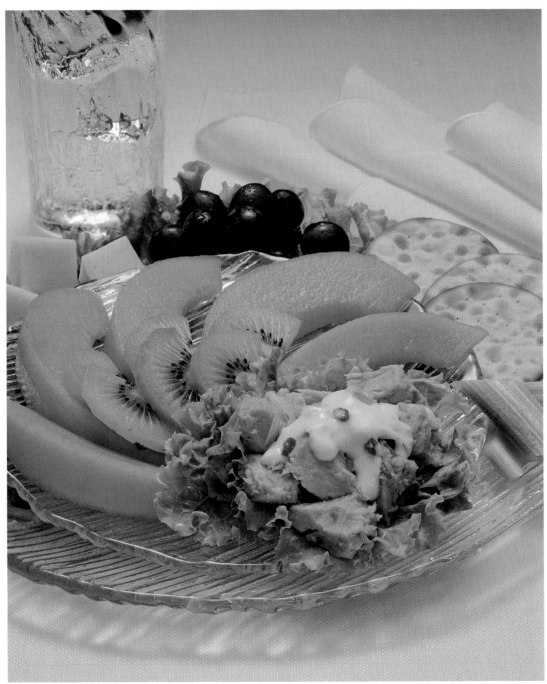

Fruit and Tuna Plate

FRUIT AND TUNA PLATE

3 tablespoons plain low-fat
   yogurt
2 tablespoons reduced-calorie
   mayonnaise *or* salad
   dressing
1 tablespoon skim milk
1 tablespoon chopped
   pimiento
⅛ teaspoon dried tarragon,
   crushed
1 medium cantaloupe
1 kiwi fruit
2 stalks celery
2 ounces Monterey Jack
   cheese
1 6½-ounce can tuna
   (water pack)
   Lettuce leaves
1 cup seedless red grapes

■ For dressing, in a small mixing bowl stir together the yogurt, mayonnaise or salad dressing, skim milk, pimiento, and tarragon. Cover and chill dressing while preparing other ingredients.

■ Cut cantaloupe in half lengthwise, then remove seeds. Cut each of the melon halves in half lengthwise again. Cut off peel. Then cut each melon quarter lengthwise into slices. Set cantaloupe aside.

■ Peel and slice kiwi fruit. Then cut kiwi slices in half. Bias-slice celery into 2-inch pieces. Cut cheese into cubes. Drain and flake tuna.

■ For salads, line four plates with lettuce leaves. Then arrange cantaloupe, kiwi fruit, celery, cheese, tuna, and grapes on the plates. Drizzle dressing on top of tuna. Makes 4 servings.

PER SERVING

Calories	231
Protein	19 g
Carbohydrate	24 g
Fat	8 g
Cholesterol	42 mg
Sodium	188 mg
Potassium	819 mg

TIMETABLE

Total preparation time:
30 minutes

---

20 minutes or less

SPICY OATMEAL MIX

Choose apple pie spice for a blend of cinnamon, allspice, nutmeg, and ginger.

2 cups quick-cooking
   rolled oats
½ cup nonfat dry milk
   powder
¼ cup raisins
2 tablespoons brown sugar
½ teaspoon ground
   cinnamon *or* apple
   pie spice
¼ teaspoon salt

■ In an airtight storage container combine the oats, dry milk powder, raisins, brown sugar, cinnamon or apple pie spice, and salt. Before using, shake the container to distribute the ingredients. Makes about 2⅔ cups cereal mixture or 5 servings.

■ *To cook 3 servings:* In a medium saucepan bring 2¼ cups *hot water* to boiling, then stir in *1½ cups* of the cereal mixture. Reduce the heat. Cook and stir for 1 minute. Let stand about 1 minute before serving.

■ *To cook 1 serving:* In a small saucepan bring ¾ cup *hot water* to boiling, then stir in *½ cup* of the cereal mixture. Reduce the heat. Cook and stir for 1 minute. Let stand about 1 minute before serving.

PER SERVING

Calories	201
Protein	9 g
Carbohydrate	38 g
Fat	2 g
Cholesterol	2 mg
Sodium	166 mg
Potassium	360 mg

TIMETABLE

Advance preparation time:
5 minutes

Final preparation time:
about 10 minutes

Seventh Day

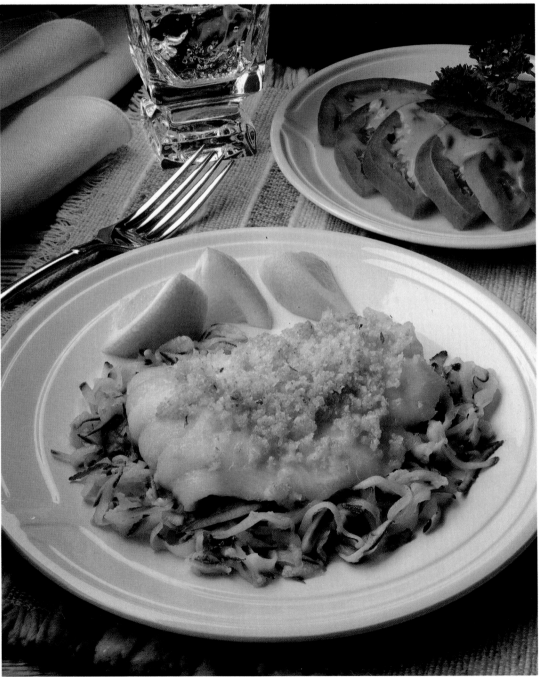

■ BREAKFAST

2 4-inch pancakes	120
2 tablespoons reduced-calorie pancake and waffle syrup	60
¾ cup unsweetened applesauce with cinnamon	80
½ cup skim milk	43
Total calories	**303**

■ LUNCH

*Souffléed Asparagus, *recipe, page 120*	250
1 cup raw carrot sticks	48
1 whole wheat roll	85
1 nectarine	65
1 cup skim milk	85
Total calories	**533**

■ DINNER

*Crumb-Topped Fish	151
1 slice whole wheat bread	70
1 tomato, sliced	25
1 tablespoon reduced-calorie Thousand Island salad dressing	30
*Raspberry Sundaes	134
Sparkling water	0
Total calories	**410**

Crumb-Topped Fish

CRUMB-TOPPED FISH

To use frozen fish, allow 6 to 8 hours for it to thaw in the refrigerator.

Nonstick spray coating
1 pound fresh skinless
    haddock fillets (½ to
    ¾ inch thick) *or* fresh
    sea scallops
¼ teaspoon finely shredded
    lemon peel (set aside)
2 teaspoons lemon juice
2 tablespoons grated
    Parmesan cheese
2 tablespoons fine dry
    seasoned bread crumbs
1 tablespoon liquid margarine
2 medium zucchini
⅛ teaspoon salt
    Lemon wedges (optional)

■ Preheat the oven to 400°. Meanwhile, spray a 10x6x2-inch baking dish with nonstick coating. Place fillets or scallops in a single layer in the dish, tucking under any thin edges of fish. Then drizzle lemon juice over fish or scallops.

■ In a small bowl combine Parmesan cheese, bread crumbs, liquid margarine, and lemon peel. Sprinkle crumb mixture on top of fish or scallops. Bake in the 400° oven for 10 to 15 minutes or till fish flakes easily with a fork or till scallops are opaque.

■ While fish or scallops are baking, in a medium saucepan bring about 1 inch of water to boiling, then reduce heat to a simmer. Meanwhile, coarsely shred zucchini (you should have about 3 cups).

■ Place zucchini in a steamer basket. Sprinkle it lightly with salt. Carefully place the basket over the simmering water. Cover and steam the zucchini for 2 to 3 minutes or till tender.

■ To serve, place the zucchini on dinner plates. Then arrange the fish fillets or scallops on top of zucchini. Serve with lemon wedges, if desired. Serves 4.

PER SERVING

Calories	151
Protein	23 g
Carbohydrate	5 g
Fat	4 g
Cholesterol	71 mg
Sodium	247 mg
Potassium	521 mg

TIMETABLE

Preparation time:
10 minutes

Cooking time:
10 to 15 minutes

20 minutes or less

RASPBERRY SUNDAES

A delicious berry topping that's also good on angel food cake.

1 cup loose-pack frozen
    red raspberries *or*
    frozen unsweetened
    whole strawberries
2 tablespoons sugar
2 tablespoons orange juice
½ teaspoon frozen, finely
    shredded orange peel
    (see tip, page 66)
2 cups vanilla ice milk

■ In a small saucepan combine frozen berries, sugar, orange juice, and orange peel. Cook and stir over medium heat till the mixture is bubbly.

■ Coarsely crush the berries. Then transfer mixture to a covered container. Slightly cool mixture, or chill till serving time or for up to 2 days.

■ To serve, scoop ice milk into dessert dishes. Spoon cooled or chilled berry mixture over ice milk. Makes 4 servings.

PER SERVING

Calories	134
Protein	3 g
Carbohydrate	25 g
Fat	3 g
Cholesterol	9 mg
Sodium	52 mg
Potassium	194 mg

TIMETABLE

Total preparation time:
20 minutes

Eighth Day

◼ BRUNCH

3 ounces cooked turkey breast slices	135
6 cooked asparagus spears	23
2 *Zucchini-Wheat Muffins	216
*Peachy Shake	130
Total calories	**504**

◼ DINNER

1 grilled salmon steak (about 4 ounces cooked)	200
*Potato-Onion Bake, *recipe, page 143*	89
1 cup cooked green beans	45
1 whole wheat roll	85
1 teaspoon margarine *or* butter	34
1 cup canned pineapple chunks (juice pack)	150
1 cup skim milk	85
Total calories	**688**

Either poach or pan-fry the turkey in a skillet sprayed with nonstick coating. Cook the turkey till it's tender and no longer pink.

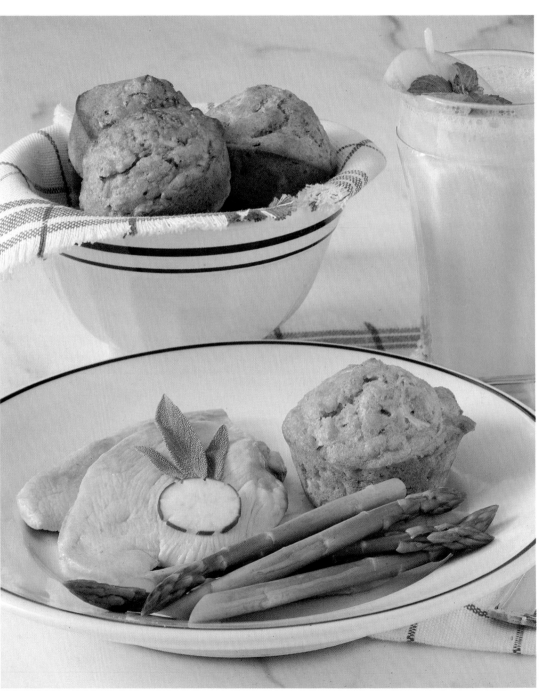

Peachy Shake, Zucchini-Wheat Muffins

PEACHY SHAKE

No ice cream? You'll find it hard to believe as you sip this thick, rich shake.

1 medium peach
⅓ cup skim milk
1 tablespoon honey
½ cup ice cubes

■ Remove pit from peach, then cut peach into large chunks (do not peel peach).

■ In a blender container combine the peach, milk, honey, and ice cubes. Cover and blend till nearly smooth. Pour into a glass. If desired, garnish with a peach slice and mint leaf. Makes 1 serving.

PER SERVING

Calories	130
Protein	3 g
Carbohydrate	31 g
Fat	0 g
Cholesterol	1 mg
Sodium	43 mg
Potassium	317 mg

TIMETABLE

Total preparation time:
5 minutes

ZUCCHINI-WHEAT MUFFINS

¾ cup whole wheat flour
¼ cup all-purpose flour
3 tablespoons sugar
1 teaspoon baking powder
⅛ teaspoon salt
⅓ cup skim milk
2 egg whites
2 tablespoons cooking oil
½ teaspoon frozen, finely
    shredded orange peel
    (see tip, page 66)
¼ of a small zucchini
    Nonstick spray coating

■ Preheat the oven to 400°. Meanwhile, in a medium mixing bowl stir together the whole wheat flour, all-purpose flour, sugar, baking powder, and salt. Set flour mixture aside.

■ In a small mixing bowl use a fork to beat together milk, egg whites, oil, and orange peel. Shred zucchini (you should have about ½ cup). Then add zucchini to milk mixture.

■ Add zucchini mixture to flour mixture, then stir just till moistened (batter should be lumpy). Spray muffin cups with nonstick coating. Fill cups ½ full. Bake in the 400° oven for 15 to 20 minutes or till golden. If desired, freeze leftover muffins in a sealed clear plastic freezer bag for up to 2 months. Makes 8.

PER SERVING

Calories	108
Protein	3 g
Carbohydrate	17 g
Fat	4 g
Cholesterol	0 mg
Sodium	89 mg
Potassium	91 mg

TIMETABLE

Preparation time:
10 minutes

Cooking time:
15 to 20 minutes

Ninth Day

■ BREAKFAST

1 cup tomato juice	**40**
1 poached egg	**80**
2 slices whole wheat bread, toasted	**140**
2 teaspoons margarine *or* butter	**67**
1 cup skim milk	**85**
Total calories	**412**

■ LUNCH

Cold beef pita sandwich (½ of a pita bread round; 2 ounces cold, sliced, cooked lean roast beef; 1 lettuce leaf; 1 teaspoon prepared mustard)	**272**
*Golden Squash Bisque	**88**
Iced tea	**0**
Total calories	**360**

■ DINNER

*Vegetable Terrine	**173**
1 cup cooked brusels sprouts	**60**
1 breadstick	**106**
¾ cup sliced fresh strawberries topped with ½ cup vanilla low-fat yogurt	**131**
Coffee *or* tea	**0**
Total calories	**470**

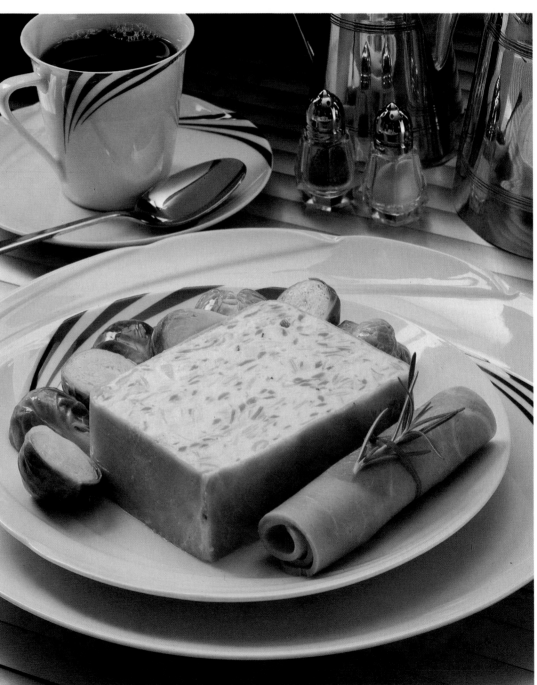

Vegetable Terrine

VEGETABLE TERRINE

An elegant make-ahead entrée.

2 large leeks
2 medium carrots
1¼ cups water
1 tablespoon instant chicken bouillon granules
¾ teaspoon dried rosemary, crushed
¼ cup cold water
1 envelope unflavored gelatin
⅔ cup packaged instant mashed potato flakes
1 8-ounce container reduced-calorie soft-style cream cheese
1 8-ounce carton plain low-fat yogurt
¼ teaspoon pepper
Nonstick spray coating
14 thin slices low-fat fully cooked ham (about 10½ ounces total)

■ Chop leeks and shred carrots. In a large saucepan combine leeks, carrots, 1¼ cups water, bouillon granules, and rosemary. Bring to boiling, then reduce heat. Cover and simmer for 10 minutes or till vegetables are tender. *Do not drain.*

■ While vegetables are simmering, in a small mixing bowl stir together cold water and gelatin. Let gelatin stand for 5 minutes to soften. Then stir the softened gelatin into vegetable mixture in saucepan. If necessary, heat vegetable mixture till gelatin is dissolved. Stir in potato flakes, then remove saucepan from heat. Cover and let stand for 1 minute. Meanwhile, in a mixing bowl stir together cream cheese, yogurt, and pepper. Stir in vegetable mixture.

■ Spray an 8x4x2-inch loaf pan with nonstick coating. Line pan with *6* of the ham slices; reserve remaining ham slices in the refrigerator. Spoon mixture into the pan. Cover and chill for 8 hours or till firm.

■ To serve, roll up remaining ham slices. Unmold terrine onto a serving platter. Slice to serve. Serve with ham rolls. Makes 8 servings.

PER SERVING

Calories	173
Protein	14 g
Carbohydrate	13 g
Fat	7 g
Cholesterol	38 mg
Sodium	777 mg
Potassium	349 mg

TIMETABLE

Advance preparation time:
20 minutes

Chilling time:
at least 8 hours

Final preparation time:
5 minutes

GOLDEN SQUASH BISQUE

1 12-ounce package frozen mashed cooked winter squash
¾ cup water
¾ cup evaporated skim milk
1 7½-ounce jar junior carrots
1 teaspoon instant chicken bouillon granules
½ teaspoon onion salt
½ teaspoon frozen, finely shredded lemon peel (see tip, page 66)
Dash ground nutmeg
Parsley sprigs

■ In a medium mixing bowl combine frozen block of squash, water, evaporated milk, carrots, bouillon granules, onion salt, lemon peel, and nutmeg. Cover and chill for 22 to 24 hours, stirring occasionally to break up squash as it thaws.

■ Before serving, stir the bisque till well combined. Ladle the bisque into individual bowls. Garnish *each* serving with a parsley sprig. Makes 4 servings.

PER SERVING

Calories	88
Protein	5 g
Carbohydrate	18 g
Fat	0 g
Cholesterol	2 mg
Sodium	374 mg
Potassium	548 mg

TIMETABLE

Advance preparation time:
10 minutes

Chilling time:
22 to 24 hours

Tenth Day

■ BREAKFAST

1 medium banana	105
1½ cups wheat flakes	150
1 cup skim milk	85
Total calories	**340**

■ LUNCH

*Turkey Tortilla	192
1 nectarine	65
1 cup skim milk	85
Total calories	**342**

■ DINNER

*All-Day Pot Roast, *recipe, page 85*	345
2½ cups tossed salad (1 cup romaine, ¼ of a green pepper, ½ of a carrot, ½ of a tomato, ¼ of a cucumber)	52
2 tablespoons reduced-calorie Italian salad dressing	12
*Orange-Yogurt Freeze	97
Coffee *or* tea	0
Total calories	**506**

Cut the vegetables for the Turkey Tortillas into julienne sticks, or coarsely shred them—either way works fine.

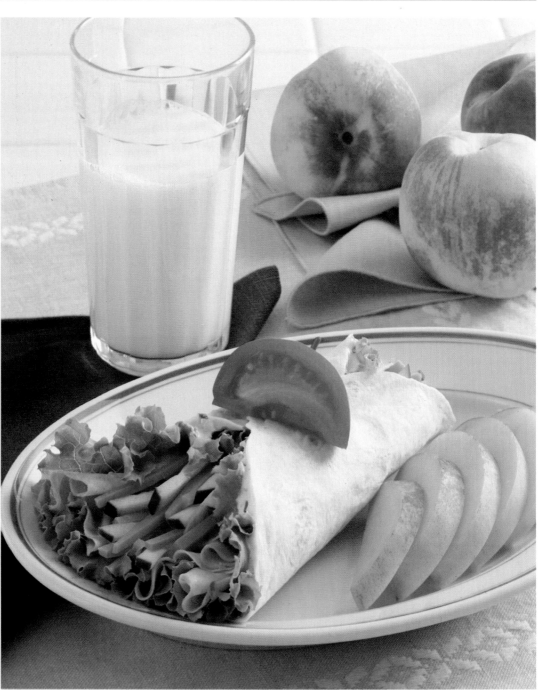

Turkey Tortilla

20 minutes or less

TURKEY TORTILLAS

Cucumber, carrot, and lettuce add a refreshing crunch to these sandwiches.

½ of a small cucumber
½ of a medium carrot
½ of a small tomato
½ of an 8-ounce container reduced-calorie soft-style cream cheese
2 tablespoons frozen snipped chives (see tip, page 39)
1 tablespoon skim milk
½ teaspoon curry powder
4 6-inch flour tortillas
4 lettuce leaves
3 2½-ounce packages very thinly sliced smoked turkey

■ Remove seeds from cucumber. Cut cucumber and carrot into julienne sticks. Cut tomato into 4 wedges. Set vegetables aside.

■ In a small mixing bowl stir together cream cheese, chives, milk, and curry powder. Spread mixture on 1 side of tortillas. Then top with lettuce leaves, turkey, cucumber, and carrot.

■ Fold *2* opposite sides of *each* tortilla over filling, overlapping in the centers. Secure with toothpicks. Garnish with tomato wedges. Makes 4 servings.

PER SERVING

Calories	192
Protein	17 g
Carbohydrate	18 g
Fat	6 g
Cholesterol	33 mg
Sodium	771 mg
Potassium	296 mg

TIMETABLE

Total preparation time:
20 minutes

ORANGE-YOGURT FREEZE

The sweetness of the oranges complements the tartness of the yogurt.

1 10½-ounce can mandarin orange sections (water pack)
2 tablespoons sugar
1 teaspoon unflavored gelatin
¼ cup orange juice
1 8-ounce carton orange low-fat yogurt
1 teaspoon vanilla
1 egg white

■ Drain orange sections, then set oranges aside. Meanwhile, in a small saucepan combine sugar and gelatin. Stir in orange juice. Heat and stir gelatin mixture till the gelatin and sugar are dissolved. Then remove from heat and cool slightly.

■ Place oranges, gelatin mixture, yogurt, and vanilla in a blender container. Cover and blend till smooth.

■ In a small mixing bowl, beat egg white with a rotary beater till stiff peaks form (tips stand straight). Fold egg white into yogurt mixture. Then transfer mixture to an 8x4x2-inch loaf dish. Cover and freeze for 3 to 24 hours or till firm.

■ To serve, scrape surface of frozen mixture. Serve in dessert dishes. Makes 5 servings.

PER SERVING

Calories	97
Protein	4 g
Carbohydrate	20 g
Fat	1 g
Cholesterol	2 mg
Sodium	38 mg
Potassium	189 mg

TIMETABLE

Advance preparation time:
15 minutes

Freezing time:
3 to 24 hours

Final preparation time:
5 minutes

Eleventh Day

■ BREAKFAST

½ of a small cantaloupe	95
1 3-inch bran muffin	125
1 cup skim milk	85
Total calories	**305**

■ LUNCH

*Meatless Chili Soup, *recipe, page 73*	312
4 saltine crackers	50
1½ cups torn fresh spinach	15
1 tablespoon reduced-calorie Italian salad dressing	6
1 cup skim milk	85
Total calories	**468**

■ DINNER

*Steamed Beef and Vegetables	247
2 round rice cakes	70
*Fruit and Yogurt	103
Sparkling water with a lime twist	0
Total calories	**420**

Steam the meatballs with the vegetables for a one-pot meal.

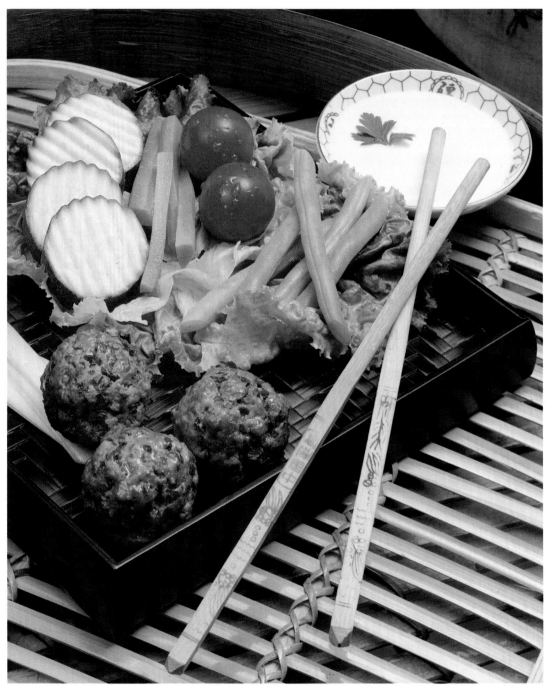

Steamed Beef and Vegetables

STEAMED BEEF AND VEGETABLES

⅓ cup frozen snipped
    parsley (see tip, page 39)
¼ cup water
3 tablespoons fine dry
    bread crumbs
¼ teaspoon salt
⅛ teaspoon pepper
12 ounces lean ground beef
2 leeks *or* 4 green onions
1 medium carrot
1 medium zucchini
4 ounces whole green beans
2 cups hot water
    Nonstick spray coating
8 cherry tomatoes
⅓ cup plain low-fat yogurt
2 tablespoons reduced-calorie
    mayonnaise *or* salad
    dressing
2 teaspoons prepared
    horseradish
1 teaspoon lemon juice
4 large lettuce leaves

■ In a medium mixing bowl stir together parsley, ¼ cup water, bread crumbs, salt, and pepper. Add beef, then mix well. Shape meat mixture into 12 meatballs; set aside. If using leeks, cut them in half lengthwise. Cut carrot into julienne sticks and zucchini into ½-inch slices. Trim beans.

■ In a wok or large skillet bring 2 cups hot water to boiling, then reduce heat to a simmer. Meanwhile, spray a steamer basket with nonstick coating. Place meatballs in a single layer on the steamer basket. Place basket over the simmering water. Cover and steam meat for 4 minutes. Add leeks, carrot, zucchini, and beans. Cover and steam for 12 minutes more. Add tomatoes and steam for 2 minutes. (If necessary, add more hot water during steaming.)

■ While meatballs and vegetables are steaming, for sauce, in a small bowl stir together yogurt, mayonnaise or salad dressing, horseradish, and lemon juice.

■ To serve, place lettuce leaves on 4 dinner plates, then arrange vegetables and meatballs on top of lettuce. Serve with the horseradish sauce. Serves 4.

PER SERVING

Calories	247
Protein	21 g
Carbohydrate	18 g
Fat	10 g
Cholesterol	61 mg
Sodium	291 mg
Potassium	618 mg

TIMETABLE

Preparation time:
20 minutes

Cooking time:
18 minutes

FRUIT AND YOGURT

Assemble the dessert before dinner, then, while you're eating, the frozen fruit will have time to thaw.

½ of a 16-ounce package
    (2 cups) frozen mixed fruit
2 tablespoons reduced-calorie
    orange marmalade
1 8-ounce carton vanilla
    low-fat yogurt
⅛ teaspoon ground coriander
1 tablespoon chopped pecans

■ Place frozen fruit into dessert dishes. In a small mixing bowl, fold orange marmalade into yogurt. Then gently stir in coriander.

■ Spoon yogurt mixture on top of fruit in dishes. Sprinkle with nuts. Let stand at room temperature about 30 minutes to allow fruit to thaw before serving. Makes 4 servings.

PER SERVING

Calories	103
Protein	3 g
Carbohydrate	19 g
Fat	2 g
Cholesterol	3 mg
Sodium	57 mg
Potassium	254 mg

TIMETABLE

Preparation time:
10 minutes

Standing time:
about 30 minutes

Twelfth Day

◼ BREAKFAST

1 English muffin	140
1 tablespoon reduced-calorie jam	24
1 cup skim milk	85
Total calories	**249**

◼ LUNCH

*Fruit and Salmon Salad	281
1 slice whole wheat bread	70
½ cup small fresh strawberries	23
10 seedless green grapes	35
Ice water	0
Total calories	**409**

◼ DINNER

*Turkey-Apple Burger	199
1 cup cooked carrots	70
1 slice whole wheat bread	70
1 teaspoon margarine *or* butter	34
1 medium pear	100
1 cup skim milk	85
Total calories	**558**

A summer luncheon special, this light, refreshing meal requires no cooking.

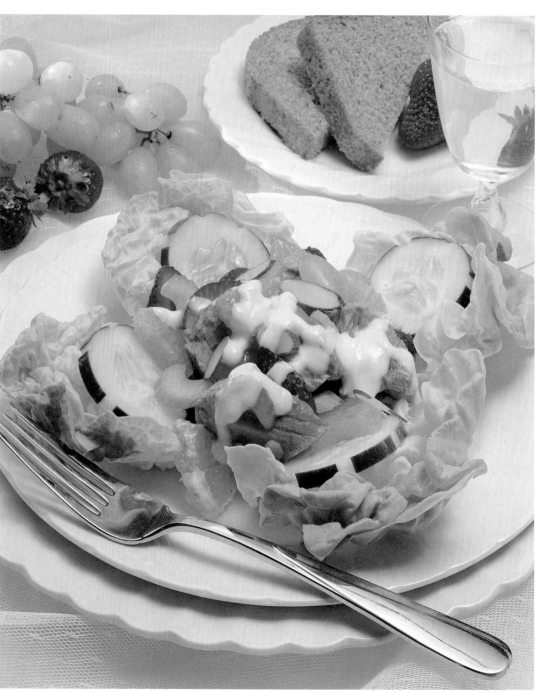

Fruit and Salmon Salad

FRUIT AND SALMON SALADS

1 **15½-ounce can salmon**
1 **medium orange**
1 **medium cucumber**
1 **stalk celery**
½ **cup strawberries**
½ **cup seedless grapes**
⅓ **cup plain low-fat yogurt**
1 **tablespoon honey**
1 **large head Bibb *or* Boston lettuce**
2 **tablespoons sliced almonds**

■ Drain the salmon. Remove skin and bones, then break salmon into chunks. Finely shred ¼ *teaspoon* peel from orange, then set peel aside. Peel orange and cut orange into bite-size pieces. Slice cucumber and celery. Cut strawberries and grapes in half. Set the cucumber slices aside.

■ For salmon mixture, in a medium mixing bowl combine salmon, orange, celery, strawberries, and grapes. Toss lightly to mix.

■ For dressing, in a small mixing bowl stir together yogurt, honey, and orange peel.

■ To serve, separate leaves from head of lettuce. Place *3 or 4* lettuce leaves on *each* of the salad plates. Arrange cucumber slices on top. Then arrange the salmon mixture on top of lettuce. Sprinkle with nuts and drizzle dressing over salmon mixture. Serves 4.

PER SERVING

Calories	281
Protein	25 g
Carbohydrate	19 g
Fat	12 g
Cholesterol	38 mg
Sodium	586 mg
Potassium	820 mg

TIMETABLE

Total preparation time: 20 minutes

TURKEY-APPLE BURGERS

Instead of using ground turkey and sage, you can substitute turkey sausage. If the sausage is frozen, remember to allow time for it to thaw.

1 **large apple**
1 **egg**
¼ **cup fine dry bread crumbs**
1 **tablespoon dried minced onion**
¼ **teaspoon salt**
⅛ **teaspoon ground sage**
1 **pound ground raw turkey**
   Nonstick spray coating
½ **of a medium tomato**
4 **lettuce leaves**
¼ **cup plain low-fat yogurt (optional)**

■ Preheat the broiler. Meanwhile, core and coarsely shred apple (you should have about 1 cup).

■ In a medium mixing bowl slightly beat egg. Then stir in apple, bread crumbs, onion, salt, and sage. Add turkey, then mix well. Shape mixture into four ½-inch-thick patties.

■ Spray the *cold* rack of an unheated broiler pan with nonstick coating. Place patties on the rack. Broil 3 to 4 inches from the heat for 4 minutes. Turn over. Broil for 4 to 5 minutes more, or till no longer pink.

■ While patties are broiling, slice tomato. Place a lettuce leaf on *each* plate. To serve, place patties atop lettuce on plates. Then top patties with tomato slices and yogurt, if desired. Makes 4 servings.

PER SERVING

Calories	199
Protein	28 g
Carbohydrate	12 g
Fat	4 g
Cholesterol	152 mg
Sodium	269 mg
Potassium	417 mg

TIMETABLE

Preparation time: 20 minutes

Cooking time: 8 to 9 minutes

Thirteenth Day

▇ BREAKFAST

1 frozen waffle	103
2 tablespoons reduced-calorie pancake and waffle syrup	60
1 cup sliced fresh strawberries	46
1 cup skim milk	85
Total calories	**294**

▇ LUNCH

*Beefed-Up Tomato Cups	185
1 slice whole wheat bread	70
1 teaspoon margarine *or* butter	34
1 medium orange	60
1 cup skim milk	85
Total calories	**434**

▇ DINNER

*Shrimp Primavera	293
1 1-inch slice French bread	100
1 teaspoon margarine *or* butter	34
1 cup fresh pineapple spears	76
Coffee *or* tea	0
Total calories	**503**

For dessert in a hurry, purchase peeled fresh pineapple.

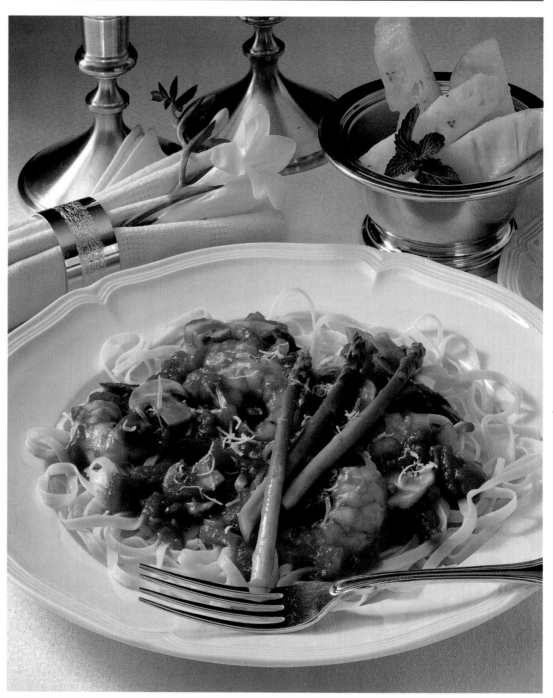

Shrimp Primavera

SHRIMP PRIMAVERA

4 ounces fettuccine
1 8-ounce package frozen
   peeled and deveined
   shrimp
1 7½-ounce can tomatoes
1 2½-ounce jar sliced
   mushrooms
3 tablespoons tomato paste
2 tablespoons frozen chopped
   onion (see tip, page 39)
2 tablespoons frozen snipped
   parsley (see tip, page 39)
1 teaspoon dried basil,
   crushed
1 teaspoon bottled minced
   garlic *or* ¼ teaspoon
   garlic powder
½ teaspoon sugar
1 pound asparagus spears
1 tablespoon finely shredded
   Parmesan cheese

■ Cook pasta according to package directions, *except* use a large saucepan and 5 cups *hot* water. Drain. Meanwhile, place frozen shrimp in a colander. Run *cool water* over frozen shrimp just till thawed. Cut up tomatoes and drain mushrooms.

■ In a medium saucepan combine *undrained* tomatoes, mushrooms, tomato paste, frozen onion, parsley, basil, garlic, sugar, ⅛ teaspoon *salt*, and dash *pepper*. Bring to boiling, then reduce heat. Simmer, uncovered, for 5 minutes. Add shrimp, then simmer about 5 minutes more or till shrimp turn pink.

■ While sauce and shrimp are cooking, cook asparagus, covered, in a small amount of boiling water for 7 to 8 minutes or till nearly tender. Drain.

■ To serve, arrange fettuccine on dinner plates. Top with shrimp mixture, then garnish with asparagus. Sprinkle with Parmesan cheese. Makes 3 servings.

PER SERVING

Calories	293
Protein	26 g
Carbohydrate	44 g
Fat	2 g
Cholesterol	115 mg
Sodium	927 mg
Potassium	1,083 mg

TIMETABLE

Total preparation time:
20 minutes

BEEFED-UP TOMATO CUPS

So colorful, these salads will brighten any luncheon.

¼ cup wine vinegar
2 tablespoons salad oil
1 teaspoon sugar
½ teaspoon dried basil,
   crushed
⅛ teaspoon pepper
½ of a 10-ounce package (1 cup)
   frozen peas and carrots *or*
   frozen mixed vegetables
6 ounces thinly sliced cooked
   lean beef
1 cup alfalfa sprouts
4 lettuce leaves
4 medium tomatoes
⅛ teaspoon salt

■ For dressing, in a screw-top jar combine vinegar, salad oil, sugar, basil, and pepper. Cover and shake well. For salad mixture, place frozen vegetables in a colander. Run *hot water* over vegetables just till thawed. Drain well, then transfer to a large mixing bowl. Trim fat from beef, then cut beef into julienne strips. Add beef and alfalfa sprouts to vegetables.

■ Line salad plates with lettuce leaves. For tomato cups, cut out ½ inch of the core from *each* tomato. Invert tomatoes onto a cutting board. For each, cut from top to, *but not quite through*, stem end, making 6 wedges. Place tomatoes on the plates. Spread wedges slightly apart, then sprinkle lightly with salt.

■ Shake dressing, then pour it over beef mixture. Toss till ingredients are well coated. Fill tomato cups with beef mixture. Makes 4 servings.

PER SERVING

Calories	185
Protein	15 g
Carbohydrate	9 g
Fat	10 g
Cholesterol	39 mg
Sodium	131 mg
Potassium	424 mg

TIMETABLE

Total preparation time:
20 minutes

Fourteenth Day

■ BREAKFAST

½ cup orange juice	55
¼ cup low-fat cottage cheese	51
1 slice whole wheat bread	70
Total calories	**176**

■ LUNCH

*Chicken-Coconut Soup	258
1 rye bagel	200
1 slice Swiss cheese (1 ounce)	105
2 tomato slices	8
Coffee *or* tea	0
Total calories	**571**

■ DINNER

*Pineapple-Ginger Chop	372
1 cup cooked broccoli spears	50
1 wedge iceberg lettuce	13
1 tablespoon reduced-calorie Italian salad dressing	6
1 cup skim milk	85
Total calories	**526**

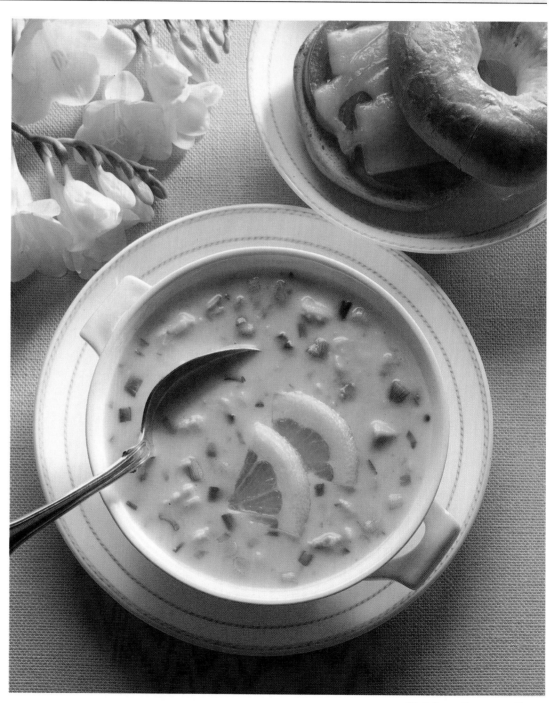

Chicken-Coconut Soup

20 minutes or less

CHICKEN-COCONUT SOUP

For an especially delicious soup-and-sandwich lunch pair, team the creamy soup with a tomato-and-cheese-topped bagel.

 2 tablespoons flaked coconut
   Nonstick spray coating
1¾ cups skim milk
 2 tablespoons frozen sliced
   green onion (see tip,
   page 39)
 1 teaspoon instant chicken
   bouillon granules
 ½ teaspoon frozen, finely
   shredded lemon peel
   (see tip, page 66)
 ¼ cup skim milk
 2 teaspoons cornstarch
 1 6¾-ounce can chunk-style
   chicken *or* 1 cup diced
   cooked chicken (see tip,
   page 109)
   Lemon slices (optional)

■ Finely chop coconut. Spray a *cold* medium saucepan with nonstick coating. Add coconut. Cook and stir over medium heat about 3 minutes or till lightly browned. Then stir in 1¾ cups milk, frozen green onion, bouillon granules, and lemon peel.

■ Stir together ¼ cup milk and cornstarch, then stir it into coconut mixture. Cook and stir till thickened and bubbly. Cook and stir mixture for 2 minutes more. Meanwhile, break canned chicken into large chunks. Add canned or diced chicken to coconut mixture. Cook just till heated through. To serve, ladle soup into individual bowls. If desired, garnish with lemon slices. Makes 2 servings.

PER SERVING

Calories	258
Protein	29 g
Carbohydrate	18 g
Fat	7 g
Cholesterol	67 mg
Sodium	385 mg
Potassium	611 mg

TIMETABLE

Preparation time:
10 minutes

Cooking time:
about 10 minutes

PINEAPPLE-GINGER CHOPS

 4 pork loin chops, cut ¾ inch
   thick (about 1½ pounds
   total)
 1 cup quick-cooking brown
   rice
 ½ cup orange juice
 1 tablespoon cornstarch
 1 8-ounce can pineapple
   tidbits (juice pack)
 2 teaspoons soy sauce
 ⅛ teaspoon ground ginger

■ Preheat the broiler. Meanwhile, trim fat from pork chops. Place chops on the unheated rack of a broiler pan. Broil chops about 4 inches from the heat for 8 minutes. Turn chops over. Then broil 7 to 9 minutes more or till meat is tender and no pink remains.

■ While chops are broiling, cook rice according to package directions. For sauce, in a small saucepan combine orange juice and cornstarch. Stir in the *un-drained* pineapple, soy sauce, and ginger. Cook and stir till thickened and bubbly, then cook and stir for 2 minutes more. To serve, transfer rice to a platter. Top with chops, then spoon sauce over chops. Serves 4.

PER SERVING

Calories	372
Protein	28 g
Carbohydrate	34 g
Fat	13 g
Cholesterol	82 mg
Sodium	365 mg
Potassium	524 mg

TIMETABLE

Preparation time:
5 minutes

Cooking time:
15 to 17 minutes

Calorie Chart

Keeping track of your daily calories? It's simple. Use this chart to find the per-serving calorie count for more than 175 foods.

A-B

ALFALFA SPROUTS, fresh; 1 cup _ 10
APPLE BUTTER; 1 tablespoon _ 33
APPLES
  fresh; 1 medium _ 80
  juice, canned; 1 cup _ 115
APPLESAUCE, canned
  sweetened; ½ cup _ 98
  unsweetened; ½ cup _ 53
APRICOTS
  canned, in syrup; ½ cup _ 108
  dried, cooked, unsweetened,
    in juice; ½ cup _ 105
  fresh; 3 medium _ 50
  nectar, canned; 1 cup _ 140
ARTICHOKE, globe, cooked,
  drained; 1 _ 55
ASPARAGUS
  cooked, drained; 4 spears _ 15
  cooked, drained; ½ cup cut _ 23
AVOCADO, peeled; ½ avocado _ 170
BACON
  Canadian-style, cooked; 2 slices _ 85
  crisp strips, medium thickness;
    3 slices _ 110
BANANA; 1 medium _ 105
BARBECUE SAUCE, bottled;
  1 tablespoon _ 10
BARLEY, pearl, light, uncooked;
  ¼ cup _ 175
BEANS
  baked, with tomato sauce and pork,
    canned; ½ cup _ 155
  garbanzo, cooked, drained; ½ cup _ 135
  green snap, cooked, drained;
    ½ cup _ 23
  navy, dry, cooked, drained; ½ cup _ 113
  red kidney, canned; ½ cup _ 115
BEAN SPROUTS, mung, fresh;
  ½ cup _ 15

BEEF, corned, canned; 3 ounces _ 185
BEEF, dried, chipped; 2.5 ounces _ 145
BEEF CUTS, cooked
  flank steak, lean only; 3 ounces _ 207
  ground beef, extra lean; 3 ounces _ 216
  ground beef, lean; 3 ounces _ 234
  ground beef, regular; 3 ounces _ 260
  pot roast, chuck, lean only;
    3 ounces _ 196
  rib roast, lean only; 3 ounces _ 204
  round steak, lean only; 3 ounces _ 165
  sirloin steak, lean only; 3 ounces _ 177
BEEF LIVER, braised; 3 ounces _ 137
BEETS, cooked, diced; ½ cup _ 28
BEVERAGES, alcoholic
  beer; 12 ounces _ 150
  dessert wine; 3.5 ounces _ 140
  gin, rum, vodka—80 proof;
    1.5 ounces _ 95
  table wine, white; 3.5 ounces _ 80
BEVERAGES, nonalcoholic
  carbonated water _ 0
  coffee _ 0
  cola; 12 ounces _ 160
  ginger ale; 12 ounces _ 125
  tea _ 0
BLACKBERRIES, fresh; ½ cup _ 38
BLUEBERRIES
  fresh; ½ cup _ 40
  frozen, sweetened; ½ cup _ 93
BOUILLON, instant granules;
  1 teaspoon _ 2
BREADS
  bagel; 1 (3½-inch diameter) _ 200
  biscuit, refrigerated; 1 _ 65
  breadstick, plain; 1 (7¾ inches long) 38
  bun, frankfurter or hamburger; 1 _ 119
  corn bread; 1 piece (2½x2½x1½
    inches) _ 161
  crumbs, dry; ¼ cup _ 98
  crumbs, soft; ¼ cup _ 30
  cubes; 1 cup _ 80

BREADS *(continued)*
  English muffin, plain; 1 _ 140
  French; 1 slice (1 inch thick) _ 100
  Italian; 1 slice (¾ inch thick) _ 85
  pita bread; 1 (6½-inch diameter) _ 165
  raisin; 1 slice _ 65
  rye; 1 slice _ 65
  white; 1 slice _ 65
  whole wheat; 1 slice _ 70
BROCCOLI
  cooked, drained; 1 medium stalk _ 50
  frozen chopped, cooked, drained;
    ½ cup _ 25
BRUSSELS SPROUTS, cooked,
  drained; ½ cup _ 30
BULGUR, uncooked; ½ cup _ 300
BUTTER
  1 pat (about 1 teaspoon) _ 35
  1 tablespoon _ 100

C

CABBAGE
  Chinese, raw; ½ cup (1-inch pieces) _ 5
  common varieties, raw, shredded;
    1 cup _ 15
  red, raw, shredded; 1 cup _ 20
CAKES, baked from mixes
  angel, no icing; 1/12 cake _ 125
  devil's food or yellow, 2 layers,
    9-inch diameter,
    chocolate frosting; 1/16 cake _ 235
  gingerbread, 8-inch square; 1/9 cake 175
CANDIES
  caramel; 1 ounce _ 115
  chocolate bar, milk; 1 ounce _ 145
  chocolate fudge; 1 ounce _ 115
  gumdrops; 1 ounce _ 100
  hard; 1 ounce _ 110
CANTALOUPE; ½ (5-inch diameter) 95

CARROTS
cooked, drained, sliced; ½ cup _____ 35
raw; 1 large _____ 30
CATSUP; 1 tablespoon _____ 15
CAULIFLOWER
cooked, drained; ½ cup _____ 15
raw, whole flowerets; 1 cup _____ 25
CELERY, raw, chopped; ½ cup _____ 10
CEREALS, cooked
oatmeal, quick; ½ cup _____ 73
wheat, quick; ½ cup _____ 70
CEREALS, ready-to-eat
bran flakes; about ¾ cup _____ 90
cornflakes; about 1¼ cups _____ 110
granola; about ⅓ cup _____ 125
rice, crisp; about 1 cup _____ 110
rice or wheat, puffed; about 1 cup _____ 50
wheat flakes; about 1 cup _____ 100
CHEESES
American, process; 1 ounce _____ 105
blue; 1 ounce _____ 100
Camembert; 1 ounce _____ 86
cheddar; 1 ounce _____ 115
cottage, cream-style, large curd;
   1 cup _____ 235
cottage, dry; 1 cup _____ 125
cottage, low-fat (2% fat); 1 cup _____ 205
cream cheese; 1 ounce _____ 100
cream cheese, reduced calorie;
   1 ounce _____ 60
Monterey Jack; 1 ounce _____ 106
mozzarella, part skim milk; 1 ounce 72
Neufchâtel; 1 ounce _____ 74
Parmesan, grated; 1 tablespoon _____ 25
ricotta, part skim milk; 1 cup _____ 340
ricotta, whole milk; 1 cup _____ 430
spread, American; 1 ounce _____ 80
Swiss (natural); 1 ounce _____ 105
CHERRIES
canned, in syrup, sweet;
   ½ cup _____ 107
canned, water pack, tart, pitted;
   ½ cup _____ 45
fresh, sweet, whole; 10 cherries _____ 50
CHICKEN
breast, skinned, roasted; ½ breast _142
canned, with broth; 5 ounces _____ 234
dark meat, skinned, roasted; 1 cup 286
light meat, skinned, roasted; 1 cup 242
thigh, skinned, roasted; 1 thigh _____ 109

CHILI SAUCE; 1 tablespoon _____ 16
CHIVES, snipped; 1 tablespoon _____ 1
CHOCOLATE
bitter; 1 ounce _____ 145
semisweet; 1 ounce _____ 143
sweet plain; 1 ounce _____ 150
syrup, fudge-type; 2 tablespoons _____ 125
syrup, thin-type; 2 tablespoons _____ 85
CHOW MEIN NOODLES, canned;
¼ cup _____ 55
CLAMS, canned; 3 ounces _____ 85
COCOA, made with milk; 1 cup _____ 225
COCOA POWDER, unsweetened;
1 tablespoon _____ 14
COCONUT, sweetened, shredded;
¼ cup _____ 118
COOKIES
chocolate chip; 1
   (2¼-inch diameter) _____ 45
cream sandwich, chocolate; 1 _____ 49
fig bar; 1 _____ 53
sugar; 1 (2½-inch diameter) _____ 59
vanilla wafer; 3
   (1¾-inch diameter) _____ 56
CORN
canned, cream style; ½ cup _____ 93
canned, vacuum pack, whole kernel;
   ½ cup _____ 83
sweet, cooked; 1 ear (5x1¾ inches) _____ 85
CORNMEAL; 1 cup _____ 435
CORNSTARCH; 1 tablespoon _____ 29
CORN SYRUP; 1 tablespoon _____ 59
CRABMEAT, canned; ½ cup _____ 68
CRACKERS
cheese; 1 (1-inch square) _____ 5
graham; 2 (2½-inch square) _____ 60
rye wafer; 2 (3½x1⅞ inches) _____ 55
saltine; 2 (2-inch square) _____ 25
CRANBERRIES, fresh; ½ cup _____ 23
CRANBERRY JUICE COCKTAIL;
1 cup _____ 145
CRANBERRY-ORANGE RELISH;
¼ cup _____ 123
CRANBERRY SAUCE, sweetened,
canned; ½ cup _____ 210
CREAM
half-and-half; 1 tablespoon _____ 20
heavy whipping; 1 tablespoon _____ 50
light (coffee); 1 tablespoon _____ 30
CUCUMBER; 6 large slices _____ 5

D-G

DATES, fresh or dried, pitted; 10 _____ 230
DOUGHNUTS
cake type, plain; 1 (3¼x1 inch) _____ 210
yeast type; 1 (3¾x1¼ inches) _____ 235
EGGNOG; 1 cup _____ 340
EGGPLANT, cooked, diced; ½ cup _____ 13
EGGS
fried; 1 large _____ 95
poached, hard- or soft-cooked;
   1 large _____ 80
scrambled, plain; made with
   1 large egg _____ 110
white; 1 large _____ 15
yolk; 1 large _____ 65
ENDIVE, raw; 1 cup _____ 10
FISH
flounder, baked; 3 ounces _____ 80
haddock, breaded, fried; 3 ounces _____ 175
halibut, broiled; 3 ounces _____ 140
herring, pickled; 3 ounces _____ 190
ocean perch, breaded, fried;
   3 ounces _____ 185
salmon, broiled or baked; 3 ounces _____ 140
salmon, canned, pink; 3 ounces _____ 120
sardines, canned, in oil, drained;
   3 ounces _____ 175
sole, baked; 3 ounces _____ 80
trout, broiled; 3 ounces _____ 175
tuna, canned, in oil, drained;
   3 ounces _____ 165
tuna, canned, in water, drained;
   3 ounces _____ 135
FLOUR
all purpose; 1 cup _____ 455
whole wheat; 1 cup _____ 400
FRANKFURTER, cooked; 1 _____ 145
FRUIT COCKTAIL
canned, in juice; ½ cup _____ 58
canned, in syrup; ½ cup _____ 93
GARLIC, peeled; 1 clove _____ 4
GELATIN, dry unflavored;
1 envelope _____ 25
GELATIN DESSERT, plain,
ready-to-serve; ½ cup _____ 70
GRAPEFRUIT
canned sections, in syrup; ½ cup _____ 75
fresh; ½ medium _____ 40

GRAPEFRUIT (*continued*)
juice, canned, sweetened; 1 cup _____ 115
juice, fresh; 1 cup _____ 95
juice, frozen concentrate, unsweetened reconstituted; 1 cup _____ 100
GRAPES
green, fresh, seedless; 10 _____ 35
juice, canned; 1 cup _____ 155

H-O

HAM, fully cooked, lean only;
2.4 ounces _____ 105
HONEY; 1 tablespoon _____ 65
HONEYDEW MELON; $1/10$
(6½-inch diameter) _____ 45
HORSERADISH, prepared;
1 tablespoon _____ 6
ICE CREAM, vanilla
ice milk; 1 cup (about 4% fat) _____ 185
regular; 1 cup (about 11% fat) _____ 270
soft-serve; 1 cup _____ 223
JAM; 1 tablespoon _____ 55
JELLY; 1 tablespoon _____ 50
KALE, cooked, drained; ½ cup _____ 20
KIWI FRUIT; 1 _____ 45
KOHLRABI, cooked, drained, diced;
½ cup _____ 25
LAMB, cooked
loin chop, lean only; 2.3 ounces _____ 140
roast leg, lean only; 2.6 ounces _____ 140
LEMON; 1 medium _____ 15
LEMONADE, frozen concentrate,
sweetened, reconstituted; 1 cup _____ 106
LEMON JUICE; 1 tablespoon _____ 5
LENTILS, cooked; ½ cup _____ 108
LETTUCE
Boston; ¼ medium head _____ 5
iceberg; ¼ medium compact head _____ 20
iceberg; 1 leaf (5 x 4 inches) _____ 3
LIME; 1 medium _____ 20
LIMEADE, frozen concentrate,
sweetened, reconstituted; 1 cup _____ 100
LIME JUICE; ½ cup _____ 33
LOBSTER, cooked; ½ cup _____ 69
LUNCHEON MEATS
bologna; 1 slice (1 ounce) _____ 90
salami, cooked; 1 slice (1 ounce) _____ 73

MACARONI, cooked tender; ½ cup _ 78
MALTED MILK; 1 cup _____ 235
MAPLE SYRUP; 1 tablespoon _____ 50
MARGARINE, soft or regular;
1 tablespoon _____ 100
MARSHMALLOWS; 1 ounce _____ 90
MAYONNAISE; 1 tablespoon _____ 100
MELBA TOAST; 1 slice _____ 20
MILK
buttermilk; 1 cup _____ 100
chocolate drink (2% fat); 1 cup _____ 180
condensed, sweetened, undiluted;
1 cup _____ 980
dried nonfat, instant; 1 cup _____ 245
evaporated, skim, undiluted;
1 cup _____ 200
evaporated, whole, undiluted;
1 cup _____ 340
low-fat (2% fat); 1 cup _____ 120
low-fat (1% fat); 1 cup _____ 100
skim; 1 cup _____ 85
whole; 1 cup _____ 150
MOLASSES, light; 2 tablespoons _____ 85
MUFFINS
blueberry; 1 _____ 135
bran; 1 _____ 125
corn; 1 _____ 145
MUSHROOMS
canned, drained; ⅓ cup _____ 12
raw, sliced; 1 cup _____ 20
MUSTARD, prepared; 1 tablespoon _ 15
NECTARINE, fresh; 1 _____ 65
NOODLES
cooked; ½ cup _____ 100
dry; 1 ounce _____ 110
NUTS
almonds; 1 ounce _____ 165
cashews, roasted in oil; 1 ounce _____ 165
peanuts, roasted in oil, shelled;
1 ounce _____ 165
pecans; 1 ounce _____ 190
walnuts; 1 ounce _____ 170
OIL; 1 tablespoon _____ 125
OKRA, cooked; 8 pods (3x⅝ inch) _____ 25
OLIVES
green; 4 medium _____ 15
ripe; 3 small _____ 15
ONIONS
green, without tops; 6 small _____ 10
mature, raw, chopped; ½ cup _____ 28

ORANGES
fresh; 1 medium _____ 60
juice, canned, unsweetened;
1 cup _____ 105
juice, fresh; 1 cup _____ 110
juice, frozen concentrate,
reconstituted; 1 cup _____ 110
OYSTERS
breaded, fried; 1 _____ 90
raw; ½ cup (6 to 10 medium) _____ 80

P-S

PANCAKE; 1 (4-inch diameter) _____ 60
PAPAYA, ½-inch cubes; 1 cup _____ 65
PARSLEY, raw; 10 sprigs _____ 5
PEACHES
canned, in juice; ½ cup _____ 55
canned, in syrup; ½ cup _____ 95
fresh; 1 medium _____ 35
frozen, sweetened; ½ cup _____ 118
PEANUT BUTTER; 1 tablespoon _____ 95
PEA PODS, cooked, drained; ½ cup _ 33
PEARS
canned, in juice; 2 halves _____ 63
canned, in syrup; ½ cup _____ 95
fresh; 1 medium _____ 100
PEAS, green, cooked; ½ cup _____ 63
PEPPERONI; 1 slice (⅛ inch thick) _ 27
PEPPERS, green, sweet, chopped;
¾ cup _____ 20
PICKLES
dill; 1 medium _____ 5
relish, sweet; 1 tablespoon _____ 21
sweet; 1 small _____ 20
PIES; ⅛ of a 9-inch pie
apple _____ 303
blueberry _____ 286
cherry _____ 308
custard _____ 248
lemon meringue _____ 268
pumpkin _____ 240
PIE SHELL, baked; one 9-inch _____ 900
PINEAPPLES
canned, in juice; ½ cup _____ 75
canned, in syrup; ½ cup _____ 100
fresh, diced; ½ cup _____ 38
juice, canned, unsweetened; 1 cup _ 140

PLUMS
canned, in juice; ½ cup _____ 73
canned, in syrup; ½ cup _____ 115
fresh; 1 (2-inch diameter) _____ 35
POPCORN
plain, air popped; 1 cup _____ 30
plain, popped in oil; 1 cup _____ 55
PORK, cooked
chop, loin center cut, lean only;
2.5 ounces _____ 165
sausage, links; 3 ounces _____ 150
shoulder, lean only; 2.4 ounces _____ 165
POTATO CHIPS; 10 medium _____ 105
POTATOES
baked; about 8 ounces _____ 220
boiled; about 5 ounces _____ 120
french fried, frozen, oven-heated;
10 medium _____ 110
hash brown; ½ cup _____ 170
mashed with milk; ½ cup _____ 80
sweet, baked; 1 medium _____ 115
PRETZELS; 10 small sticks _____ 10
PRUNE JUICE, canned; 1 cup _____ 180
PRUNES, dried
cooked, unsweetened; ½ cup _____ 113
uncooked, pitted; 5 large _____ 115
PUDDINGS, cooked
chocolate; ½ cup _____ 150
vanilla; ½ cup _____ 145
PUMPKIN, canned; 1 cup _____ 85
RADISHES, raw; 4 medium _____ 5
RAISINS; 1 cup (not packed) _____ 435
RASPBERRIES
fresh; ½ cup _____ 30
frozen, sweetened; ½ cup _____ 128
RHUBARB
cooked, sweetened; ½ cup _____ 140
raw, diced; 1 cup _____ 26
RICE
brown, cooked; ½ cup _____ 115
white, cooked; ½ cup _____ 113
white, quick-cooking, cooked;
½ cup _____ 93
ROLLS
cloverleaf; 1 (2½-inch diameter) _____ 85
hard; 1 (3¾-inch diameter) _____ 155
sweet; 1 medium _____ 220
RUSK; 1 (3⅜-inch diameter) _____ 38
RUTABAGAS, cooked, drained,
cubed; ½ cup _____ 30

SALAD DRESSINGS
blue cheese; 1 tablespoon _____ 75
French; 1 tablespoon _____ 85
Italian; 1 tablespoon _____ 80
mayonnaise; 1 tablespoon _____ 100
mayonnaise, reduced-calorie;
1 tablespoon _____ 45
mayonnaise-type; 1 tablespoon _____ 60
Russian; 1 tablespoon _____ 76
Thousand Island; 1 tablespoon _____ 60
SAUERKRAUT, canned; ½ cup _____ 23
SCALLOPS, breaded; 6 _____ 195
SHERBET, orange; ½ cup _____ 135
SHORTENING; 1 tablespoon _____ 115
SHRIMP
canned; 3 ounces _____ 100
French fried; 3 ounces _____ 200
SOUPS, condensed, canned
(diluted with water unless
specified otherwise)
bean with bacon; 1 cup _____ 170
beef bouillon, broth, consomme;
1 cup _____ 15
beef noodle; 1 cup _____ 85
chicken noodle; 1 cup _____ 75
clam chowder, Manhattan-style;
1 cup _____ 80
cream of chicken,
diluted with milk; 1 cup _____ 190
cream of mushroom,
diluted with milk; 1 cup _____ 205
pea; 1 cup _____ 165
tomato; 1 cup _____ 85
tomato, diluted with milk; 1 cup _____ 160
vegetable beef; 1 cup _____ 80
SOUR CREAM, dairy; ½ cup _____ 248
SOY SAUCE; 1 tablespoon _____ 10
SPAGHETTI, plain, cooked tender;
½ cup _____ 78
SPINACH
canned, drained; ½ cup _____ 25
frozen, cooked, drained; ½ cup _____ 28
raw, torn; 1 cup _____ 10
SQUASH
summer, cooked, drained, sliced;
½ cup _____ 18
winter, baked, cubed; ½ cup _____ 40
STRAWBERRIES
fresh, whole; ½ cup _____ 23
frozen, sweetened, sliced; ½ cup _____ 123

SUGARS
brown, packed; ½ cup _____ 410
granulated; 1 tablespoon _____ 45
powdered; ½ cup _____ 193

T-Z

TANGERINE; 1 medium _____ 35
TAPIOCA, dry; 1 tablespoon _____ 30
TARTAR SAUCE; 1 tablespoon _____ 74
TOFU; 1 piece (2¾ x 2½ x 1 inch) _____ 85
TOMATOES
canned; ½ cup _____ 25
fresh; 1 medium _____ 25
juice, canned; 1 cup _____ 40
paste, canned; 1 cup _____ 220
puree; 1 cup _____ 105
sauce; 1 cup _____ 75
TORTILLA, corn; 1 _____ 65
TURKEY
bologna; 1 ounce _____ 57
canned, with broth; 5 ounces _____ 231
ham; 2 ounces _____ 75
roasted, light and dark; 1 cup _____ 240
salami; 1 ounce _____ 56
TURNIPS, cooked, diced; ½ cup _____ 15
VEAL, cooked, cutlet; 3 ounces _____ 185
VEGETABLE JUICE COCKTAIL;
1 cup _____ 45
VINEGAR; 1 tablespoon _____ 0
WAFFLE; 1 section
(4½ x 4½ x ⅝ inch) _____ 140
WATER CHESTNUTS, canned;
½ cup _____ 35
WATERCRESS, raw, chopped;
½ cup _____ 12
WATERMELON; 1 wedge
(8x4 inches) _____ 155
WHIPPED DESSERT TOPPING,
thawed; 1 tablespoon _____ 15
**WHIPPED DESSERT TOPPING
MIX,** prepared; 1 tablespoon _____ 10
WILD RICE, raw; ½ cup _____ 283
YOGURT
low-fat, fruit-flavored;
8 ounces _____ 230
low-fat, plain; 8 ounces _____ 145
ZWIEBACK; 1 piece _____ 30

*I*ndex